CASE STUDIES IN

Critical Care
Nursing

CASE STUDIES IN

Critical Care Nursing

EDITED BY
BARBARA CLARK MIMS, RN, MSN, CCRN

Coordinator
Critical Care and Trauma Nurse Internship
Parkland Memorial Hospital
Dallas, Texas

Director
Barbara Clark Mims Associates
Lewisville, Texas

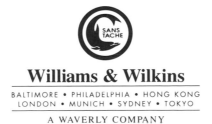

Williams & Wilkins

BALTIMORE • PHILADELPHIA • HONG KONG
LONDON • MUNICH • SYDNEY • TOKYO

A WAVERLY COMPANY

Editor: Susan M. Glover
Associate Editor: Marjorie Kidd Keating
Copy Editors: Klemie Bryte, Bill Cady, Tom Lehr, Michelle Crawley
Designer: Wilma Rosenberger
Illustration Planner: Ray Lowman
Production Coordinator: Anne Seitz

Copyright © 1990
Williams & Wilkins
428 East Preston Street
Baltimore, Maryland 21202, U.S.A.

Accurate indications, adverse reactions, and dosage schedules for drugs are provided in this book, but it is possible that they may change. The reader is urged to review the package information data of the manufacturers of the medications mentioned.

Printed in the United States of America

Library of Congress Cataloging-in-Publication Data

Case studies in critical care nursing / edited by Barbara Clark Mims.
     p.   cm.
   ISBN 0-683-06051-7
    1. Intensive care nursing—Case studies.   2. Emergency nursing—
–Case studies.   I. Mims, Barbara Clark.
RT120.I5C37   1990
610.73′61—dc20   89-38845
                                     CIP

94
4 5 6 7 8 9 10

To my colleagues, past and present,
in recognition of your compassion, commitment,
and quest for excellence in caring for the critically ill.

FOREWORD

During the past two decades, critical care nursing has undergone dramatic changes. One of the most significant changes relates to the complex technological advances that have forced critical care nurses to master increasing numbers of machines and devices. The "high tech" component of the critical care environment often overwhelms the novice critical care nurse and even can become the focus of seasoned critical care nurses who are weary of simple routines.

Another significant change is the expanded role of the critical care nurse. No longer does the nurse simply execute physicians' orders. Today, the critical care nurse is a patient advocate who collaborates with the physician and other health team members. The critical care nurse plays a vital role in coordinating and focusing the efforts of the many health care workers toward realistic patient-oriented goals.

Yet another change in critical care nursing involves the massive amount of information needed to deliver expert, skilled care to critically ill patients. The nurse can no longer simply complete a basic arrhythmia course or a critical care orientation program to become proficient in the world of critical care. Rather, the critical care nurse must be involved in a lifelong learning process to stay abreast of rapidly changing medical advances and to acquire and maintain clinical skills essential for safe patient care. With short staffing and long hours, however, it is difficult to find adequate time to attend continuing education courses, to read current research journals, and to practice infrequently used skills.

The critical care nurse is challenged to integrate new knowledge with previous experiences to continue professional growth. With experience, the critical care nurse learns to analyze vast bits of information, evaluate their significance, and integrate them into a total picture of the patient and his or her problems. Such critical analysis and decision-making skills are not developed overnight, but are acquired gradually through study and experience.

Case Studies in Critical Care Nursing is an exciting book for the critical care nurse who is striving to develop skills in analyzing the complex needs of critically ill patients. The text, as described by the editor Barbara Clark Mims, RN, MSN, CCRN, is designed for the experienced critical care nurse. The 56 case studies compiled in the volume present realistic patient cases, large quantities of data, and descriptions of medical, surgical, and nursing management. The patient problems described are from the world of critical care today, not yesterday. Many involve multiple organ injury, system failure, and life-threatening metabolic problems. The scope of clinical situations addressed is extensive and includes common problems, such as adult respiratory distress syndrome and myocardial infarction, and more unusual conditions, such as rhabdomyolysis and air transport of the critically ill. I commend the efforts of the editor and the many contributing authors for presenting realistic case studies with clinically useful information in an easy-to-read format.

To conclude, I would like to share a short story with you. Three men, all engaged in the same employment, were asked what they were doing. One said he was making fifteen dollars an hour. Another replied that he was cutting stone. The third said that he was building a cathedral. The difference was not in what they were actually doing. They were all earning the same wage; they were all cutting stone; but, only one saw his work as helping to build a great edifice. Some nurses see their work as simply earning so many dollars an hour; others see their work as a series of specific tasks performed during the shift; yet, some view their work as the delivery of expert, safe nursing care to the critically ill patient. For these nurses who value their work, their professional focus will guide them to seek opportunities for continued learning and applied critical thinking. This book is for professional critical care nurses who are building a cathedral.

Vee Rice, RN, PhD
Program Coordinator
Critical Care Program
The University of Tennessee
Nashville, Tennessee

PREFACE

Case Studies in Critical Care Nursing is a book for the experienced critical care nurse. Organized by core systems, the book includes 56 case studies covering nearly every major clinical condition commonly encountered in critical care practice. The case studies have been written by expert critical care nurses across the country; in many instances these describe actual patients cared for by the authors. However, no patient names or identifying features have been used.

Each case study includes a patient scenario, followed by questions and answers. Rather than focusing on generalities, and therefore being limited in actual practice value, these cases are specific and focus on circumscribed types of pathophysiologic processes. Space constraints do not permit a comprehensive presentation of all aspects of each condition, so the questions address the most clinically relevant aspects of each case. The intent is to facilitate critical thinking and advanced decision making in the nurse practicing at the bedside of the critically ill.

Nurses who will benefit from the book include those studying for the CCRN examination; those working in specialty units who wish to update, reinforce, or verify their knowledge base; those enrolled in critical care graduate programs; and hospital-based critical care nurse educators. The book is not intended for use by student nurses or those without critical care experience.

In order to approximate actual patient charts and to increase the readability of the clinical data, units of measurement (mm Hg, mEq/liter, gm/dl, etc.) are not given each time a parameter is mentioned. Unless otherwise specified, the units used throughout the book are listed in Appendix A, as are normal values for each.

My deepest appreciation goes to the contributors, whose energy and enthusiasm provided the impetus for moving swiftly forward with the production of this book. In addition, special thanks go to the many expert nurse and physician reviewers, whose critical analysis and thoughtful comments added immeasurably to the accuracy and scope of the book.

Barbara Clark Mims, RN, MSN, CCRN
P.O. Box 9019
Suite 201–320
Lewisville, Texas 75067
(817) 430-0483

CONTRIBUTORS

Wendy L. Baker, RN, MS, CCRN
Trauma Clinical Nurse Specialist
Vanderbilt University Hospital
Nashville, Tennessee

Rochelle Logston Boggs, RN, MS, CCRN, CEN
Trauma/Critical Care Clinical Nurse
 Specialist
Surgical, Trauma, and Critical Care
 Associates
Parkersburg, West Virginia

Leslie Borcherding, RN, MS
Education Specialist
Irving Healthcare System
Irving, Texas

Mary Ellen Cafiero, RN, MA, CCRN
Education Specialist
Mount Sinai Medical Center
New York, New York

Venita Dasch, RN, BSN
Critical Care Nurse
Surgical ICU
Parkland Memorial Hospital
Dallas, Texas

Dorie M. Gates, RN, MS, CCRN
Supervisor, Surgical ICU
University of California, San Diego
Medical Center
San Diego, California

Diane L. Gilworth, RN, BSN, CCRN
Critical Care Nurse
Coronary Care Unit
Brigham and Women's Hospital
Boston, Massachusetts

Connie Glass, RN, MSN, CCRN
Critical Care Clinical Nurse Specialist
Medical College of Virginia Hospitals
Richmond, Virginia

Barbara Hackett, RN, BSN, CCRN
Critical Care Nurse
Special Care Unit
Good Samaritan Hospital
West Islip, New York

Marsha Halfman-Franey, RN, MSN
Director
Cardiovascular Nurse Specialist Program
Arizona Heart Institute Foundation
Phoenix, Arizona

Virginia Byrn Huddleston, RN, MSN, CCRN
Associate
Barbara Clark Mims Associates
Lewisville, Texas
Critical Care Nurse
Metropolitan Nashville General Hospital
Nashville, Tennessee

Kimmith M. Jones, RN, BS, CCRN
Critical Care Nurse
Neurotrauma Center
Maryland Institute for Emergency Medical
 Services Systems
Baltimore, Maryland

Terry L. Jones, RN, BSN, CCRN
Assistant Head Nurse
Medical Respiratory ICU
Parkland Memorial Hospital
Dallas, Texas

Meredith King, RN, MA, CEN
Clinical Supervisor
Department of Neurosurgery
Mount Sinai Medical Center
New York, New York

Lynda Lane, RN, MS
Clinical Nurse Specialist
Department of Cardiovascular Physiology
 and Space Medicine
University of Texas Southwestern Medical
 Center at Dallas
Flight Nurse Director
Alpha Aviation
Dallas, Texas

Laura E. Luecke, RN, BSN, CCRN
Nurse Educator
Coronary Care Unit and Medical
 Respiratory ICU
Parkland Memorial Hospital
Dallas, Texas

Kathleen Martin, RN, MSN, CCRN
Clinical Research Associate
Hoffman-La Roche
Nutley, New Jersey

Lisa Morra Martin, RN, BSN, CCRN
Burn Nurse Clinician
Parkland Memorial Hospital
Medical-Legal Analyst
Vial, Hamilton, Koch, and Knox
Attorneys and Counselors
Dallas, Texas

Barbara Clark Mims, RN, MSN, CCRN
Coordinator
Critical Care and Trauma Nurse Internship
Parkland Memorial Hospital
Dallas, Texas
Director
Barbara Clark Mims Associates
Lewisville, Texas

Susan Nevins, RN, MA, CNRN
Nurse Clinician, Neurosurgical Specialty
Mount Sinai Medical Center
New York, New York

Susan Nussle, RN, BSN, CCRN
Renal Nurse Educator
Parkland Memorial Hospital
Dallas, Texas

Susan L. Oskins, RN, MS, CCRN, CS
Medical-Surgical Clinical Nurse Specialist
Grant Medical Center
Columbus, Ohio

Jacquelyne V. Prince, RN, MSN
Continuing Education Coordinator
Norton Community Hospital
Norton, Virginia

Mary K. Roberts, RN, MSN, CCRN
Critical Care Instructor
Critical Care and Trauma Nurse Internship
Parkland Memorial Hospital
Dallas, Texas

Cathy H. Rosenthal, RN, MN, CCRN
Clinical Nurse Specialist, Pediatric Critical
  Care
National Institutes of Health
Bethesda, Maryland

Kathleen H. Toto, RN, MSN, CCRN
Critical Care Education Coordinator
Parkland Memorial Hospital
Dallas, Texas
Associate
Barbara Clark Mims Associates
Lewisville, Texas

Margaret A. Wegner, RN, BSN, CCRN
Assistant Head Nurse
Coronary Care Unit
Parkland Memorial Hospital
Dallas, Texas

Linda Weld, RN, MSN, CCRN
Cardiovascular Clinical Nurse Specialist
Robert H. Dedman Memorial Medical
  Center
Dallas, Texas

CONTENTS

PART I
Cardiovascular System

xiii

PART II
Pulmonary System

PART III
Neurological System

PART IV
Renal System

PART V
Endocrine System

PART VI
Gastrointestinal System

PART VII
Multisystem Involvement

APPENDICES

Part I

Cardiovascular System

CHAPTER 1

Abdominal Aortic Aneurysm

Virginia Byrn Huddleston, RN, MSN, CCRN

Leonard Ash is a 68-year-old man admitted to the ICU for preoperative pulmonary artery catheterization for an abdominal aortic aneurysm (AAA) repair the next day. He has a positive history of coronary artery disease, peripheral vascular disease, and mild emphysema. He suffered an inferior MI 3 years prior to admission. He has been taking antihypertensive medications since his MI and was admitted to the hospital for one incident of left-sided congestive heart failure 2 years prior to admission.

The pulmonary artery catheter and radial arterial line were placed without incident. Using the Starling curve, optimum filling pressures and cardiac output were established. Preoperative teaching was completed, and Mr. Ash successfully underwent AAA repair the next day. A bifurcated Dacron graft was placed, and the aneurysmal sac was wrapped around the graft and anastomoses. Upon arrival in the ICU, the following data were obtained:

Hemodynamic Parameters		Ventilator Settings	
CVP	10	Mode	Assist Control
PAP	38/18	Rate	12
PAWP	15	FIO$_2$	0.40
CO	3.8	Tidal volume	900
BP	210/110		
HR	100		

Mr. Ash was lethargic upon arrival, but his pupils were equal and reactive to light. His temperature was 95°F, and a warming blanket was applied. His ECG monitor showed normal sinus rhythm with rare PVCs. Both the dorsalis pedis and posterior tibial pulses were audible bilaterally with the Doppler. His extremities were cool and pale, but capillary refill was less than 3 sec. Mr. Ash was orally intubated and connected to the ventilator at the charted settings. Arterial blood gases (ABGs) were adequate. Auscultation of the chest revealed bilateral breath sounds with mild expiratory wheezes. The patient's nasogastic tube (NGT) was connected

1

to low wall suction with minimum return of dark green aspirate and his Foley catheter drained large amounts of pale, yellow urine. Examination of the abdomen revealed a midline incisional dressing that was dry and intact. Sodium nitroprusside was administered at 0.3 μg/kg/min for Mr. Ash's hypertension and aggressive monitoring was begun.

QUESTIONS AND ANSWERS

1. Describe the etiology and development of Mr. Ash's aneurysm.

The development of Mr. Ash's AAA is most likely due to his existing atherosclerosis, the presumed cause of over 95% of AAAs. Other causes include trauma, arteritis, congenital abnormalities, and syphilis. The majority of AAAs (>90%) are infrarenal and fusiform (involvement of entire aortic circumference) in presentation. Because the infrarenal segment of the aorta is also more prone to development of atherosclerotic disease, it has been classically held that the development of aneurysms are causally related to the presence of atherosclerosis. While this tenet is still widely supported, several recent studies have advanced the idea of metabolic and enzymatic abnormalities as also contributing to the development of a weakened vascular wall. Increased collagenase activity and medial layer deterioration have both been implicated in the progression of wall weakness, as well as age-related decreases in aortic elasticity. The decreased tensile wall strength, increased turbulence at the bifurcation, and increased systolic pressure waves all lead to further dilatation of the aortic wall and increased likelihood of rupture. Changes in laminar blood flow occur as dilatation increases, and laminar thrombi develop on the interior wall of the aneurysm.

According to the law of Laplace, tension on the vessel wall is directly proportional to the radius of the wall. As the aneurysm increases in size, the wall is under an increasing amount of tension; therefore, the larger the aneurysm and the higher the systemic blood pressure, the more likely the aneurysm is to rupture.

2. What major risk factors should be evaluated in Mr. Ash preoperatively?

Cardiac disease
Peripheral vascular disease
Pulmonary disease
Renal disease
Age

The majority of patients presenting with an AAA are also suffering from other chronic disease states involving the cardiac, vascular, pulmonary, and renal systems. History of hypertension, occlusive disease, CVA, and renal insufficiency are common. Cardiovascular disease is the major factor in perioperative morbidity and mortality in AAA repair. Over 50% of postoperative mortality is attributed to myocardial infarction. While these factors contribute to increased operative morbidity, the risk of rupture usually outweighs the risk of surgery, so asymptomatic aneurysms >4–6 cm are usually electively repaired. All symptomatic AAAs are repaired.

Pulmonary function tests, arteriography, and renal evaluation may be performed to maximize perioperative management. Many patients are admitted to the ICU the day prior to surgery for preoperative pulmonary artery catheterization. Baseline cardiovascular status is established and optimal fluid loading is begun.

Many of the complications a patient experiences postoperatively are directly related to preexisting disease states and risk factors. Knowledge of the patient's past medical history is important for more effective monitoring of the patient postoperatively. The admission of the patient to the ICU prior to surgery enhances the nurse's familiarity with the patient and allows the patient to become familiar with the staff and the ICU environment. Preoperative teaching and baseline assessment can be performed in the unit. Because fear and anxiety can contribute greatly to postoperative hypertension, interventions to decrease their potential ill effects may aid in preventing future problems after surgery.

3. **What major complications is Mr. Ash at risk for postoperatively?**

Distal thrombosis/embolization	Hemorrhage
Acute MI	Renal failure
Graft occlusion	Pulmonary dysfunction
Bowel ischemia	Aortoenteric fistula
GI stress ulceration	Graft infection
Sexual dysfunction	CVA

4. **Aortic cross-clamping with graft placement is a frequent source of complications in the patient, both intra- and postoperatively. What impact may it have on the cardiovascular, pulmonary, and renal organ systems, and how may this affect Mr. Ash postoperatively?**

The aorta is usually cross-clamped just inferior to the renal arteries. Both iliac arteries are also clamped. The clamping of the aorta causes an immediate increase in vascular resistance (afterload), increased myocardial workload and oxygen demands, decreased cardiac output, and hypoperfusion to the lower extremities. Hypotension may ensue, but is more common as the cross-clamp is removed.

Cross-clamping, even infrarenally, has been shown to decrease renal cortical flow and predispose the patient to renal embolization. This phenomenon may be related to alterations in afterload and cardiac output, but other undefined mechanisms are also thought to be affecting renal hemodynamics during aortic cross-clamping. Prerenal oliguria or frank ATN may then result. Adequate circulating volume must be maintained intra- and postoperatively to prevent further coronary stress, increased oxygen demands, and renal insult. Fluid status, serial laboratory tests, and urine output must be judiciously monitored.

Hypotensive events and vigorous volume replacement may predispose the lung to pulmonary edema or ARDS. Once again, aggressive pulmonary hygiene and assessment are required to maintain optimal pulmonary function. Manipulation of the lesion and reinstitution of flow may cause release of emboli to distal extremities; therefore, pedal pulses, skin temperature and color, and capillary refill should be frequently assessed to aid in the early identification of embolic phenomena.

5. **Prior to cross-clamping, Mr. Ash is systemically heparinized with 5000 units intravenously. What is the purpose of heparinization? What implications does it have for the critical care nurse caring for Mr. Ash postoperatively?**

During aortic cross-clamping, the distal extremities are severely hypoperfused. Systemic heparinization is instituted to prevent small vessel thrombosis in the distant vasculature. Protamine sulfate is given to reverse the heparinization, but prolonged clotting times may still occur in the early postoperative period. While postoperative bleeding and hematoma formation are more commonly associated with anastomotic leak or vessel tear, coagulopathies must still be considered. PT/PTT studies should be sent with the other routine labs when the patient is admitted to the unit from the Operating Room.

6. **What is the reason for Mr. Ash's early postoperative hypertension? What is the recommended treatment?**

Several factors may be responsible for the hypertension seen postoperatively in AAA repair. Hypothermia with its concomitant peripheral vasoconstriction is common. Cases are lengthy due to the complexity of the surgery, and a major portion of the viscera remains exposed during the procedure.

Pain and anxiety lead to an increase in the circulating catecholamines, which precipitates vasoconstriction, tachycardia, and increases in myocardial oxygen demands. Withdrawal of antihypertensive medications preoperatively may also predispose the patient to postoperative hypertension.

These factors, either in isolation or in concert with each other, place an additional workload on an already compromised heart, thus increasing the risk of cardiac decompensation, failure, and acute MI.

7. **Approximately 4 hr after admission to the unit, Mr. Ash's blood pressure decreased to 90/50, his PAWP and CVP increased to 18, and his CO decreased to 1.9. His calculated SVR was 1895 dyn/sec/cm^{-5}. He became tachycardic and extremely anxious. Dopamine was begun at 4 μg/kg/min. Why did Mr. Ash become hypotensive?**

There are numerous causes of hypotension in the early postoperative period. As the patient rewarms, peripheral vessels dilate and pooling occurs. Third spacing of fluid occurs secondary to extensive manipulation of the bowel and other abdominal viscera intraoperatively.

Blood loss may be an additional source of hypovolemia and hypotension. Unreplaced operative losses, leakage from the anastomotic site, or coagulopathies provide avenues for blood loss. Previously controlled vessel bleeders in the operative site may rebleed secondary to uncontrolled hypertension in the immediate postoperative period and must be surgically corrected.

Mr. Ash's hypotension occurred secondary to cardiac dysfunction, which is one of the most life-threatening causes of hypotension in this patient population. Mr. Ash's heart was already compromised preoperatively, and intraoperative insults such as increased systemic vascular resistance (SVR) or hypotension could have led to cardiac ischemia and damage. As Mr. Ash's heart fails to pump effectively, his ejection fraction decreases, wedge increases, and SVR increases, thus further increasing the workload of the heart. An acute MI could ensue if prompt measures are not taken to remedy the failing heart and maintain adequate loading and perfusion pressures. A combination of fluids, dopamine, and sodium nitroprusside are often used to maximize cardiac function and output.

8. **What is the rationale for using nitroprusside and dopamine in combination with each other?**

Nitroprusside is used to decrease SVR by dilating the venous and arterial beds (primarily arterial). With the afterload decreased, the heart has less resistance to work against in ejecting its stroke volume. Dopamine, a β-agonist at low doses, is infused for its positive inotropic effects. Low dose dopamine also increases perfusion to the renal parenchyma by dilating the renal vascular bed, thus decreasing the potential for renal complications.

The nurse at the bedside must perform meticulous hemodynamic monitoring, including frequent measurements of HR, BP, PAWP, CO, and CVP. Optimum preload (the PAWP producing the best CO), assessed preoperatively using the Starling curve, should be maintained to provide an adequate ejection fraction and prevent the onset of left-sided CHF and pulmonary edema.

Tachycardia can be a disastrous side effect with dopamine infusion, requiring the use of dobutamine in isolation or as an adjunct to lowered doses of dopamine. Dobutamine, also a β-agonist, may decrease SVR, so careful titration of the nitroprusside is absolutely necessary to prevent a hypotensive event. If adequate diastolic pressures are not maintained, coronary filling may be greatly hampered, placing further stress on the damaged myocardium.

Fluid shifts and large swings in hemodynamic parameters continue to complicate the clinical picture even further. The goal of early postoperative care, therefore, is to minimize hemodynamic and electrolyte lability.

9. **On day 2, Mr. Ash's urine output decreases to inadequate levels. A fluid challenge is unsuccessful, and the PAWP begins to rise. Furosemide administration is tried with fair results, and laboratory results reveal levels of: potassium, 5.2; BUN, 30; and serum creatinine, 2.3. Over the next 24 hr, Mr. Ash's output remains decreased, and his weight increases. His potassium, creatinine, and BUN continue to rise. A diagnosis of acute renal failure is made. What are the possible factors predisposing Mr. Ash to renal failure?**

    Mr. Ash's renal failure may be attributed to several causes. Hypotensive episodes during and after surgery may result in renal failure. As discussed previously, aortic cross-clamping may lead to diminished renal cortical blood flow or renal embolization. The use of radiopaque dyes in preoperative arteriography also may predispose the patient to an increased risk of renal failure, especially if renal insufficiency previously existed. Before the patient is taken to surgery, adequate renal function must be established after arteriography.

    The risk of renal failure is much higher in the patient with a ruptured aneurysm because of the increased time of systemic hypotension, the more frequent placement of the cross-clamp suprarenally, and the increased risk of renal embolization.

10. **On day 3, the critical care nurse caring for Mr. Ash notices multiple punctate lesions on both of Mr. Ash's feet. The lesions are necrotic**

and the feet are extremely painful. Pedal pulses remain audible with the Doppler, but the feet are cooler to touch and mottled, and capillary refill is sluggish. What is occurring and why?

Manipulation of the aorta during surgery loosened atherosclerotic debris, which then embolized to the distal extremities. In Mr. Ash's case, the major arteries have not been blocked (pedal pulses remain audible), but the smaller, more distal arteries have been occluded. This syndrome, often labeled "trash foot," leads to small areas of decreased perfusion, necrosis, and gangrene. Catheter embolectomy may be attempted, but is often unsuccessful due to the amount of debris and the small size of the vessels involved. Systemic heparinization is begun to arrest further thrombosis and hopefully preserve limb viability. Frequent assessment for further damage must be performed, and pain control also becomes a priority. The extremities are usually not elevated unless edema is significant, because elevation would not enhance increased arterial flow to the area.

11.   **Bowel ischemia, while not common, can be a devastating complication in a patient following aortic surgery. Describe the etiology and presentation of this dangerous complication.**

Predisposing factors to mesenteric ischemia include improper inferior mesenteric artery ligation or reinstitution of arterial flow, manipulative surgical trauma to the colon, hypotension, congenital alterations in the mesenteric collateral circuits, and surgical sacrifice of existing collaterals. The inferior mesenteric artery arises from the left anterolateral aspect of the abdominal aorta, and it supplies most of the blood to the left colon. Upon resection of the AAA, the inferior mesenteric artery back pressures must be assessed. If the pressures are inadequate (poor collateral supply), the artery must be reimplanted into the prosthetic graft rather than tied off.

The clinical picture varies with the degree of ischemia, which can range from small areas of mucosal ischemia to transmural necrosis. Ischemia leads to submucosal edema, inflammation, and hemorrhage. Colonic bacterial invasion occurs, which may lead to mucosal slough and ulceration. If the ischemia is too severe, ulceration of the muscularis and transmural necrosis develop, leading to acute perforation. Sepsis, DIC, ARDS, ATN, and liver failure may then ensue with disastrous consequences in an already compromised patient. Signs and symptoms of bowel ischemia include:

Pain	Fever
Diarrhea	Rebound tenderness
Abdominal distention	Acidosis
Leukocytosis	Oliguria

12. What nursing diagnoses apply in this case?

Alteration in tissue perfusion related to aortic cross-clamping, distal embolic phenomena, and hypotension

Decreased cardiac output related to cardiac ischemia secondary to aortic cross-clamping and hypotension

Anxiety related to critical care environment and severity of condition

Fluid volume excess related to acute renal failure

Impaired physical mobility: imposed related to hemodynamic instability

SUGGESTED READINGS

Bernhard VM, Towne JB, eds. Complications in vascular surgery. 2nd ed. New York: McGraw-Hill, 1985.

Dalsing MC, Dilley RS, McCarthy M. Surgery of the aorta. Crit Care Q 1985; 8(2):25–38.

Gelman S, McDowell H, Varner PD, et al. The reason for cardiac output reduction after aortic cross-clamping. Am J Surg 1988;155:578–586.

Hollier LH. Surgical management of abdominal aortic aneurysm in the high-risk patient. Surg Clin N Am 1986;66:269–279.

Hotter AN. Preventing cardiovascular complications following AAA surgery. Dimens Crit Care Nurs 1987;6(1):10–18.

Oman KS. Sequelae to ruptured aortic aneurysm. Crit Care Nurs 1985;5(6):15–19.

Wilson SE, Veith FJ, Hobson RW, Williams RA, eds. Vascular surgery: Principles and practice. New York: McGraw-Hill, 1987.

CHAPTER 2

Cardiac Transplantation

Connie Glass, RN, MSN, CCRN

Bob Harley is a 59-year-old married man who has had cardiac disease since his initial myocardial infarction in 1976. Seven years later he had a second infarction and was found to have inoperable diffuse three-vessel disease. Cardiac catheterization in 1983 revealed:

RAP	8	CO	3.0
PAP	40/26	CI	1.5
PAWP	24	Ejection fraction	10%

Medical management was somewhat effective, although he was unable to work and had chronic unstable angina. In November 1988, he had an episode of ventricular fibrillation at home, which converted after three countershocks. Subsequent electrophysiologic study showed reproducible ventricular tachycardia/ventricular fibrillation (VT/VF) with circulatory collapse. Mr. Harley was placed on inotropic, diuretic, afterload reduction and antiarrhythmic therapy and discharged from his local hospital. On December 12, 1988, Mr. Harley was admitted to the transplant center to be evaluated for a cardiac transplant. His physical examination showed a well-nourished, 5-foot 10-inch, 74-kg man in no acute distress. He was neurologically intact with clear lungs and no peripheral edema. Murmurs of aortic insufficiency and mitral regurgitation grade III/VI were present.

Vital Signs

BP	90/60
HR	60
Resp	18
Temp	99°F

Cardiac Cath Results

RAP	0
RVP	40/0
PAP	40/12
PAWP	8
CO	3.36
CI	1.76

Laboratory Values

Na	143	ALT	24
K	5.0	AST	21
Cl	104	BUN	74
CO_2	31	Digoxin level	1.3
Gluc	54	PT	12/12
Creat	1.6	PTT	28/27
Hgb	12.4	RBC	4.75
Hct	37.2	T bili	0.4
WBC	8.4	TP	7.2
Albumin	3.7		

After an extensive evaluation, Mr. Harley's name was placed on the organ procurement computer on December 26, 1988. Donor weight range for Mr. Harley was 61–86 kg. His ABO group was B+ with no atypical antibodies.

On January 22, 1989, Mr. Harley was placed on gown and glove isolation and medicated with cyclosporine, methylprednisolone, and azathioprine and sent to the Operating Room to receive a heart transplant. After 8 hr in surgery he was admitted to the ICU.

Hemodynamic Parameters		Vital Signs		
CVP	10	BP		112/67
PAP	36/16	HR	109	junctional
PAWP	13			tachycardia
CO	4.6			
CI	2.4			
SVR	1252			
$S_{\bar{v}}O_2$	63%			

Laboratory Values		ABGs	
Na	136	pH	7.45
K	4.7	$PaCO_2$	36
Cl	100	PaO_2	315
CO_2	28	SaO_2	98%
Gluc	141	HCO_2	25
Creat	1.5	**Ventilator Settings**	
Hgb	12.0		
Hct	36.8	Mode	SIMV
Plat	99,000	FIO_2	0.8
BUN	26	Tidal volume	700
PT	14/12	Rate	10
PTT	41/27		

Medications: Dobutamine, 5 μg/kg/min
              Nitroprusside (Nipride), 0.3 μg/kg/min
              Isoproteronol (Isuprel), 0.67 μg/min
Chest tube drainage: 15–30 ml/hr for first 24 hours total = 520 ml

FIO_2 was decreased to 0.4 with the following ABGs:

pH	7.41
$PaCO_2$	37
PaO_2	130
SaO_2	98%
HCO_3	25

On January 24, 1989, 24 hours postoperatively, Mr. Harley was extubated and placed on 2 liters per minute nasal oxygen. His blood pressure, temperature, and respiratory rate were all within normal limits, but his heart rate had slowed to the low 80s, and his ECG monitor showed normal sinus rhythm with remnant P waves. The Isuprel infusion was increased to 1.3 μg/min to maintain a heart rate of 100.

The immunosuppression begun before surgery was continued, with cyclosporine being given PO, azathioprine administered every evening, and ATG given daily for 12 doses. Mr. Harley's steroids were being tapered. He had good bowel sounds and was started on oral feedings. By the third postoperative day, he was weaned off of dobutamine and Nipride. Subsequently, his hemodynamic parameters were:

CI	1.2
SVR	3500
$S_{\bar{v}}O_2$	37%

The dobutamine was restarted at 2.3 μg/kg/min and the cardiac index improved to 2.0 liters/min/m^2. Isuprel administration remained at 1.3 μg/min with a heart rate of 90–100. Pulmonary artery and arterial lines were discontinued the evening of January 25 and Mr. Harley was assisted out of bed to a reclining chair.

Laboratory Values

TP	5.4
Albumin	3.3
Cholesterol	83

On January 28, Mr. Harley's heart rate was remaining at 90–100 and he was weaned off of Isuprel. The patient was ambulatory in the room without difficulty and by January 30, he was ready for transfer to the telemetry floor. A transvenous endomyocardial biopsy on February 8 showed acute early rejection and methylprednisolone was started. Mr. Harley continued to improve clinically, and a biopsy the next week was negative. The patient was discharged from the hospital February 23, 1 month posttransplantation. His discharge medications included cyclosporine, azathioprine, ferrous sulfate, and multivitamins.

QUESTIONS AND ANSWERS

1. **What are the major steps in evaluating a patient for cardiac transplantation? Which specific criteria did Mr. Harley meet? Were there contraindications for transplantation?**

    Cardiac transplantation is the only therapy now available to prolong life in the patient with end-stage heart disease. When the decision was made that no additional medical therapy or conventional surgical procedures could offer help to Mr. Harley, he was referred for evaluation for transplant. Evaluation protocols vary depending on the transplant center but usually include:

Complete medical history and physical examination
Laboratory workup including
  Biochemical
  Hematologic
  Immunologic
  Radiologic
  Microbiologic and virologic
Pulmonary function evaluation
Complete cardiac workup
Psychosocial, pulmonary, renal, infectious disease, and other consultations as needed

Eligibility is based on the information obtained from this extensive evaluation if the following criteria are met:

End-stage cardiac disease with maximum medical therapy for which no conventional surgery can offer help
<55–60 years of age
Stable psychologically with ability to understand procedure, risks, need for lifetime compliance.

Mr. Harley met all of the criteria.

Contraindications for transplantation usually include any of the following:

Irreversible multiorgan failure
Systemic infection or disease
Active bleeding
Neurologic deficits
Current drug or alcohol abuse
Pulmonary hypertension or recent pulmonary embolus

Mr. Harley's decreased renal function (demonstrated by a potassium of 5.0, BUN 74, and creatinine 1.6) was the only concern. This was most likely prerenal and was not considered serious enough to prevent transplantation.

2. **Once the patient has been accepted as a candidate for transplantation, he or she may have to wait for weeks or months for a donor heart. Describe the psychological impact of this period on the patient and his or her family.**

Acceptance after the evaluation procedure usually brings hope and excitement to the end-stage cardiac disease patient. However, the knowledge that someone else must die for the patient to receive the organ so desperately needed is often difficult to deal with and may bring guilt feelings. As holidays or weekends approach, hope may be countered with sadness, fear, and anxiety. Progressive symptoms, hemodynamic deterioration, hospitalization, and maintenance on inotropic IV therapy, intraaortic balloon counterpulsation, or even a ventricular assist device compound the psychological trauma of waiting. Recipient priority classifications have been established and range from working or attending school to dire need where death is imminent without transplant. The decision of who will receive the available heart is often made on the basis of priority, although it is known that patients in better preoperative condition have a significantly better chance for recovery. This may have ethical implications for the patient and his family. Another consideration is the travel distance required to access the donor heart.

3. How is a cardiac donor selected?

Selection of a donor for the waiting patient is made on the basis of ABO group, general weight and size, and how far the donor is from the transplant center. Human lymphocyte antigen (HLA) matching is done if time allows. HLA typing is completed posttransplant for retrospective research if it cannot be done before the patient receives the transplant. Ischemic time cannot be >4 hr in most centers. Certain criteria must be met before a person declared brain dead can become a heart donor:

> Absence of systemic infection or transmissible disease
> Absence of malignancy (excluding primary, nonmetastatic brain tumor)
> Absence of heart disease, cardiac trauma (no CPR, intracardiac injections, or defibrillation)
> <35 years of age for males, <40 years of age for females
> Requiring minimal inotropic support

4. What is an orthotopic transplant procedure?

The recipient's diseased heart is excised and the posterior walls of both atria are left in place. The donor heart is trimmed to fit the recipient atria and sutured in place. The pulmonary arteries and aorta of donor and recipient are anastomosed (Fig. 2.1). The recipient's right atrium retains its SA node. Although the recipient's SA node fires, impulses originating there are not conducted. The donor heart's SA node is also present, and because of the intact conduction system of the donor heart, it transmits electrical impulses normally to the ventricles. The ECG will show P waves from both recipient and donor SA nodes. The P waves originating from the recipient's right atrium are termed "remnant" P waves (Fig. 2.2).

5. What is the leading cause of death within the first 3 months after cardiac transplantation? What puts Mr. Harley at risk?

The leading cause of early death (<3 months) following cardiac transplantation is infection. Most infections are bacterial with viral,

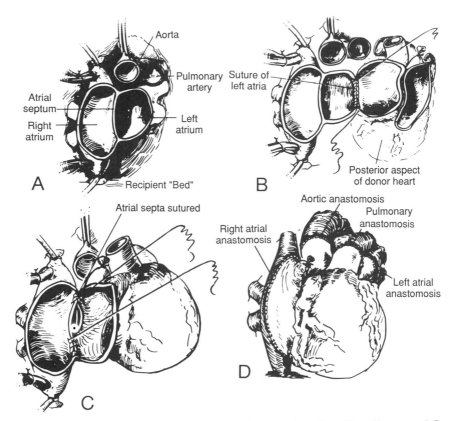

Figure 2.1. Surgical technique of orthotopic cardiac transplantation. (From Futterman LG. Cardiac transplantation: A comprehensive nursing perspective. Part I. Heart Lung 1988;17(5):499–507.)

fungal, and protozoal in smaller percentages and occurring later in the recovery period. Sites of early bacterial infections are pulmonary, central nervous system, and urinary tract. Mr. Harley is at risk for infection because of his weeks of hospitalization prior to transplantation, immunosuppressive therapy, multiple invasive lines, and the surgical procedure itself.

6. **Mr. Harley was on dobutamine and Isuprel IV infusions postoperatively. How do these drugs help overcome the hemodynamic effects of the denervated donor heart?**

Once the donor heart is implanted, it must adjust to the absence of balanced autonomic innervation. Catecholamines, which have inotropic, chronotropic, and dromotropic effects on cardiac function,

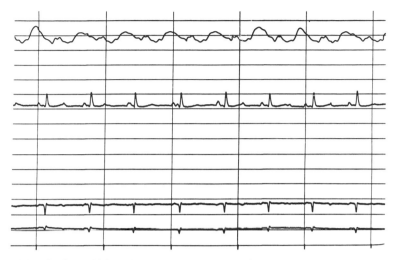

Figure 2.2. Surface ECG and venous pulse tracing demonstrating characteristic dissociation between donor and recipient P wave activity. Recipient P wave remains electrically isolated and thus ineffective in transmission of sinus impulses. (From Futterman LG. Cardiac transplantation: A comprehensive nursing perspective. Part II. Heart Lung 1988;17(6): 631–638.)

must now come from intravenous drug administration or normal circulating catecholamines released from the adrenal medulla. Because of the stress of end-stage cardiac disease and the stress of surgery, Mr. Harley's circulating catecholamines may be depleted. Therefore, replacement with dobutamine for the inotropic effect and Isuprel for the chronotropic and dromotropic effects is necessary. With increased oxygen demand, the normally innervated heart increases rate and contractile force. The response of the denervated heart is controlled by increases in preload and circulating plasma catecholamines, which increase contractility and rate, respectively. In addition, vagal parasympathetic stimulation such as Valsalva maneuvers, carotid sinus massage, or abrupt posture changes have no effect on the denervated heart. On January 25, Mr. Harley's cardiac index decreased because the dobutamine had been discontinued. His systemic vascular resistance increased because the afterload-reducing drug Nipride had been discontinued. The second factor contributing to the increased SVR may have been a compensatory increase in preload to augment the patient's cardiac index. He needed the inotropic support a little longer as seen by the increase in his cardiac index when the dobutamine was restarted.

7. **How much postoperative bleeding did Mr. Harley have? Why is medi-astinal bleeding of concern in the cardiac transplant patient?**

    Mr. Harley's chest tube drainage was not excessive. It is important to monitor chest tube drainage and cardiac function (cardiac index and output, left and right ventricular filling pressures, and blood pressure) frequently because tamponade is a potential complication of any cardiac surgery. Chronic congestive heart failure and right ventricular failure can lead to decreased liver function and abnormal coagulation. Heparinization during cardiopulmonary bypass may not be reversed totally and may lead to bleeding. Because of Mr. Harley's ischemic cardiomyopathy, his pericardium had stretched to accommodate his enlarged heart. When the smaller, donor heart was implanted, a pericardial space was left, which could collect and conceal this postoperative bleeding. Turning the patient side to side and assuring patency of the mediastinal chest tubes can usually avoid concealed blood collection.

8. **Mr. Harley converted from a junctional tachycardia to "sinus rhythm with remnant P waves" on the second postoperative day. Explain the meaning of this rhythm and the reason the patient needs a heart rate greater than 80.**

    Because Mr. Harley's posterior atrial wall was not excised during the orthotopic transplant procedure, his SA node continued to re-spond to sympathetic and parasympathetic stimuli and produce P waves. These remnant P waves are unable to cross the scar line to reach the myocardium and therefore are evidence of electrical activ-ity only. The donor heart's SA node, unaffected by autonomic ner-vous system stimulation or the recipient's SA node, controls conduc-tion, depolarization, and contraction. In order for the transplanted heart to increase in rate, it must be stimulated by an increased pre-load and circulating catecholamines. A slightly elevated resting heart rate will help ensure adequate tissue perfusion.

9. **As with other transplanted organs, rejection may occur. How does hyperacute rejection differ from acute rejection?**

    Hyperacute rejection is an immediate catastrophic rejection of the donor heart by the immune system of the recipient. There is evidence that it can occur in the absence of ABO incompatibility or any HLA antidonor antibodies. Antidonor vascular endothelial cell antibodies may be responsible. Damage occurs within minutes, causing throm-bosis of coronary arteries and ischemic failure. Acute rejection oc-curs most frequently within the first 2 months after transplantation and is diagnosed by endomyocardial biopsy. The interstitium and myocardium become edematous, with infiltration of lymphocytes and other immunoactive cells. Acute rejection is classified as early and moderate, both of which are reversible, and severe rejection, which is very difficult or impossible to reverse. Severe rejection involves interstitial hemorrhage and myocyte necrosis. Clinical signs of rejection include fatigue, low grade fever, shortness of breath, and weight gain.

10. **Immunosuppression therapy varies with physician and transplant center. What are the drugs most commonly used and the method of determining toxicity of each?**

Methylprednisolone (Solu-Medrol)

Primary Action—impairs recognition of antigens and the resulting macrophage response, antibody synthesis, and T-cell proliferation.

Method of Monitoring—Large doses of steroid therapy are usually administered at the time of transplant with doses tapered over several weeks. Some centers discontinue steroid therapy before discharge if possible. Drug levels or specific laboratory tests to determine toxicity are not used.

Major Side Effects—prolonged healing, masking of infection, glucose intolerance.

Azathioprine (Imuran)

Primary Action—inhibits purine and DNA synthesis, thereby preventing the proliferation of immunologically active cells, especially white blood cells.

Method of Monitoring—monitor WBC and platelet count. Leukopenia and thrombocytopenia are dose dependent and usually reversible with dose reduction.

Major Side Effects—bone marrow suppression and hepatotoxicity.

Cyclosporine (Sandimmune)

Primary action—inhibits helper T-cell production of interleukin-2 thereby selectively providing cell-mediated immunosuppression without suppression of the total immune system.

Method of Monitoring—Serum or blood trough levels are monitored every 12 hr at first, then less frequently as the risk of rejection decreases and the dose is lowered.

Major Side Effects—vasoconstriction causing nephrotoxicity and hypertension, and hepatotoxicity.

Anti-human Thymocyte Globulin (ATG)

Primary Action—coats targeted T-cells making them more easily phagocytosed

Method of Monitoring—usually given immediately before and/or after transplantation for a limited number of doses. Also given in response to moderate to severe rejection episodes not suppressed by steroids.

Major Side Effects—hypersensitivity and anaphylaxis, pain at injection site or cellulitis.

11. How was Mr. Harley's acute rejection on February 8 treated and why was this regimen chosen?

Mr. Harley's endomyocardial biopsy on February 8 showed early acute rejection. He received the standard therapy of methylprednisolone 1 g IV followed by 500 mg daily for 2 days. High dose steroid therapy causes failure of antigen recognition, and lymphocytes are no longer drawn to the donor organ. The lymphocytes already aggregated in the organ redistribute. These effects inhibited the progression of Mr. Harley's rejection episode. A clear biopsy does not rule out rejection, as it is possible that the tissue sample was not in the specific area of rejection.

12. Nutrition is a vital part of recovery. What was Mr. Harley's nutritional status preoperatively and on the third postoperative day?

Pretransplantation Mr. Harley's nutritional status was adequate, based on height, weight, total protein, and albumin. Because he was not malnourished at the time of surgery as some end-stage cardiac disease patients may be, nutrition was not a significant problem. After his transplant, it was not necessary for Mr. Harley to have tube feedings or hyperalimentation because he was extubated on the second postoperative day and began to eat on day 3. The best diet for him was a low cholesterol, low fat, low sugar diet. Because of the risk of sugar intolerance when on steroids, complex carbohydrates are much better than simple carbohydrates. Some centers omit raw unpeeled fruits and vegetables from the diet for 6–8 weeks because the risk of infection is increased.

13. On January 29, Mr. Harley was 7 days postop and planning to transfer to the telemetry floor the next day. What psychological concerns would the nurse expect to deal with at this time?

Dependency, excitement at improvement, fear of change and decreased nursing support, fear of organ rejection, and a desire for more independence can all be present in some form. Ambivalent feelings as well as steroid-induced mood swings may make it difficult for the family to understand and support Mr. Harley. Frank discussions of feelings and fears in an accepting atmosphere often help the patient to sort out thoughts and emotions. Listening to Mr. Harley may be the best therapy the nurse can give.

14. **Mr. Harley was discharged from the hospital 32 days after his transplant. What patient teaching was necessary before discharge in order for him to care for himself at home?**

Mr. Harley was encouraged to learn about and participate in his own care. He was given information at every stage of the treatment. The nurse made sure he knew how to care for himself as he was recovering in the hospital. Information was given to him on:

Symptoms of infection, rejection, and drug toxicity
Medication administration and side effects
Cardiac biopsy procedure and meaning of results
Exercise, activity, and the effects of the denervated heart on activities of daily living
Methods of preventing infection
Transplant team members to call with questions or problems

Mr. Harley was provided with a notebook containing important information plus pages for personal record keeping. Compliance is enhanced when patients participate in and understand their care.

15. **What nursing diagnoses would apply to Mr. Harley's cardiac transplantation?**

Potential for infection related to surgery and immunosuppression
Potential for injury related to rejection
Decreased cardiac output related to decreased heart rate
Impaired verbal communication related to endotracheal intubation
Sleep pattern disturbance related to environment
Powerlessness
Knowledge deficit related to self-care posttransplantation
Fear related to rejection episode
Alteration in body image related to donor heart
Pain

16. **One year after his transplant, Mr. Harley was admitted to a community hospital with abdominal pain. What basic understanding of heart transplantation must the staff have in order to care for Mr. Harley?**

Transplanted hearts are denervated, therefore:

Resting heart rate will be above normal.
Slow response in heart rate is seen with hypovolemia, exercise, fever, or hypoxemia.

There is no vagal response so anticholinergic drugs (atropine) will not increase heart rate.

No heart rate response occurs with change in posture so care must be taken to prevent orthostasis.

Any chest pain comes from the chest wall, pleura, or is referred pain. Infarctions present with dyspnea, hypotension, or conduction changes. Mr. Harley is unable to experience anginal pain.

Immunosuppression therapy must continue for life, therefore:

Current medication regimen must be followed carefully.

Cyclosporine is given even when Mr. Harley is taking nothing by mouth.

Method of storage, measurement, and administration are very important with cyclosporine.

Immunosuppression predisposes to infection, therefore:

Mr. Harley should not be admitted to an area adjacent to infected patients.

Strict handwashing is imperative and masks should be worn by all caregivers.

Sterile gloves should be worn for all invasive procedures, and nonsterile gloves should be worn when working with the patient.

Lines and tubes should be put in only when absolutely necessary and removed as early as possible.

At the first sign of infection, Mr. Harley should be thoroughly cultured and antibiotics should be administered. Response to infection may be suppressed due to immunosuppression and the normal signs may be absent.

Viral and fungal infections, as well as bacterial, impose a threat.

SUGGESTED READINGS

Barnhart GR, Richard R. Lower cardiac transplantation. In: Cerilli GJ, ed. Organ transplantation and replacement. Philadelphia: JB Lippincott, 1988:493–510.

Futterman LG. Cardiac transplantation: A comprehensive nursing perspective. Part I. Heart Lung 1988;17(5):499–510.

Futterman LG. Cardiac transplantation: A comprehensive nursing perspective. Part II. Heart Lung 1988;17(6):631–638.

Living with heart transplantation. Sandoz Pharmaceuticals Corp., 1988.

McGregor CGA. Cardiac and cardiopulmonary transplantation. In: Catto RGRD, ed. Clinical transplantation Boston: MTP Press, 1987:211–226.

Metzger JT, Hoffman LA. Cardiac transplantation: The changing faces of immunosuppression. Heart Lung 1988;17(4):414–425.

CHAPTER 3

Cardiogenic Shock in Anterior Myocardial Infarction

Margaret A. Wegner, RN, BSN, CCRN

Charles Case is a 65-year-old man who was admitted to the Coronary Care Unit with a diagnosis of acute anterior myocardial infarction (MI). He complained of severe substernal chest pain lasting over 4 hr that was accompanied by a "choking feeling," severe shortness of breath, and diaphoresis. He described the pain as a deep pressure that was unrelieved by rest, antacids, or three sublingual nitroglycerin tablets.

Significant medical history included stable exertional angina for 7 years, adult-onset diabetes mellitus for 3 years, and recently diagnosed hypertension. He had a 45-year history of cigarette smoking averaging 1½–2 packs/day. He was not taking any routine daily medications and took less than one sublingual nitroglycerin tablet a month for anginal chest pain.

In the Emergency Department, Mr. Case's initial examination revealed a moderately overweight male in obvious distress. Vital signs were:

BP	164/100
HR	122
Resp	34
Temp	36°C

His mentation was clear, and he was able to move all extremities spontaneously with purpose. His skin was cool, pale, and diaphoretic. No peripheral edema was noted. A normal S_1 and S_2 were auscultated without murmurs, gallops, or rubs. Respirations were slightly labored but all lung fields were clear to auscultation.

Mr. Case complained of continued shortness of breath and chest pain and he was given supplemental oxygen at 2 liters/min/nasal cannula. Cardiac monitoring revealed sinus tachycardia (120 beats/min) without ectopy. An intravenous line was placed and 3 mg of morphine sulfate was administered IV push with a decrease in chest pain noted within minutes. A 12-lead ECG revealed sinus tachycardia, no ectopy, and normal QRS complexes. The ST segments were elevated in leads V_{1-4}, and Q waves were noted in leads V_{2-4}.

Laboratory results were significant for an elevated creatine kinase (CK) and MB isoenzymes with normal serum concentrations of lactate dehydrogenase (LDH) and aspartate aminotransferase (AST)—formerly termed serum glutamic oxaloacetic transaminase (SGOT). Serum concen-

21

trations of glucose, cholesterol, and triglyceride were elevated, and serum electrolytes and CBC were within normal limits. An arterial blood gas revealed a respiratory alkalosis with adequate oxygenation.

QUESTIONS AND ANSWERS

1. How is the diagnosis of anterior myocardial infarction made?

The diagnosis of an MI is usually determined by three factors:

> The patient's history and physical assessment
> Elevation of specific cardiac enzymes and isoenzymes
> Serial ECG changes in specific leads

The patient presenting with an MI usually complains of chest pain, with or without radiation, that is more severe than his or her typical angina and of greater duration, frequently lasting more than 30 min. The patient may also complain of nausea, shortness of breath, dyspnea, dizziness, or weakness and may appear restless, diaphoretic, ashen, or cyanotic. Cardiac auscultation may reveal an S_3, S_4, murmur, or rub. The patient will frequently deny he or she could be having an MI.

Elevation of serum cardiac enzymes is a result of myocardial cell damage. This occurs when myocardial ischemia, due to an imbalance in the myocardial oxygen supply/demand ratio, results in myocardial tissue infarction. With progressive myocardial cell damage, there is leakage of intracellular enzymes into the blood with a subsequent rise and peak in serum concentration of the cardiac enzymes—first CK, then AST, and finally LDH. Quantification of these enzymes during the first 24–48 hr after an MI can be used to estimate the amount of cellular damage that has occurred. However, these enzymes may also be elevated due to other kinds of muscular injury or following cardioversion/defibrillation. CK-MB is a "myocardial-specific" isoenzyme of CK. Its presence in the blood is an indication of myocardial injury.

ECG changes that reflect a transmural anterior myocardial infarction will be noted in the precordial leads V_{1-4}. These may include: (*a*) Q waves, (*b*) loss of R wave voltage, and (*c*) ST elevation with initially peaked and later inverted T waves. (For more details on the diagnostic value of 12-lead ECGs in the setting of MI, see Chapter 11, "Inferior Myocardial Infarction with Right Ventricular Myocardial Infarction.")

A variety of noninvasive techniques may be used to identify, localize, or estimate the size of a myocardial infarction and assess residual myocardial function. These tests include: technetium 99m stannous pyrophosphate scintigraphy (also called PYP scan), thallium-201 myocardial scintigraphy, radionuclide ventriculography, echocardiography, and magnetic resonance imaging (MRI).

Admission orders included 12-lead ECG and cardiac enzyme levels q 6 hr for the first 24 hr, strict bedrest, and continuous cardiac monitoring. With patient complaints of chest pain, nurses were to obtain a 12-lead ECG and notify the physician.

Medications ordered included:

> Morphine sulfate, 2–5 mg IV push PRN chest pain not relieved by nitroglycerin
>
> Propranolol, 10 mg slow IV push now
>
> Propranolol, 40 mg PO q 6 hr; start 1 hr after IV dose is given (hold for systolic BP < 90, HR <40)
>
> Nitroglycerin (NTG), per continuous IV infusion; start at 5 μg/min and increase by 5 μg/min q 5 min for relief of chest pain; hold for systolic BP ≤100
>
> Regular insulin, SC q 6 hr PRN per sliding scale for glucose >200
>
> Colace, 100 mg PO BID
>
> Heparin, 5000 units SC BID

2. **What is the goal of treatment for a myocardial infarction? What methods are employed to meet this goal?**

The goal of treatment is to minimize the amount of myocardial damage and preserve the maximum amount of functional myocardium. This is accomplished through mechanical, pharmacological, and nursing interventions that increase myocardial oxygen supply and decrease myocardial oxygen demand.

In the setting of an acute MI, mechanical interventions such as percutaneous transluminal coronary angioplasty or coronary artery revascularization may be employed to restore coronary blood flow rapidly. (For more details, see Chapter 16, "Unstable Angina and Percutaneous Transluminal Coronary Angioplasty" and Chapter 7, "Coronary Artery Bypass Graft.")

Coronary blood flow may also be restored by administration of thrombolytic agents, as >90% of acute transmural infarctions occur secondary to occlusive coronary artery thromboses. Thrombolytic agents include streptokinase, urokinase, and tissue plasminogen activator. (For further details, see Chapter 15, "Thrombolytic Therapy for Acute Myocardial Infarction.")

Medications may also be given in the acute stage of an MI to attempt to beneficially affect the balance between myocardial oxygen supply and demand. Morphine sulfate, which acts as a sedative and an analgesic, reduces myocardial oxygen demand by alleviating the anxiety with resultant tachycardia and hypertension that frequently occur in the patient who is having an MI. Furthermore, morphine sulfate also causes peripheral venodilatation, which reduces oxygen demand by decreasing preload. It is given intravenously in increments of 2–4 mg q 5 min until chest pain is relieved, with careful monitoring of heart rate (morphine should not be given if the patient is bradycardic), and with frequent assessments for respiratory depression, nausea, or urinary retention.

Nitroglycerin may be given both to decrease preload (by increasing venous capacitance) and to increase coronary blood flow (by dilating the coronary arteries). Nitroglycerin therefore decreases oxygen demand and increases oxygen supply simultaneously. (For information on nitroglycerin, see Chapter 16, "Unstable Angina and Percutaneous Transluminal Coronary Angioplasty.") While Nipride is also used in the post-MI period for its vasodilating effects, it may occasionally prove detrimental. As a result of its nonpreferential vasodilatation, blood may actually be distributed away from the ischemic myocardium. This phenomenon is known as coronary "steal" syndrome.

β-Adrenergic blocking agents such as propranolol, atenolol, and metoprolol may be administered in the first hours after MI to reduce myocardial oxygen demand by decreasing sympathetic stimulation of the myocardium. This causes a decrease in heart rate, myocardial contractility, cardiac output, and blood pressure. Several studies have demonstrated that the administration of β-adrenergic blockers early in the setting of an MI may reduce infarct size. This may be the result of decreased myocardial oxygen demand, redistribution of blood from the epicardium to the ischemic areas of the subendocardium, or antagonism of the direct and indirect cardiotoxic effects of elevated catecholamine levels. β-Blockers have also been shown to decrease the occurrence of complex ventricular dysrhythmias (i.e., ventricular fibrillation), reinfarction rate, and post-MI mortality. Typically, a 5–15-mg dose would be given intravenously over 5–10 min, while carefully monitoring for hypotension and bradycardia, followed 30–60 min later with an oral dose. Total recommended daily oral dose of each agent would be:

Propranolol	160–480 mg/day
Atenolol	50–100 mg/day
Metoprolol	100–200 mg/day

Administration is contraindicated in patients with hypotension, bradycardia, severe heart failure, AV block, or bronchial asthma.

A decrease in myocardial contractility, heart rate, and afterload may be achieved by administration of calcium-channel blocking agents (i.e., verapamil, diltiazem, nifedipine). These medications prevent the flow of calcium ions into the cells, resulting in smooth muscle relaxation and vasodilatation of both coronary and peripheral vessels. The benefits of calcium-antagonist administration include both decreased myocardial oxygen demand and increased blood flow to the ischemic areas. (For more details, see Chapter 17, "Vasospastic (Prinzmetal's) Angina.")

Other agents under study for use in limiting infarct size include: nonsteroidal anti-inflammatory drugs, hyaluronidase, free-radical scavengers (i.e., mannitol, allopurinol, catalase), prostacyclin, and a glucose, insulin, and potassium infusion.

Nursing interventions to minimize myocardial oxygen demand and maximize myocardial oxygen supply include encouraging bedrest, administering supplemental oxygen per orders, and maintaining a calm, quiet environment. Antianxiety medications (i.e., diazepam) may be administered as needed.

On admission to the CCU, Mr. Case's vital signs were:

BP	150/100
HR	112
Resp	30
Temp	36°C

Mr. Case stated that his chest pain was a mild, dull ache, and he appeared to be in no acute distress. Propranolol was given as ordered, and nitroglycerin infusion was maintained at a rate of 30 μg/min with complete relief of chest pain. A Foley catheter was placed.

One hour later, Mr. Case experienced the sudden onset of shortness of breath. Auscultation of his lungs revealed diffuse crackles. Within 10 min, he complained of severe substernal pressure, and a change in his heart rate was noted. Vital signs at this time were:

BP	140/100
HR	126
Resp	36

He was placed on a 40% oxygen facemask, a 12-lead ECG was obtained, and the physician was notified immediately. The nitroglycerin infusion was increased with no improvement in chest pain, so morphine (2 mg) was administered intravenously. Twelve-lead ECG revealed sinus tachycardia without ectopy and a new left bundle branch block.

3. **What are the potential complications of an acute myocardial infarction?**

The potential complications include:

Dysrhythmias (i.e., tachyarrhythmias, heart block, ectopy)
Congestive heart failure
Cardiogenic shock
Left ventricular rupture
Infarct extension
Pericarditis
Papillary muscle dysfunction or rupture
Ventricular septal defect
Left ventricular aneurysm/pseudoaneurysm
Sudden death

4. **What is the significance of left bundle branch block occurring in the setting of an acute anterior MI?**

Most anterior MIs are due to an occlusion of the left anterior descending coronary artery, which supplies blood to the anterior surface of the left ventricle, ⅔ of the right bundle, the bundle of His, the anterior fascicle of the left bundle branch, and a part of the posterior fascicle of the left bundle branch. With an anterior myocardial infarction, necrosis may occur in these conducting tissues, resulting in bundle branch block (right, left, bifascicular), and/or atrioventricular block (second and third degree).

Left bundle branch block (LBBB) is the most common complication of acute anterior MI. It occurs when electrical conduction through the bundle of His or both fascicles of the left bundle branch is blocked. When LBBB occurs, a temporary transvenous pacemaker should be placed prophylactically, as the onset of a LBBB in the setting of an acute anterior MI signifies extensive left ventricular damage and may progress to a higher degree (i.e., third degree) heart block. (For ECG criteria, see Chapter 4, "Cardiomyopathy.")

Mr. Case continued to complain of severe chest pain and shortness of breath and he became increasingly agitated and restless. His skin was cool, ashen, and diaphoretic. He was placed on 100% oxygen and the nitroglycerin infusion increased without relief of his pain. An arterial blood gas on 100% oxygen revealed a mixed respiratory and metabolic acidosis with hypoxemia. Mr. Case's systolic blood pressure fell to 40 mm Hg and then improved to 80 mm Hg after successful intubation. The nitroglycerin infusion was discontinued due to hypotension.

A physical examination at this time revealed jugular venous distention, an S_3, rales in all lung fields, and depressed neurologic function with responsiveness only to painful stimuli. A chest x-ray showed the endotracheal tube in proper position, pulmonary vascular congestion, and an enlarged heart. Cardiogenic shock was suspected.

A temporary transvenous pacing wire was placed due to the new left bundle branch block. A balloon-tipped, flow-directed pulmonary artery catheter was inserted for hemodynamic monitoring. A radial arterial catheter was placed for continuous blood pressure monitoring and frequent blood sampling.

5. **What is cardiogenic shock? Why does it occur after myocardial infarction?**

   Cardiogenic shock is a circulatory state in which cardiac output fails to provide adequate perfusion to tissues and organs to fulfill metabolic requirements. Because the left anterior descending coronary artery ordinarily supplies the largest amount of myocardium, cardiogenic shock occurs most commonly in the setting of an anterior myocardial infarction and has a mortality rate of >80%. The pathogenesis of cardiogenic shock following myocardial infarction is:

   Infarction of myocardium → loss of myocardial functioning → abnormal, inadequate left ventricular functioning → decreased stroke volume → decreased cardiac output → increased left ventricular end-diastolic volume and pressure → increased myocardial oxygen demand and decreased tissue perfusion → systemic lactic acidosis → decreased myocardial functioning. This cycle repeats and the shock state exists until reversed by interventions.

6. **Most signs and symptoms of cardiogenic shock are reflections of inadequate tissue perfusion. These include:**

	Early Manifestations	Late Manifestations
Neurological:	Irritability	Lethargy
	Anxiety	Confusion
	Restlessness	Coma
Cardiovascular:	Tachycardia	Peripheral edema
	Normal or slightly decreased blood pressure	Jugular venous distention
		Angina
	S_3 gallop	Tachycardia
		Hypotension
		S_3 gallop
Pulmonary:	Tachypnea (due to chemoreceptor stimulation)	Pulmonary congestion
		Tachypnea (to compensate for metabolic acidosis)

Gastrointestinal/	Oliguria	Hypoactive bowel
genitourinary:		sounds
		Oliguria
		Anuria

The laboratory values in cardiogenic shock typically reflect:

Serum—Metabolic acidosis with respiratory compensation (i.e., decreased bicarbonate, increased lactate, decreased arterial CO_2) hypoxemia, increased creatinine, increased BUN, increased potassium

Urine—increased specific gravity and osmolality, decreased creatinine clearance

Mr. Case's initial vital signs and hemodynamic parameters were:

CVP	16	BP	90/58
PAP	50/24	HR	128
PAWP	30		
CO	2.0		
CI	1.03		
SVR	2120		

Urine output at this time was 15–20 ml/hr.

7. **What are the normal hemodynamic parameters? What are the typical hemodynamic findings in cardiogenic shock?**

Normal		**Cardiogenic Shock**
CVP	2–6	Elevated
PAP	20–30/8–15	Elevated
PAWP	6–12	Elevated (>20)
CO	4–8	Decreased
CI	2.5–4	Decreased (<1.8)
SVR	900–1200	Elevated

Continuous intravenous infusions of dopamine and dobutamine were initiated at 2.5 µg/kg/min each.

8. **What are the therapeutic benefits of dopamine and dobutamine administration in cardiogenic shock?**

Dopamine is the metabolic precursor of norepinephrine. Its pharmacologic effects are dose related. In low doses (<5 µg/kg/min), it stimulates the dopaminergic receptors, resulting in increased renal blood flow and increased urine output. At an infusion rate of 5–10 µg/kg/min, cardiac β-adrenergic receptors are stimulated, resulting in an increased contractility and cardiac output. Dopamine stimulates the α-adrenergic receptors at doses >10 µg/kg/min causing vasoconstriction in all vascular beds. This may result in an increased arterial blood pressure and systemic vascular resistance and decreased urine output. Dopamine is administered as a continuous intravenous infusion through a central venous access, using an infusion pump to carefully regulate the flow rate. Infusions are usually started at 2.5 μg/kg/min and maintained at 5–20 μg/kg/min, titrating to a mean arterial pressure of 70–80 mm Hg or a systolic BP of 90–100 mm Hg. The side effects associated with dopamine infusion include tachycardia and ventricular dysrhythmias.

Dobutamine is a synthetic catecholamine that stimulates the β-adrenergic receptors. The effects of dobutamine administration include: (*a*) increased myocardial contractility, (*b*) improved stroke volume, (*c*) decreased systemic vascular resistance (in higher doses), and (*d*) decreased ventricular filling pressure resulting in improved coronary perfusion. These changes result in an increased cardiac output, decreased pulmonary congestion, and decreased myocardial oxygen consumption, usually without any significant change in heart rate, blood pressure, or frequency of dysrhythmias. Dobutamine is administered as a continuous intravenous infusion through a central venous access, using an infusion pump to carefully regulate the flow rate. Infusions are usually started at 2.5 μg/kg/min and maintained at 5–10 μg/kg/min (30 μg/kg/min maximum).

Dopamine and dobutamine may be used alone or in combination in patients in cardiogenic shock. Given in approximately equal doses, the benefits of combined infusion include: (*a*) improved myocardial contractility, (*b*) maintenance of adequate systemic arterial pressure, (*c*) enhanced renal perfusion (maintaining an adequate urine output), and (*d*) decreased pulmonary artery wedge pressure.

To calculate the amount of dopamine or dobutamine the patient is receiving, the following formula is used:

$$\frac{\mu\text{g drug}}{\text{ml diluent}} \times \frac{\text{infusion rate (ml/hr)}}{60 \text{ min/hr}} \times \frac{1}{\text{weight (kg)}} = x \ \mu\text{g/kg/min}$$

The dopamine infusion was titrated to maintain a systolic blood pressure of 100 mm Hg. The dobutamine was titrated to establish and maintain a cardiac output of 4–6 liters/min.

Many hours later, vital signs and hemodynamic parameters had improved to:

CVP	12	BP	126/54
PAP	40/18	HR	103
PAWP	22		
CO	4.1		
CI	2.1		
SVR	1288		

Urine output improved to 60–80 ml/hr.

Over the next 2 days, the dobutamine and dopamine infusions were weaned without hemodynamic compromise. Intravenous furosemide was administered to improve diuresis and help relieve pulmonary congestion. Oxygenation improved and mechanical ventilatory support was also weaned. Urine output was >80–100 ml/hr. The intravenous nitroglycerin infusion was resumed and titrated to a maintenance dose of 30 μg/min.

9. **What is the rationale for administering a nitroglycerin infusion in cardiogenic shock?**

    Intravenous nitroglycerin infusion causes a decrease in both preload and afterload. Nitroglycerin causes peripheral venodilatation, which reduces venous return to the right side of the heart thereby decreasing preload. At high doses, intravenous nitroglycerin infusion may cause arterial dilatation and a reduction in systemic vascular resistance thereby decreasing afterload. The beneficial effects on preload and afterload decrease the left ventricular workload and myocardial oxygen demand. (For more details on intravenous nitroglycerin infusions, see Chapter 16, "Unstable Angina and Percutaneous Transluminal Coronary Angioplasty.")

10. **What mechanical interventions are available for the treatment of cardiogenic shock?**

    Intraaortic balloon pump (IABP) counterpulsation and left ventricular assist devices may be used successfully in the treatment of cardiogenic shock. Counterpulsation with the intraaortic balloon pump is carefully timed so that inflation of the balloon occurs with diastole, thereby increasing blood flow to the coronary arteries. Deflation of the balloon occurs during systole, thereby decreasing left ventricular outflow resistance (i.e., afterload). (See Chapter 4, "Cardiomyopathy," for futher information regarding IABP.) A left ventricular assist device may be used to aid the damaged left ventricle in providing an adequate cardiac output. Systemic circulation is augmented while viable areas of the left ventricle recover from ischemia and injury.

By the fifth hospital day, Mr. Case was successfully extubated. He remained lethargic and confused. Hemodynamic parameters at this time were all within normal limits. The nitroglycerin infusion was discontinued, and the pulmonary artery and radial artery catheters were removed. Maintenance medications included captopril, 12.5 mg PO TID, digoxin, 0.125 mg PO q day, and furosemide, 40 mg PO BID. As the LBBB persisted, Mr. Case was scheduled for permanent pacemaker placement and transferred to a general medical ward.

11. What are other potential complications of cardiogenic shock?

Cerebral infarction
Disseminated intravascular coagulation
Dysrhythmias
Gastrointestinal ulcers and ischemia
Liver dysfunction
Myocardial infarction
Renal failure

12. What nursing diagnoses apply in this case?

Decreased cardiac output related to cardiogenic shock and dysrhythmias
Altered cardiac tissue perfusion related to inadequate myocardial oxygen supply during MI
Altered peripheral tissue perfusion related to decreased cardiac output with cardiogenic shock and dysrhythmias
Pain related to myocardial ischemia during MI
Anxiety related to ICU environment and treatment regimen
Knowledge deficit regarding diagnosis and treatment
Potential infection related to invasive lines
Alteration in mental status related to inadequate cerebral perfusion with hypotension and cardiogenic shock
Alteration in acid/base balance related to inadequate tissue perfusion with hypotension and cardiogenic shock

SUGGESTED READINGS

Alspach JG, Williams SM. Core curriculum for critical care nursing. 3rd ed. Philadelphia: WB Saunders, 1985:162–163, 168–174.

Ayres SM. The prevention and treatment of shock in acute myocardial infarction. Chest 1988;93(1 Suppl):17–21.

Cane RD, Shapiro BA. Case studies in critical care medicine. Chicago: Year Book, 1985:147–160.

Gold HK, Leinbach RC. Thrombolysis in acute myocardial infarction. Chest 1988;93(Suppl 1):10–16.

Hillis LD, Firth BG, Winniford MD, Willerson JT. Manual of clinical problems in cardiology. 3rd ed. Boston: Little, Brown & Co, 1988:36–45, 48–49, 76–94, 114–115, 309–311.

Kenner CV, Guzetta CE, Dossey BM. Critical care nursing: Body, mind, spirit. 2nd ed. Boston: Little, Brown & Co, 1982:82.

Lange RA, Hillis LD. Southwestern Internal Medicine Conference: Evolving concepts in the treatment of acute myocardial infarction. Am J Med Sci 1988;296(2):143–152.

Misinski M. Pathophysiology of acute myocardial infarction: A rationale for thrombolytic therapy. Heart Lung 1988:17(6) (Part 2):743–750.

Misinski M. Role of conventional management and alternative therapies in limiting infarct size in acute myocardial infarction. Heart Lung 1987;16(6)(Part 2):746–755.

Rippe JM, Csete ME, eds. Manual of intensive care medicine. 1st ed. Boston: Little, Brown & Co, 1983:56–57, 67–85.

Roberts R. Enzymatic diagnosis of acute myocardial infarction. Chest 1988;93 (Suppl 1):3–6.

Roberts R. Inotropic therapy for cardiac failure associated with acute myocardial infarction. Chest 1988;93(Suppl 1):22–24.

Willerson JT. Radionuclide assessment and diagnosis of acute myocardial infarction. Chest 1988;93(Suppl 1):7–9.

Yusaf S. The use of Beta-adrenergic blocking agents, intravenous nitrates, and calcium-channel blocking agents following acute myocardial infarction. Chest 1988; 93(Suppl 1):25–28.

CHAPTER 4

Cardiomyopathy

Diane L. Gilworth, RN, BSN, CCRN

Albert Davis is a moderately obese 55-year-old man with a history of hypertension and coronary artery disease. He had his first episode of angina on March 3, 1988, at which time he was admitted to a community hospital and a myocardial infarction was ruled out. He underwent a cardiac catheterization, which revealed a 90% occlusion of the left main coronary artery, 100% occlusion of the left anterior descending coronary artery, and a normal right coronary artery. A left ventriculogram was performed, revealing an ejection fraction of 20%. On March 7, 1988, Mr. Davis had a coronary artery bypass graft of the left anterior descending and left circumflex coronary arteries. He had no postoperative complications and was discharged on March 15, 1988 on the following medications: aspirin, Persantine, Inderal, digoxin, and Lasix.

Mr. Davis was pain free until October 1, 1988, when he had an episode of fever, diaphoresis, and shortness of breath. He was admitted to a community hospital and a myocardial infarction was again ruled out. He underwent a second cardiac catheterization, which revealed patent coronary artery grafts but severe congestive heart failure with pulmonary artery pressures of 60/50. Four hours after the catheterization, he became hypotensive and required aggressive inotropic support. He was discharged 4 weeks after admission on the following medications: Vasotec, digoxin, Lasix, potassium, and tocainide. Subsequently, he was referred for cardiac transplantation and placed on a waiting list.

After discharge, Mr. Davis was assisted by a housekeeper, home health aide, and a visiting nurse. He was able to participate in minimal activities of daily living, but his activity tolerance was severely limited by exertional angina and dyspnea. On November 2, 1988 he developed extreme shortness of breath, vomiting, abdominal pain, and severe angina. Upon arrival at an outlying hospital, his BP was 82/60, heart rate 120, and respiratory rate 44. He required the intraaortic balloon pump (IABP) and vasopressors. After stabilization, he was transferred to our facility with a diagnosis of ischemic cardiomyopathy and cardiogenic shock.

On admission, Mr. Davis was on 20 μg/kg/min of dopamine, 20 μg/kg/min of dobutamine, and 16 μg/min of Levophed. He was on the IABP with 1:1 assist, maintaining a BP of 94/60, heart rate 131, respiratory rate 32, on 100% face mask. He was alert and oriented, but anxious. His ECG was most notable for a left bundle branch block and biventricular hypertrophy.

Hemodynamic Parameters		Laboratory Values			
CVP	15	Na	128	LDH	352
PAP	49/28	K	5.1	CK	8
PAWP	32	Gluc	117	Alk Phos	231
CO ·· •	3.6	Creat	1.9	AST	137
		BUN	42		

QUESTIONS AND ANSWERS

1. What is cardiomyopathy?

The term cardiomyopathy refers to a group of diseases that involve the heart muscle itself. They are classified by common pathyophysiological abnormalities and grouped into three functional categories: dilated cardiomyopathy, hypertrophic cardiomyopathy, and restrictive cardiomyopathy.

2. How does ischemic cardiomyopathy fit into the three categories of cardiomyopathies?

Ischemic cardiomyopathy is a type of dilated cardiomyopathy that develops in the setting of severe multivessel coronary artery disease. After multiple infarctions and prolonged ischemia, the myocardial cells remodel, hypertrophy, and produce a large, dilated heart with very poor contractile properties. As a result, most cardiomyopathy patients suffer repeated episodes of biventricular congestive heart failure. Mr. Davis presented with the typical picture of shortness of breath, chest pain, peripheral edema, hypotension, and dysrhythmias.

3. What are the major pathophysiological alterations in ischemic cardiomyopathy?

Four-chamber dilatation resulting in impaired contractility, reduced stroke volume, and increased end-diastolic pressure

Papillary muscle dysfunction resulting in mitral and tricuspid regurgitation

Blood stasis within the chambers with mural thrombus formation and the potential for arterial and venous emboli

Alterations in pulmonary vascularity resulting in various degrees of pulmonary congestion

Decreased systemic perfusion resulting in renal dysfunction and confusion

Passive congestion of the liver and peripheral edema

4. **What are the most common symptoms of ischemic cardiomyopathy?**

Dyspnea	Nausea
Orthopnea	Right upper quadrant
Fatigue	pain
Dizziness	Angina
Syncope	Peripheral edema

5. **Shortly after admission to the CCU, Mr. Davis complained of nausea and shortness of breath. His respiratory rate was 38, he was diaphoretic, his BP decreased to 82/60, and his heart rate increased from 110 to 140. What should the first nursing intervention be?**

    The nurse should calmly reassure Mr. Davis while doing an ECG and contacting the physician. Vital signs should be checked repetitively. Measures must be taken to determine if this episode is ischemic and, if so, treatment must begin immediately.

6. **What are the usual ECG manifestations of cardiomyopathy?**

    Most ischemic cardiomyopathy patients present with right and left ventricular hypertrophy. Left bundle branch block is also common, and a variety of other conduction disturbances may occur.

7. **What are the ECG indicators of hypertrophy?**

    Left ventricular hypertrophy (LVH) is evidenced by a deep S wave in V_1 and V_2 and tall R waves in V_5 and V_6. If the voltage in V_1 or V_2 is added to V_5 or V_6 and is >35 mm, this is usually a strong indicator of left ventricular hypertrophy. (For more specific criteria for LVH, see Chapter 9, "Hypertensive Crisis.") Right ventricular hypertrophy produces a tall R wave in V_1 and a deep S wave in lead V_6. Biventricular hypertrophy is more difficult to detect, because the left-sided changes may obscure the right-sided changes. Biventricular hypertrophy may produce a shallow S wave in V_1 when compared to V_2, with an associated right axis in the limb leads. Most physicians today rely on echocardiograms to diagnose the degree of hypertrophy, because echocardiograms are more sensitive in right and left ventricular enlargement.

8. **Why do cardiomyopathy patients have conduction abnormalities? What are the criteria for right and left bundle branch blocks?**

    Conduction abnormalities may arise because the conduction tissue has been stretched from extensive hypertrophy. More commonly, however, the conduction system is necrotic from previous infarctions. While left bundle branch block is typical, right bundle block may also occur, as may first, second, and third degree blocks. The ECG criteria for bundle branch blocks are as follows:

Left Bundle Branch Block

> QRS ≥0.12 sec wide
> rS or QS in V_1
> No Q wave with wide R or RSR' in V_6

Right Bundle Branch Block

> QRS ≥0.12 sec wide
> RSR' in V_1
> Deep, wide S wave in V_6

Ischemia is not only difficult to detect on ECG in patients with cardiomyopathy, but also may produce less pain in this population. Many patients experience chest pain initially, but as CHF worsens angina often becomes a secondary symptom. If the patient does not have angina, the first clinical signs of ischemia may be those of right and left ventricular failure.

11. What are the signs of right and left ventricular failure?

As left ventricular contractility deteriorates with ischemia, left ventricular end-diastolic volume increases and is reflected in an elevated PAWP. As fluid backs up into the lungs, pulmonary edema develops and manifests with dyspnea and tachypnea. When the right ventricle fails, the right atrial pressure increases, and blood backs up into the peripheral venous bed. Neck vein distention, peripheral edema, and liver engorgement commonly occur. Additional signs of failure include tachycardia, diaphoresis, and dysrhythmias.

12. Why is it particularly important in the ischemic cardiomyopathy patient to prevent episodes of ischemia?

At rest, the hypertrophied myocardium has a higher myocardial oxygen demand than a normal myocardium. The heart compensates for this increased oxygen demand by increasing heart rate, increasing contractility, and dilating the coronary arteries. When the myocardium is then subjected to ischemia, the heart cannot compensate for this additional insult because the normal compensatory mechanisms are already in use. Ischemic tissue does not contract, resulting in a reduction of coronary artery blood supply and worsening of ischemia. This sets in motion a vicious cycle of ischemia, congestive heart failure, and more ischemia.

Note the evidence of ventricular failure in Mr. Davis' clinical data. His liver function tests are elevated due to liver engorgement and his CVP is 15 (right-sided failure). His left ventricle is also in failure, as evidenced by a PAWP of 32, respiratory rate of 32, and rales throughout all lung fields. His CO is only 3.6 and his sodium is low due to poor renal perfusion and resultant fluid retention.

13. **Mr. Davis had a Foley catheter inserted, received 40 mg of IV Lasix, and passed 750 ml of urine in 2 hr. Shortly thereafter, a 12-beat run of multifocal ventricular ectopy was seen on the monitor. What is the appropriate nursing intervention?**

    The nurse should check the vital signs, confirm that the patient is hemodynamically stable, obtain a print-out of the event, and notify the physician. She or he should obtain the latest ABG and electrolyte results and assess Mr. Davis for clinical symptoms of hypoxia.

14. **What is the treatment of choice for ventricular ectopy in this setting?**

    The most likely etiology for this run of ventricular ectopy is hypokalemia resulting from Lasix administration. The serum potassium should be checked, and potassium supplements administered as indicated. A low magnesium level can also cause ventricular ectopy, so the magnesium level should also be checked. Generally, cardiomyopathy patients are very sensitive to low potassium and magnesium levels, so these electrolytes should be monitored closely to prevent ventricular ectopy.

15. **Despite supplemental KCl and Mg, Mr. Davis continued to have multifocal ventricular ectopy. During the runs of ventricular ectopy, Mr. Davis had a decrease in blood pressure, so lidocaine was started. What are the nursing responsibilities in monitoring antiarrhythmic medications?**

    While antiarrhythmic therapy may be lifesaving, it also carries associated risks. The enlarged ventricle is more sensitive to these medications, and administration of antiarrhythmics may result in a decrease in cardiac output and an increase in ventricular ectopy. The nurse's role in monitoring ventricular ectopy is to note the frequency, type (unifocal or multifocal), and associated symptoms such as hypotension, palpitations, or chest pain. While administering antiarrhythmic therapy, the nurse should observe for an increase or change in the pattern of the ventricular ectopy, as well as any changes in vital signs, and communicate this information to the physician.

16. **Mr. Davis required intraaortic balloon counterpulsation. What are the common indications for IABP?**

> Angina, which is refractory to intravenous nitroglycerine, especially in the setting of severe coronary artery disease
>
> Complications resulting from an acute myocardial infarction, including papillary muscle dysfunction, mitral regurgitation, and ventricular septal defect
>
> Congestive heart failure, which cannot be successfully treated with dopamine and dobutamine
>
> Prior to cardiac surgery, an IABP may be indicated for those patients with severe coronary artery disease who are pain free but have great potential for a catastrophic event.
>
> After cardiac surgery, an IABP may be indicated for those patients who experience difficulties when the cardiac bypass pump is removed, and also for those patients who have a greater potential for a postoperative myocardial infarction.

17. **Why was the IABP inserted in this case?**

The IABP was inserted to augment circulation in the setting of cardiogenic shock. Physiological effects of the IABP include augmentation of coronary artery blood flow and reduction of left ventricular afterload. The IABP is a palliative measure that should only be used in acute conditions that can be medically reversed or surgically corrected.

18. **Is cardiogenic shock caused by ischemic cardiomyopathy a potentially reversible event?**

Yes. In fact, recent studies indicate that ischemic tissue exhibits contractile reserve. While ischemic tissue does not participate in contraction, it does have the capability to contract once an adequate oxygen supply is restored. The IABP can help to restore the oxygen supply to ischemic tissue and thereby restore contractility and reverse the cardiogenic shock. This ischemic contractile reserve is clearly illustrated by Mr. Davis, as he was successfully weaned off the IABP.

19. **What are the possible complications and associated nursing responsibilities for a patient on an IABP?**

Complications

> Distal extremity ischemia, either from balloon impedance to flow or thrombus formation on the tip of the balloon with subsequent embolization

Balloon migration (*a*) toward the aortic arch with occlusion of the subclavian arteries, or (*b*) toward the renal arteries with occlusion of those arteries

Potential perforation of the aorta during insertion or with inadvertent patient movement. This is a rare complication and usually occurs during insertion of the balloon when the guidewire is used. However, if the patient were to sit up abruptly, or bend the leg in such a way that the catheter is rapidly forced upward, there is potential for perforation.

Inappropriate timing causing hypotension and dysrhythmias

Psychological consequences including increased anxiety, loss of control, alteration in sleep, and pump psychosis

Nursing Responsibilities

Palpate dorsalis pedis and posterior tibial pulses every hour, mark the location of pulses, and note the quality of pulses on both feet.

Check IABP dressing every hour, note any oozing, and circle any area of bleeding with a black marker.

Firmly secure the IABP, check stability of sutures, and restrain the IABP extremity to maintain it in a straight position. Keep the head of the bed lower than 30°. All these measures prevent inadvertent migration of the balloon.

Note any sudden decrease in urinary output or any differences in blood pressure between the right and left arms. Both of these signs may indicate IABP migration and a chest x-ray may be necessary to check placement.

Maintain appropriate timing, check timing after a 10-beat change in heart rate, and frequently observe the balloon pressure waveform to ensure appropriate inflation/deflation and position of the IABP (Fig. 4.1). Correct timing occurs when the IABP inflates during diastole, forcing the blood in the aorta retrograde into the coronary arteries. Deflation creates a dead space in the aorta and is timed to occur just prior to systole. This maneuver results in afterload reduction, as there is less resistance for the left ventricle to pump against. Timing is done with the central lumen or radial arterial pressure waveform. Inflation is set to occur on the aortic notch, which signifies the beginning of diastole, and deflation is set to occur just prior to the next upstroke of the waveform.

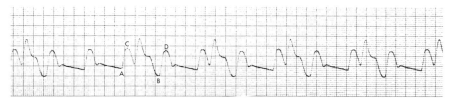

Figure 4.1. IABP tracing showing correct timing. (Reproduced by permission from Quaal SJ. Comprehensive intra-aortic balloon pumping. St. Louis, 1984, The C.V. Mosby Co.)

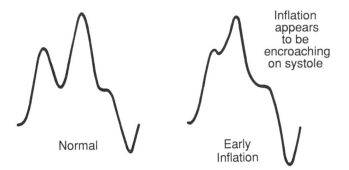

Figure 4.2. IABP tracing showing early inflation. (Reproduced by permission from Quaal SJ. Comprehensive intra-aorta balloon pumping. St. Louis, 1984, The C.V. Mosby Co.)

The most detrimental kinds of inappropriate timing include early inflation and late deflation. Early inflation occurs when the IABP inflates prior to the dicrotic notch or prior to the end of systole (Fig. 4.2). This causes displacement of blood toward the open aortic valve and may cause premature closure of the aortic valve, decreasing cardiac output and impeding blood flow to the periphery. Late deflation occurs past the upstroke of the next systole (Fig. 4.3). Late deflation is the most dangerous, because ventricular contraction now occurs against an inflated 40-ml balloon. This dramatically increases afterload, decreases cardiac output, and increases myocardial oxygen demand. Fortunately, most IABP models are manufactured with complex computerized algorithms capable of tracking rhythms and preventing inflation during systole. Some models even boast of "automatic timing," but automatic timing is a misnomer. Assisted timing is a much more appropriate description for this type of computerized timing. Computers routinely approximate the timing interval but a

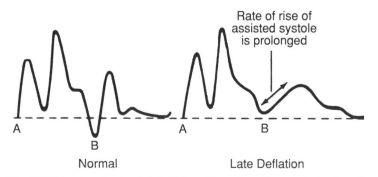

Figure 4.3. IABP tracing showing late deflation. (Reproduced by permission from Quaal SJ. Comprehensive intra-aortic balloon pumping. St. Louis, 1984, The C.V. Mosby Co.)

nurse's expertise is always necessary for validation and fine tuning of the individualized IABP timing.

20.   What additional complications can occur with IABP use?

There is always potential for infection and air embolization with any indwelling catheter, and the IABP is certainly no exception. Sterile technique should be used for line and dressing changes. The prevention of air embolization cannot be overemphasized, because the central lumen lies in the aorta and an air embolus has the potential to produce a massive CVA. A physician should connect the pressure tubing to the central lumen catheter. The line should be flushed thoroughly prior to attachment, expelling all air bubbles, and an air filter should be attached to the pressure tubing. The tubing should be clearly marked with caution stickers to prevent accidental flushing or drawing blood from the line.

21.   What are the contraindications to IABP insertion?

Aortic aneurysm, aortic dissection, and aortic valvular insufficiency are absolute contraindications to IABP insertion. If the aorta is weakened from an aneurysm or dissection, placement of the IABP could perforate the aorta and result in death of the patient. If the aortic valve is not competent, the blood displaced from the IABP will increase end-diastolic volume and exacerbate congestive heart failure.

The IABP slightly reduces blood flow peripherally. This normal reduction in blood flow may result in a complete loss of peripheral blood flow in patients with severe peripheral vascular disease. These patients also have a greater risk for embolization of atherosclerotic plaques in the aorta. As a result, severe peripheral vascular disease also precludes insertion of the IABP.

22.   Mr. Davis was gradually weaned off dopamine, dobutamine, and the IABP. His cardiac ouput improved, but his activity tolerance was limited by exertional angina. Low dose intravenous nitroglycerin (NTG) helped alleviate most of his exertional angina, and prophylactic sublingual NTG was added when he ambulated, used the commode, or consumed large meals. What kinds of medications will Mr. Davis need to resume his activities of daily living, and what are the nursing responsibilities associated with discharge teaching?

Most cardiomyopathy patients experience progressive congestive heart failure, so treatment is aimed toward maximizing cardiac output, eliminating peripheral edema formation, preventing ischemic episodes, and controlling symptomatic dysrhythmias.

Digitalis is the only positive inotrope available in oral preparation. Patients should be carefully instructed about the effects and side effects of digitalis and cautioned against overdosing on digitalis. Patients should be taught to take their pulse daily and notify the physician if the pulse slows or becomes irregular. While digitalis increases cardiac output, Lasix is concomitantly administered to decrease preload, minimize pulmonary congestion, and reduce myocardial workload. The potential for digitalis toxicity is increased when patients are also on Lasix, because Lasix depletes potassium and magnesium stores. Digitalis and potassium compete for the same receptor site on the cell membrane, so when the potassium level drops, digitalis is able to occupy more receptor sites and exert a greater influence on cardiac activity. To prevent this from happening, supplemental potassium tablets are also prescribed. Patients should have a basic understanding of the synergistic activity of these medications so as to minimize possible complications.

In addition to these three medications, patients may also be discharged on captopril or hydralazine. These afterload reducers help decrease myocardial oxygen demand but may also cause severe hypotension. Patients are tested on these medications prior to discharge, but should be cautioned to report light-headedness or dizziness to the physician. Patients should also be instructed about postural hypotension and ways it can be minimized. Calcium channel blockers such as nifedipine and diltiazem may also be prescribed to prevent coronary artery spasm and subsequent angina, but their use may have deleterious effects on left ventricular function. Adverse effects from these medications include hypotension, headache, nausea, and vomiting.

Antiarrhythmic agents such as mexilitene, quinidine, and procainamide may also be agents of choice to control symptomatic ventricular ectopy. Any antiarrhythmic carries the risk of potentiating dysrhythmias, especially in the setting of a low potassium level. Patients should be instructed about side effects and be cautioned to report increased palpitations, increased shortness of breath, or dizziness. Ideally, spouses should be trained in CPR. The risk of sudden death from a dysrhythmia is great, as nearly one-half of patients with moderate to severe CHF succumb to ventricular dysrhythmias.

Prophylactic sublingual nitroglycerin is also prescribed, and ischemic cardiomyopathy patients should be taught to take nitroglycerin prior to physical activity. When these patients have chest pain, they should rest and take up to three nitroglycerin tablets at least 5 min apart. If the chest pain continues after 15–20 min, the patient should be instructed to seek medical attention.

The personal stress associated with a rigorous drug regimen, the drastic change in life-style, and the morbid prognosis have grave psychological consequences for most cardiomyopathy patients. The family unit is also disturbed by this disease and has special needs as well. Thus, these patients and their families need: (*a*) extensive discharge teaching on medications, nutrition, cardiac pathology, and activity level at home; (*b*) knowledge of community services such as Visiting Nurses' Association (VNA), regional support groups, and professional psychological services; (*c*) close follow-up with a cardiologist with regular clinic visits; and (*d*) appropriate patients should be referred for cardiac transplantation.

23. What are the associated nursing diagnoses?

Alteration in cardiac output: decreased, related to impaired myocardial contractility

Fatigue related to low cardiac output

Altered peripheral tissue perfusion secondary to presence of IABP

Potential for injury related to presence of IABP with possible abrupt changes in patient's position

Impaired physical mobility related to presence of IABP

Potential for infection related to presence of invasive lines

Disturbance in self concept related to the patient's and significant others' response to chronic illness.

SUGGESTED READINGS

Becker AE. Pathology of cardiomyopathies. In: Shaver JA, Brest AN, eds. Cardiomyopathies: Clinical presentation, differential diagnosis, and management. Philadelphia: FA Davis, 1988:11–25.

DeAngelis R. The cardiovascular system. In: Alspach JG, Williams SM, eds. Core curriculum for critical care nursing. 3rd ed. Philadelphia: WB Saunders, 1985:191–192.

Goldberger AL. Myocardial infarction, electrocardiographic differential diagnosis. 3rd ed. St. Louis: CV Mosby, 1984:85–93.

Goodwin JF. Overview of the cardiomyopathies. In: Shaver JA, Brest AN, eds. Cardiomyopathies: Clinical presentation, differential diagnosis, and management. Philadelphia: FA Davis, 1988:1–9.

Marriott HJ. Practical electrocardiography. 7th ed. Baltimore: Williams & Wilkins, 1983:69.

Quaal SJ. Comprehensive intra-aortic balloon pumping. St. Louis: CV Mosby, 1984:87–234.

Rahko PS, Orie JE. The clinical presentation and laboratory evaluation of congestive and ischemic cardiomyopathy. In: Shaver JA, Brest AN, eds. Cardiomyopathies: Clinical presentation, differential diagnosis, and management. Philadelphia: FA Davis, 1988:75—114.

Rutherford JD, Cohn PF, Braunwald E. Chronic ischemic heart disease. In: Braunwald E, ed. Heart disease a textbook of cardiovascular medicine. Philadelphia: WB Saunders, 1988:1366.

Uretsky BF. Diagnostic considerations in the adult patient with cardiomyopathy or congestive heart failure. In: Shaver JA, Brest AN, eds. Cardiomyopathies: Clinical presentation, differential diagnosis, and management. Philadelphia: FA Davis, 1988:37–42.

Vitello-Cicciu J, Johantgen M. Cardiomyopathy. In: Kinney MR, Packa DR, Dunbar SB, eds. AACN's clinical reference for critical-care nursing. 2nd ed. New York: McGraw-Hill, 1988:682–688.

Vitello-Cicciu J, Stewart SL, Griffin EL. Coronary artery disease. In: Kinney MR, Packa DR, Dunbar SB, eds. AACN's clinical reference for critical-care nursing. 2nd ed. New York: McGraw-Hill, 1988:595–598.

Wynne J, Braunwald E. The cardiomyopathies and myocarditis. In: Braunwald E, ed. Heart disease a textbook of cardiovascular medicine. Philadelphia: WB Saunders, 1988:1410–1435.

CHAPTER 5

Carotid Endarterectomy

Linda Weld, RN, MSN, CCRN

Lillie Hamilton, a 68-year-old woman, is admitted to the ICU after having two transient ischemic attacks (TIAs) over the last 3 days. She is admitted for observation and a diagnostic workup. She has a history of adult-onset diabetes and mild hypertension, which is controlled by a low salt diet and furosemide (Lasix). At this time, she is slightly anxious, alert, and oriented ×3. Her pupils are equal and reactive bilaterally. She moves all extemities and has equal strength bilaterally. She states that her TIAs lasted approximately 10–15 min and resulted in slurred speech and right-sided weakness. Her symptoms were the same during both TIAs.

Vital Signs

BP	136/90
HR	88
Resp	18
Temp	98.6°F

Her monitor shows NSR with rare PACs. She has no rubs, murmurs, or gallops on auscultation. All other findings are normal, as are her electrolytes, serum glucose, BUN, and creatinine.

A diagnostic workup is done, including Doppler flow studies, CT scan, and digital subtraction angiography (DSA). 90% occlusion is found at the left carotid bifurcation, and the patient is scheduled for a left carotid endarterectomy.

Mrs. Hamilton returns from the Operating Room with the following vital signs:

Vital Signs

BP	130/100
HR	98
Resp	20
Temp	99.8°F
CVP	10

She is alert and oriented ×3 and moving all four extremities to command.

QUESTIONS AND ANSWERS

1. **List the possible causes of carotid artery lesions.**

   Atherosclerosis
   Fibromuscular dysplasia
   Irradiation
   Arterial kinking
   Extrinsic compression
   Traumatic occlusion
   Takayasu's arteritis

2. **Describe the clinical manifestations of carotid artery disease.**

   The manifestations of carotid disease vary with the extent of the disease and collateral blood supply. Many patients will have a bruit, which sounds like a high-pitched systolic murmur, heard best with a stethoscope placed at the angle of the jaw. Bruits occur when the artery is narrowed by at least 50% and disappear when there is total occlusion. Patients with significant carotid artery disease may be asymptomatic, or may manifest with TIAs, RINDs, amaurosis fugax, or stroke.

3. **Define the terms TIA, RIND, and amaurosis fugax.**

   A transient ischemic attack (TIA) is a focal neurological deficit lasting <24 hr, with complete neurological recovery. When the TIA results from occlusion of the carotid artery, the typical symptoms include paralysis, motor weakness, and sensory abnormalities contralateral to the diseased vessel. Speech may be affected if the dominant hemisphere is affected.

   RIND stands for reversible ischemic neurologic deficit. This is defined as a neurologic deficit lasting >24 hr but no more than several days. A RIND is considered an ominous neurological sign. Amaurosis fugax is a phenomenon produced by microemboli to the retina, resulting in monocular blindness described as if a window shade is slowly pulled across the field of vision. This is usually temporary in nature.

4. **What observations should be made after DSA?**

   During DSA, an intravenous injection of contrast material is given intraarterially, and the major arteries are visualized using computed fluoroscopic techniques. After the procedure, the patient should be observed for dye reactions, signs and symptoms of nephrotoxicity, and symptoms of stroke. Fluids should be encouraged to facilitate excretion of the dye.

5. If Mrs. Hamilton decided to be managed medically, what are the usual treatments?

At present, there is considerable controversy regarding the efficacy of carotid endarterectomy in the prevention of stroke. There are randomized prospective studies presently under way to identify which patients should be operated on and which may be managed medically.

Patients who select medical management will be instructed in risk factor modification, have aspirin prescribed in a dose of approximately one tablet per day, and be discharged home. While control of hypertension is one important aspect of risk factor modification, the blood pressure should be lowered gradually to avoid worsening the cerebral ischemia.

6. What other tests may be included in Mrs. Hamilton's preoperative workup?

Most centers perform a complete angiographic evaluation of the aortic arch, carotid artery, and the posterior cerebral circulation if the patient's symptoms are vertebrobasilar. A preoperative CT scan of the brain is done to identify patients whose symptoms are caused by other intracranial problems. The CT scan also serves as a baseline in case the patient has a postoperative neurological deficit.

Because of the high incidence of associated coronary artery disease, these patients receive an in-depth cardiac evaluation. An ECG is done routinely. Many patients require further cardiac evaluation, which may include a treadmill exercise test or myocardial perfusion scan. If the patient has coronary disease, the carotid endarterectomy may be done under local rather than general anesthesia. When patients have symptomatic coronary artery disease, staged or combined myocardial revascularization and carotid endarterectomy may be done.

7. Postoperatively Mrs. Hamilton's BP is 160/100. What are the possible causes and treatments of her hypertension?

After carotid endarterectomy, either hyper- or hypotension may be seen. With the removal of plaque from the carotid artery, the baroreceptors in the carotid sinus are exposed, subjected to new flow, and stimulated. Impulses are transmitted to the medulla, resulting in inhibition of the vasomotor center and peripheral vasodilatation. This creates a relative hypovolemia, which causes hypotension. Stimulation of the baroreceptors may also result in decreased cardiac rate and strength of contraction, which contributes to the decrease in BP.

The mechanism causing postoperative hypertension is unclear, but may be due to cerebral renin release. Patients with a history of diabetes and hypertension have an increased risk for postoperative hypertension. Treatment is usually started if the systolic BP exceeds 180 mm Hg. Sodium nitroprusside (Nipride) is the drug of choice. Extreme caution during Nipride administration is necessary as patients with marked fluctuations in BP have an increased incidence of postoperative stroke.

8. Describe the neurological assessment done after surgery.

The patient is assessed every hour for the first 24 hr. The neurological assessment includes: orientation, pupils, extremity movement and strength, speech, fine hand movements, visual acuity, and cranial nerve function. Visual acuity may be tested by having the patient read or state the time by looking at a clock or watch. Temporal pulses are checked every hour.

9. Cranial nerve injuries can occur from inadvertent transection or retractor injuries. Which nerves are most often injured, and what are the clinical manifestations?

Cranial Nerve	Clinical Manifestations of Injury
Facial, VII	Drooping of ipsilateral corner of lip, inability to smile
Glossopharyngeal, IX	Difficulty in swallowing
Superior laryngeal (branch of vagus, X)	Minor problems with swallowing and easy fatigability of voice
Recurrent laryngeal (part of vagus, X)	Ipsilateral cord paralysis and hoarseness
Hypoglossal, XII	Deviation of tongue to operative side; difficulty with speech and mastication

The great auricular nerve is not a cranial nerve, but is part of the cervical plexus. It may also be injured during carotid endarterectomy and cause paresthesias of portions of the face and ear.

10. What are the other potential complications?

Wound complications
Perioperative stroke
Recurrent carotid stenosis
Pulmonary complications from surgery
Operative death

11. **Twelve hours after surgery, the nurse notices a hematoma around the incision site. What can cause a hematoma following carotid endarterectomy and what is the danger of this finding?**

   Possible causes of hematoma formation following carotid endarterectomy include the heparin received during surgery and coughing during extubation. While hematomas in this setting are not uncommon, they should be observed closely and reported to the physician. The potential for tracheal compression and airway obstruction exists. In the case of a large or rapidly expanding hematoma, reoperation will be performed to rule out a potential suture-line bleed.

12. **Describe measures to promote pulmonary hygiene after surgery.**

   These patients are turned every 2 hr and encouraged to deep breathe. Vigorous coughing is not encouraged. Incentive spirometers and other devices are used to encourage lung expansion. Adequate oxygenation must be maintained, because hypoxemia can lead to fluctuations in the blood pressure.

13. **Are there any restrictions on movement of the neck after surgery?**

   The patient may move her neck any way that is comfortable.

14. **What nursing diagnoses apply in this case?**

   Altered cerebral perfusion related to vascular narrowing
   Potential for injury related to changes in neurological status
   Potential for ineffective breathing patterns related to tracheal compression
   Potential for infection related to nonintact skin and presence of invasive lines
   Potential fluid volume deficit related to volume losses during surgery and inadequate oral intake
   Sleep pattern disturbance related to environmental stimuli

SUGGESTED READINGS

Baum PL. Carotid endarterectomy: One strike against stroke. Nursing 1983; 13(3):50–59.

Cote R, Caron J. Management of carotid artery occlusion. Curr Concepts Cerebrovasc Dis Stroke 1988;23:25–29.

Del Zappo GJ. Thrombolytic therapy in cerebral vascular disease. Curr Concepts Cerebrovasc Dis Stroke 1988;23:7–11.

Fahey VA. Vascular nursing. Philadelphia: WB Saunders, 1988.

Friedman SG, Riles TS, Lamparelle PJ, Imparato AM, Sakwa MP. Surgical therapy for the patient with internal carotid occlusion and contralateral stenosis. J Vasc Surg 1987;5:856–861.

Guzzetta CE, Dossey BM, eds. Cardiovascular nursing: Bodymind tapestry. St. Louis: CV Mosby, 1984.

Mitchell S, Yates R. Cerebral vascular disease. In: Kenner CV, Guzzetta CE, Dossey BM, eds. Critical care nursing: Body-mind-spirit. 3rd ed. Boston: Little Brown & Co, 1985.

Pearce W, Mill MR, Marsch JG. Cerebrovascular insufficiency. Crit Care Q 1985; 8:11–20.

White RA. Diagnosis and therapy of emergent vascular diseases. In: Shoemaker WC, Ayres S, Grenvik A, Holbrook PR, Thompson WL, eds. Textbook of critical care. 2nd ed. Philadelphia: WB Saunders, 1989.

CHAPTER 6

Congestive Heart Failure/ Pulmonary Edema

Leslie Borcherding, RN, MS

Sarah Martin, a 61-year-old woman, was admitted to the CCU at 4:00 AM, after being briefly evaluated in the Emergency Department. Her admitting diagnosis was congestive heart failure (CHF). She had come to the hospital after suddenly awakening around midnight to "breathlessness." Previously, she had required two to three pillows in order to sleep comfortably. Sitting upright with her legs dangling from the bedside helped, but she still remained short of breath. Pertinent assessment data included the following:

History and Patient Interview. Previous medical records document coronary artery disease (CAD) with a large anterior MI 6 months ago; left ventricular ejection fraction 30%; noncompliance with medication and diet protocols (medication regime included digoxin, Lasix, and a potassium supplement); weight gain of "several pounds" over past 2 months; shortness of breath with household duties; and increasing fatigue.

Physical Examination. Patient appears tired and in moderate distress; skin cool and moist; nailbeds dusky; capillary refill slow; peripheral pulses weak; JVD at 45°; inspiratory crackles; laterally displaced point of maximal impulse (PMI); irregular heart sounds; constant grade II/VI harsh pansystolic murmur loudest at cardiac apex; hepatomegaly; and mild pitting lower leg edema.

Clinical Parameters and Diagnostic Studies

Vital Signs		Weight	Laboratory Values	
BP	100/70	154 pounds (70 kg)	Na	134
HR	120, irregular	**Height**	K	3.9
Resp	24, shallow		Hgb	12.5
Temp	38.1°C	5 feet 6 inches	Hct	33%
			AST	45
ABGs (room air)		**ECG**	Digoxin level	0.6
pH	7.48	Sinus tachycardia; 6–8	Creat	1.9
PaCO₂	30	multifocal PVCs/min		
PaO₂	80			
SaO₂	95%	**Chest X-ray**		
HCO₃	24	Bilateral pulmonary congestion; slightly enlarged cardiac silhouette		

An IV line of D_5W was running at a keep open rate and a Foley catheter had been inserted. Oxygen was being administered at 2 liters/min via nasal cannula. Lidocaine at 70 mg IV push had been given initially, followed by 35 mg IV push in 10 min and a maintenance drip at 2 mg/min. Lasix, 40 mg IV push, had been given in the Emergency Department. Ms. Martin's CCU admission orders included digoxin, Lasix, oxygen, and a potassium supplement routinely, with morphine and NTG as needed.

By the afternoon of day 1, Ms. Martin's status had deteriorated. The nurse noted increased fatigue, crackles throughout all lung fields, pulsus alternans, an occasional cough that produced frothy sputum, and a faint S_3 gallop audible at the cardiac apex. The monitor showed sinus tachycardia, rate 125, with frequent PVCs. Ms. Martin had received a total dose of 20 mg of morphine intravenously for anxiety and dyspnea. Urine output had dropped to <20 ml/hr. 80 mg of Lasix was given IV push. A thermodilution balloon-tipped flow-directed pulmonary artery catheter was inserted via the right subclavian vein and a left radial arterial catheter was placed.

Hemodynamic Parameters		ABGs (2 liters/min Nasal O_2)	
PAP	45/28	pH	7.24
PAWP	25	$PaCO_2$	60
CVP	20	PaO_2	60
CO	2.5	SaO_2	88%
CI	1.4	HCO_3	24
BP	94/70		
MAP	78		

Ms. Martin's O_2 delivery system was changed to a Venti-mask at 40%. A dobutamine infusion was initiated, to be titrated from 2.5 to 10.0 μg/kg/min. Nitroprusside (Nipride) was initiated at 3 μg/kg/min. The therapeutic goal was to titrate the infusions to lower Ms. Martin's PAWP to the 17–18 mm Hg range while maintaining her systolic BP in the 90–100 mm Hg range. Oral medications were changed to IV ones.

Two days later, assessment findings were as follows:

Physical Examination. Patient is alert and cooperative; skin warm and dry; peripheral pulses stronger and equal; respirations 14–16/min, nonlabored; absence of cough and sputum production; fine crackles present in bases bilaterally; heart sounds essentially regular; absence of S_3; grade II/VI systolic murmur still present; and minimal peripheral edema.

Total urine output had exceeded 8000 ml since admission. ECG monitor showed sinus rhythm with 2–4 PVCs/min.

Hemodynamic Parameters		ABGs (40% Venti-mask)	
PAP	25/17	pH	7.44
PAWP	16	$PaCO_2$	35
CVP	14	PaO_2	88
CO	3.8	SaO_2	95%
CI	2.1	HCO_3	25
BP	108/62		
MAP	77		

All infusions were tapered. Ms. Martin was placed on 0.125 mg of oral digoxin q day, 16 mEq of potassium q day, 12.5 mg of captopril TID, and 40 mg of Lasix q day. On day 4, all invasive monitoring lines and catheters were discontinued, and the patient began eating small, light, low sodium meals. Although still very cautious about cardiac workload, the nurses allowed Mrs. Martin to assist minimally with her bath and to sit in a bedside chair for meals. At this point, the staff also gradually introduced the educational component of a rehabilitation plan designed for Ms. Martin and on day 5, she was transferred to the telemetry unit to continue her cardiac rehabilitation program.

QUESTIONS AND ANSWERS

1. **Describe the typical pathophysiological process of CHF and pulmonary edema.**

   Heart failure is the inability of the heart to pump sufficient blood to meet the body's demands. Failure may begin with the left or right ventricle or occur simultaneously in both ventricles, depending upon etiology.

   A common presentation is left ventricular failure leading to pulmonary edema and subsequent right ventricular failure. Left ventricular stroke volume falls due to disease or injury. The right ventricle continues to pump blood into the pulmonary circulation as left ventricular volumes and pressures rise. Rising pressures soon occur in the left atrium and pulmonary circulation causing dyspnea. Pulmonary edema begins as pulmonary capillary oncotic pressure is exceeded and fluid extravasates into the interstitial spaces, generally causing cough and sputum production. Continued high pressures cause fluid to move into the alveoli, resulting in frank pulmonary edema. Elevated pressures eventually occur in the right ventricle, causing right ventricular failure. Right atrial pressure rises, which results in systemic venous congestion and the presence of edema.

   As this process develops and cardiac output falls, the following compensatory mechanisms may be activated:

Decreased blood pressure stimulates the sympathetic nervous system to increase heart rate and contractility by increases in circulating norepinephrine and epinephrine.

Decreased blood pressure also causes the sympathetic nervous system to initiate peripheral vasoconstriction so that blood pressure rises and oxygenated blood is shunted to vital organs (brain, heart) and away from the skin, skeletal muscle, and abdominal organs.

Impaired renal perfusion results in: (*a*) sodium and fluid retention to increase intravascular volume; and (*b*) release of renin, the enzyme that converts angiotensinogen to angiotensin I, which is then converted into the potent vasoconstrictor angiotensin II.

Increased preload, which causes ventricular dilatation. Within limits, this causes increased stretch of myocardial muscle fibers, resulting in longer, more efficient contractions.

Ventricular hypertrophy occurs, over time, due to increased systemic vascular resistance (peripheral vasoconstriction). Although contraction is less for each individual muscle unit, the larger mass of myocardium can increase cardiac output.

Compensatory mechanisms provide beneficial effects as long as they remain within normal physiological limits. However, once left ventricular end-diastolic volume and stretch exceed these limits, fibers can no longer shorten adequately during systole. Contractility decreases, cardiac output decreases, and the typical cycle of heart failure ensues.

2. What are the signs and symptoms of heart failure?

Right Heart Failure

JVD
Peripheral edema
Weight gain (fluid retention)
Increased right atrial pressure
Hepatomegaly
Anorexia
Nausea
Vomiting

Left Heart Failure

Paroxysmal nocturnal dyspnea
Shortness of breath/dyspnea
Fatigue
Cool moist skin
Slow capillary refill
Dusky nailbeds
Weak pulses
Laterally displaced PMI

Decreased breath sounds
Cough
Frothy sputum
Tachypnea
Decreased $PaCO_2$ (early)
Increased $PaCO_2$ (later)
Decreased PaO_2
Increased PAP, PAWP

Systolic murmur of mitral insufficiency	Decreased CO
S$_3$	Pulsus alternans
Tachycardia	Dizziness/syncope

3. Ms. Martin's digoxin level was 0.6 ng/ml upon admission. What is the normal value?

The normal digoxin level is 0.8–2.0 ng/ml. With Ms. Martin's digoxin level of 0.6 ng/ml, it is unlikely that she has been taking the medication as prescribed. This has important nursing implications, as she should receive patient teaching regarding the importance of her medications once she is stabilized. She is subsequently prescribed 0.25 mg of digoxin PO q 6 hr for a total of 1 mg loading dose. Because of her decreased renal function, she is then prescribed 0.125 mg PO q day.

4. What factors contributed to Ms. Martin's heart failure?

History of coronary artery disease[a]
History of hypertension[a]
History of anterior MI
Noncompliance with medication and diet protocols

5. What other etiologies or precipitating factors are associated with heart failure?

Acute MI	Cardiomyopathies
Valvular heart disease	Septal defects
Cardiac tamponade	Constrictive pericarditis
Infiltrative diseases	Systemic hypertension
Sustained tachycardia	Pulmonary hypertension
Sustained bradycardia	High output states (i.e., anemia
Increased blood volume (i.e., pregnancy or renal failure)	or hyperthyroidism)

6. What are the major determinants of cardiac output?

Preload is the degree of stretch on the myocardial muscle fibers just prior to systole (left ventricular end-diastolic pressure). It is clinically measured as the PAWP.

Afterload is the resistance to blood flow out of the left ventricle into the aorta. The left ventricle must overcome this resistance to eject blood during systole. It is clinically measured as systemic vascular resistance (SVR).

[a] Currently a leading cause of CHF.

Contractility refers to the mechanical shortening of muscle fibers as they respond to electrical stimulation. There is no direct measure of cardiac contractility, so the clinician must rely on clinical indicators in evaluation of contractility.

Heart Rate

$$\text{cardiac output} = \text{heart rate} \times \text{stroke volume}$$

Therefore, an increase in heart rate will have a beneficial effect on cardiac output up to a point. An increased heart rate after an acute MI is usually an indicator of severe left ventricular damage. As the heart rate increases, myocardial oxygen consumption increases significantly. In addition, because the coronary arteries fill during diastole, as do the ventricles, shortening diastolic filling time at rapid heart rates can result in myocardial ischemia and a decrease in cardiac output.

7.   Calculate Ms. Martin's cardiac index using the initial data following pulmonary artery catheter insertion. How is this parameter useful?

The cardiac index is simply the cardiac output divided by the body surface area (BSA). The BSA is obtained by inserting the patient's height and weight into a nomogram. (See Appendix D.) Ms. Martin was 5 feet 6 inches tall and weighed 154 pounds, so her BSA was 1.8.

$$\text{CI} = \frac{\text{CO}}{\text{BSA}} = \frac{2.5}{1.8} = 1.4$$

The CI is a more precise parameter than CO because it takes into account the patient's size. The normal CI is 2.5–4.0 liters/min.

8.   How are pharmacologic agents used to improve cardiac performance in the patient with congestive heart failure?

The two major ways drugs are used to influence cardiac performance in this setting are by reducing preload and/or afterload, or by improving the inotropic state of the heart. A reduction in preload will decrease pulmonary congestion, while a reduction in afterload will increase cardiac output. Remember, preload has to do with the stretch on the left ventricle prior to systole, is determined primarily by the venous return, and is measured by PAWP. Afterload has to do with impedance to left ventricular ejection, is determined by arteriolar vasoconstriction, and is measured by the SVR. Preload reducing agents are venodilators, and afterload reducing agents are arteriolar dilators. Some agents affect both arteriolar dilatation and venodilatation.

Vasodilators

Hydralazine (Apresoline)

Hydralazine is the prototype arteriolar dilator. By reducing arteriolar resistance, it decreases the work of the left ventricle, decreases myocardial oxygen requirements, and increases cardiac output. It can be given IV or PO. When given PO for chronic CHF, it may cause a slight increase in heart rate and contractility and may induce angina pectoris in patients with ischemic heart disease. It is frequently given in combination with nitrates. Chronic administration of this combination has been shown to prolong survival in patients with mild to moderate CHF. Side effects include GI upset, fluid retention, peripheral neuropathy, and lupus erythematosus.

Minoxidil

The effects of minoxidil are similar to those of hydralazine. However, it is of limited use in patients with CHF because of a tendency to cause severe fluid retention.

Nifedipine (Procardia)

Nifedipine is a calcium channel blocker that inhibits flow of calcium ions into cardiac and vascular smooth muscle cells, resulting in decreased muscle tone. It decreases afterload and increases cardiac output, but may cause hypotension, tachycardia, and fluid retention. Calcium channel blockers have significant negative inotropic effects and may actually worsen ventricular function.

Nitroglycerin and Other Nitrates

Nitroglycerin is a venodilator at low dosages but an arteriolar dilator at higher dosages. When administered intravenously in the acute setting, NTG may increase cardiac output. When nitrates are administered chronically, they are primarily venodilators. For afterload reduction, an arteriolar dilator is added to the regimen.

The primary side effects of nitrates include headache and hypotension.

Sodium Nitroprusside (Nipride)

Nipride has a balanced effect on arteriolar dilatation and venodilatation. It is given IV, and is frequently used in the patient with acute CHF in the ICU. The advantages of Nipride include its immediate onset, short half-life, ease of titration, and absence of effects on heart rate. Thiocyanate toxicity may occur with high dosages (>15 μg/kg/min) or prolonged administration (>48 hr).

Captopril

Captopril is a balanced arteriolar and venous vasodilator. It works by blocking the enzyme that is required for angiotensin I to be converted to angiotensin II. Other actions include an enhancement of the action of vasodilator kinins and prostaglandins E and I_2, all of which are known vasodilators. Captopril is especially useful in the chronic management of CHF. In addition to its primary effects, it also has been shown to produce a reduction in heart rate, a normalization of serum sodium and potassium concentrations, a reduction in circulating catecholamines, and a reduction in ventricular dysrhythmias. Major side effects include hypotension and bradycardia, which may occur with the first dose. Other adverse effects may include taste alterations, skin rash, fever, hypotension, and a persistent "captopril cough."

Enalapril

Enalapril works by the same mechanism as captopril (blocks the enzyme required for converting angiotensin I to angiotensin II). The effects and side effects are similar to captopril, but it has a much longer half-life. It's use has been shown to prolong survival in patients with severe heart failure. It should be used cautiously in patients with marginal renal perfusion, as the longer duration of action could result in prolonged hypotension if renal excretion is impaired.

Positive Inotropes

Digoxin

Digoxin is the most commonly used cardiac glycoside. It increases myocardial contractility, thereby increasing cardiac output. It also slows atrioventricular conduction and is particularly useful in the setting of atrial fibrillation. It should be noted that hypokalemia, hypercalcemia, and hypomagnesemia may sensitize the heart to digitalis preparations. Because Lasix may result in hypokalemia, it is extremely important to monitor the serum potassium in patients receiving both digoxin and Lasix.

Dopamine

The effects of dopamine are dose related.

Dose	Receptor Specificity			
	α	B_1	B_2	Dopaminergic
2–5 µg/kg/min	0	+	0	++++
6–10 µg/kg/min	0	++++	++	+
10–20 µg/kg/min	+++	++++	+	0

Dobutamine (Dobutrex)

Dobutamine is a sympathomimetic that possesses both α- and β-adrenergic receptor activity; however, it is relatively specific for cardiac β_1-adrenergic receptors. The result is enhanced cardiac contractility with minimal or no α or β_2 stimulation at low dose range (2.5–10 μg/kg/min). Higher doses are more likely to cause tachycardia and ventricular dysrhythmias.

Amrinone (Inocor)

Amrinone acts directly on the myocardial fibers to slightly increase contractility. Its major action is to cause both arteriolar and venous vasodilatation, thus reducing afterload and preload.

9. Discuss the drug regimen used in Ms. Martin's case.

Preload Reduction

Lasix was given for diuresis.
Morphine was given for venous dilatation.
Nipride caused reduction in both preload and afterload.

The therapeutic goal was to decrease the PAWP from 25 to 17–18 mm Hg. This would maximize the Starling forces and improve cardiac output.

Afterload Reduction

Nipride

Nipride caused arteriolar vasodilatation, a reduction in afterload, a decrease in myocardial oxygen consumption, and an increase in cardiac output.

Morphine

Morphine also decreased afterload, with less pronounced but similar effects to those of Nipride. Morphine also lessened Ms. Martin's anxiety and dyspnea.

Captopril

Captopril decreased both preload and afterload while preserving blood pressure. Ectopy also decreased.

Positive Inotropes

Digoxin

Digoxin was given to improve myocardial contractility.

Dobutamine

Ms. Martin received dobutamine in the range of 2.5–10 μg/kg/min. This provided stimulation of cardiac β_1-receptors, resulting in increased myocardial contractility, and improved peripheral perfusion with increased urine output. Higher dosages are sometimes used, but careful monitoring of HR, BP, and cardiac rhythm is essential in such cases.

10. **The SVR is a clinical calculation that is useful in evaluating the effects of afterload reducing drugs. Calculate Ms. Martin's SVR both before and after unloading therapy.**

$$SVR = \frac{MAP - CVP}{CO} \times 80$$

$$MAP = \frac{Systolic\ BP - diastolic\ BP}{3} + diastolic\ BP$$

SVR is expressed in dyn/sec/cm^{-5}. Normal is 900–1200.

Before Therapy

$$MAP = \frac{94 - 70}{3} + 70 = 78$$

$$SVR = \frac{78 - 20}{2.5} \times 80$$

$$SVR = \frac{58}{2.5} \times 80 =$$

$$1856\ dyn/sec/cm^{-5}$$

After Therapy

$$MAP = \frac{108 - 62}{3} + 62 = 77$$

$$SVR = \frac{77 - 14}{3.8} \times 80$$

$$SVR = \frac{63}{3.8} \times 80 =$$

$$1326\ dyn/sec/cm^{-5}$$

11. **What is the significance of Ms. Martin's extra heart sounds?**

The third heart sound, referred to as S_3, is usually considered pathologic in adults. It is a low pitched sound heard in early diastole, which is the phase of rapid ventricular filling. Vibrations occur due to this rapid filling and become audible when the ventricle is overdistended or noncompliant, as in congestive heart failure. An S_3 is best auscultated at the cardiac apex when originating from the left ventricle, and at the fourth intercostal space along the left sternal border when originating from the right ventricle.

A pansystolic (holosystolic) murmur means that the sound occurs throughout the systolic cycle; therefore, it begins with S_1 and ends with S_2. When a ventricle becomes volume overloaded, muscle fibers stretch to promote stronger contractions and better emptying. Over time, the ventricle enlarges and becomes permanently distended. This prevents the leaflets of the atrioventricular valve (mitral or tricuspid) from closing sufficiently during systole. Blood then regurgitates into the atrium during systole. Blood flowing backwards through this incompetent, normally one-way valve creates the harsh, blowing sound referred to as a murmur. The murmur of mitral regurgitation is best heard at the cardiac apex, while tricuspid regurgitation is best heard along the lower left sternal border. The intensity of a murmur is graded on a scale of I to VI:

I	Barely audible; faint
II	Soft; can be heard without straining
III	Moderately loud
IV	Loud
V	Very loud, but requires stethoscope chestpiece on chest
VI	Extremely loud; heard with stethoscope chestpiece off chest

The murmur is recorded as the grade assessed over the highest grade in the scale, i.e., II/VI.

12. What nursing diagnoses apply in this case?

Decreased cardiac output related to myocardial dysfunction
Impaired gas exchange related to pulmonary edema
Activity intolerance related to reduced peripheral oxygenation
Anxiety related to a feeling of impending doom
Potential for infection related to presence of invasive lines
Noncompliance with medication regimen
Potential impaired skin integrity related to bedrest and altered tissue perfusion

SUGGESTED READINGS

Canobbio MM. Cardiovascular system. In: Thompson J, McFarland G, Hirsch J, Tucker S, Bowers A, eds. Clinical nursing. St. Louis: CV Mosby, 1986:3–108.

DeAngelis R. The cardiovascular system. In: Alspach J, Williams S, eds. AACN core curriculum for critical care nurses. 3rd ed. Philadelphia: WB Saunders, 1985:102–217.

Di Piro J, Talbert RL, Hayes PE, et al. Pharmacotherapy: A pathophysiologic approach. New York: Elsevier, 1989:220–221.

Dossey BM. The person with heart failure. In: Guzzetta CE, Dossey BM, eds. Cardiovascular nursing: Bodymind tapestry. St. Louis: CV Mosby, 1984:516–547.

Gawlinski A. Congestive heart failure and pulmonary edema. In: Swearingen PL, Sommers MS, Miller K, eds. Manual of critical care. St. Louis: CV Mosby, 1988:85–90.

Hillis, LD, Firth BG, Winniford MD, Willerson JT. Manual of clinical problems in cardiology. 3rd ed. Boston: Little, Brown & Co, 1988.

Hindle P, Wallace AG. Complications of coronary artery disease. In: Andreoli K, ed. Comprehensive cardiac care. St. Louis: CV Mosby, 1987:114–130.

Holloway, N. Nursing the critically ill adult. 3rd ed. Menlo Park, CA: Addison Wesley, 1988.

McCauley KM, Isacson LM, Schulz KJ. Congestive heart failure: A step by step guide to better nursing management. Nurs Life 1984;4(3):34–39.

Ryan AM. Stopping CHF while there's still time. RN 1986;August:28–33.

Van Parys E. Assessing the failing state of the heart. Nursing 1987;17(2):42–49.

CHAPTER 7

Coronary Artery Bypass Graft

Marsha Halfman-Franey, RN, MSN

Richard Hall, a 65-year-old man with known coronary artery disease, was admitted for coronary artery bypass surgery. His risk factors for atherosclerosis include a strong family history, high cholesterol (>300 mg/dl), and an unfavorable HDL/LDL ratio. He has not suffered a myocardial infarction, but has been admitted to the CCU several times with angina. Cardiac catheterization demonstrated a high grade (>90%) stenosis of the left anterior descending (LAD) coronary artery just proximal to the first diagonal branch. Good ventricular function was noted, with a left ventricular ejection fraction (LVEF) of >50% and good septal motion. He appeared to be a good surgical candidate, and a left internal mammary artery (LIMA) graft was planned.

Following the usual surgical preparation and drape, a median sternotomy incision was accomplished without incident. The right atrial appendage was cannulated for venous drainage and the ascending aorta for arterial return. Cardiopulmonary bypass was instituted with moderate hypothermia and cardioplegic arrest. The left internal mammary artery was dissected and anastomosed to the LAD. Adequate hemostasis was obtained and the patient returned to the Cardiovascular Thoracic ICU (CVTICU) in satisfactory condition (total pump time, 56 min; total blood administered, none).

Upon admission to the CVTICU, the following information was recorded:

BP	120/80
HR	100 (normal sinus rhythm)
Resp	12
Temp	98°F
LAP	12
CVP	6

Mr. Hall was somewhat responsive, moving all extremities. He had several lines, including a CVP, left atrial (LA), and arterial line and was normotensive without pharmacologic support. He remained intubated on a Servo ventilator with adequate blood gases on an FIO_2 of 0.40. Chest tubes were connected to underwater seal drainage, and several hundred milliliters of urine were noted in the Foley bag. A chest x-ray was ordered. The most recent laboratory work from the Operating Room included:

K	4.1
Hgb	12
Hct	35

QUESTIONS AND ANSWERS

1. Describe the anatomical placement of a LIMA graft.

The LIMA is usually left attached to the left subclavian artery and is dissected away from the posterior ribs. When only the LAD is done, it is an end to side anastomosis. The LIMA can be left attached to the left subclavian and then used as a "jump" or "sequential" graft to more than one area. The LIMA can also be detached from the left subclavian and used as a "free" graft (like in saphenous vein bypass graft (SVBG).

2. What are the advantages and disadvantages to the use of a LIMA graft as compared to a SVBG?

Advantages

Superior patency (96% at 5 years versus 80–85% at 5 years for SVBG)
Can enlarge to meet increased myocardial oxygen requirements
More compatible in size to coronary artery
Not subject to atherosclerosis and/or intimal hyperplasia (decreased need for future reoperation)
No valves
Intact blood supply
Only alternative in cases of previous vein stripping or previous CABG

Disadvantages

Technically difficult (increased time and skill to dissect LIMA)
Potential for spasm
Insufficient length to reach distal circumflex and posterior descending coronary artery (PDCA)

3. What nursing considerations are specific to the patient undergoing LIMA graft?

Pulmonary Considerations

Early extubation is recommended to avoid hyperinflation and stretching of the graft. While ventilatory support is required, smaller tidal volumes should be used and PEEP should be avoided if possible. This is because of the proximity of the LIMA graft to the lung. Pulmonary hyperinflation can result in mechanical dislodgment of the artery from the heart.

Avoid vigorous stripping of chest tubes due to close proximity of the tip of the tube to the LIMA graft. Vigorous stripping may damage the graft.

There is an increased incidence of atelectasis and intrapulmonary shunting. The pleural space has been entered, and pleural effusions frequently occur. Also, transient paresis of the phrenic nerve may occur secondary to the iced saline lavage of the pericardium. Since the iced saline is directed toward the left ventricle, the left phrenic nerve is most commonly involved. This manifests as an elevated left hemidiaphragm and left lower lobe atelectasis.

Bleeding

There may be an increased need for blood or blood products due to extensive dissection.

Pain Control

Pain is increased due to complex nerve supply in the pleura, stretching of the intercostals, and manipulation of the sternum.

Acute Graft Spasm

There have been several reports in the literature concerning catastrophic LIMA spasm necessitating reopening the chest and direct application of papaverine-soaked gauze to alleviate spasm. This dreaded complication manifests as profound hemodynamic instability. Fortunately, this only appears to happen in the early postoperative period.

4. **What are the specific nursing considerations regarding the LA line? Why is it in?**

The LA line is placed directly into the left atrium to monitor the pressure in that chamber. The LAP should reflect left ventricular end-diastolic pressure (because the mitral valve is open during diastole, allowing pressure to be transmitted from the left ventricle to the left atrium). The LA line can be placed only intraoperatively so its use is restricted to the cardiac surgical patient. A pulmonary artery (PA) catheter can also measure LVEDP via PAWP, but it is an indirect measurement and may be subject to respiratory variation and distortion by PEEP.

The LA line, unlike the PA line, is in the arterial system and is subject to all the risks inherent with arterial cannulation. The line must be kept free of air and should not be irrigated, as either could result in embolization to the heart or brain. The line generally dampens after the first day and is removed. The surgeon simply clips the suture and pulls the line through the chest wall. (Removal should occur before chest tube removal so that any bleeding can be noted.)

5. A CVP/RA line is also used. For what purpose?

The CVP/RA line measures RVEDP. In a normal heart, it may be sufficient to look at CVP/RA pressure to evaluate cardiac function. In the diseased heart, CVP/RA pressure only reflects right heart function and needs to be evaluated in conjunction with LA/PAWP. This line can also be used for central fluid or drug administration.

6. Other than hemodynamic pressures, what other information can be gained from RA/CVP and LA/PA lines?

Although pressure readings are important, the value of observing the waveform configuration should not be overlooked. (See Chapter 12, "Mitral Valve Replacement.") Elevations in "a" waves in either of the two waveforms may suggest increasing resistance to RV or LV filling. This resistance to ventricular filling can occur secondary to a change in ventricular compliance or ventricular failure. Elevated "v" waves would indicate valvular insufficiency, either as a primary problem or secondary to ventricular chamber dilatation (with the resultant distortion of the valve annulus and its relationship to the papillary muscles and chordae tendinae). Elevation of both components of the waveform might be indicative of hypervolemia or tamponade.

7. Mr. Hall's blood pressure begins to drop rapidly and is unresponsive to fluid challenge. A pulmonary artery catheter is inserted. What additional information can be obtained from this line?

The most important parameter is that of cardiac output (CO). Once CO is measured, one can derive any number of important values (systemic vascular resistance, pulmonary vascular resistance, cardiac index, left ventricular stroke work index, etc.), as well as determine PA pressures and obtain mixed venous blood gases. If the catheter also has oximetry capabilities, $S_{\bar{v}}O_2$ can be monitored and various oxygen delivery and consumption variables can be assessed. (See Appendix B.)

8. Given the following information, what is Mr. Hall's problem?

BP	90/60	RAP	6	CT drainage	30–50
HR	130	PaO_2	90		ml/hr
PAWP	25	SaO_2	98%	Urine output	15
CO	3.2	$S_{\bar{v}}O_2$	50%		ml/hr
SVR	2400	Hgb	12		

Arterial oxygen content $(CaO_2) = (Hgb \times 1.39 \times SaO_2) = 16$ vol % (normal is 20 vol %). Oxygen delivery $(CaO_2 \times CO \times 10)$ is

512 ml O_2/min (normal is 1000 ml O_2/min). O_2 content is slightly below normal, and O_2 delivery is significantly below normal.

The body's response to inadequate O_2 delivery is to increase CO or to increase O_2 extraction at the tissue level. As this patient has a limited cardiovascular reserve, the only compensatory mechanism available to him is to increase O_2 extraction, thereby accounting for his decreased $S_{\bar{v}}O_2$ value. (The body also increases SVR and increases heart rate to redistribute blood flow to vital organs and to increase oxygen delivery.) This increased SVR further compounds the problem, as the increased afterload increases myocardial oxygen consumption and decreases CO. The increased heart rate also increases myocardial oxygen consumption. The imbalance between oxygen supply and demand is critical, as indicated by the $S_{\bar{v}}O_2$ of 50%. Further deterioration will lead to lactic acidosis.

9. **What therapy is indicated?**

Several options exist. One way to increase O_2 delivery is to increase arterial O_2 content. Because SaO_2 is >95%, further respiratory interventions are not indicated. The Hgb of 12 (probably secondary to hemodilution from cardiopulmonary bypass and postoperative bleeding) could be raised with blood transfusion. However, blood transfusions carry significant risks, and 1 unit of blood typically increases the Hgb by about 1 gm. Therefore, 2 units of blood would bring the Hgb up to 14, which would only raise the O_2 transport to 600 ml/min.

$$CaO_2 = 14 \times 1.39 \times 0.98 = 19 \text{ vol } \%$$

$$O_2 \text{ transport} = 3.2 \times 19 \times 10 = 608 \text{ ml } O_2/\text{min}$$

In contrast, increasing CO to 5.0 liters/min would make a substantial difference.

$$O_2 \text{ transport} = CaO_2 \times CO \times 10$$
$$= 16 \times 5 \times 10$$
$$= 800 \text{ ml } O_2/\text{min.}$$

10. **How would this therapy affect the myocardial muscle?**

All therapies used to manipulate cardiac output affect the heart muscle, generally in terms of their effect on the myocardial oxygen supply/demand balance. Orders are usually written to titrate drugs to effect while keeping the mean arterial pressure (MAP) around 70 mm Hg. The MAP represents the perfusion pressure in the systemic circuit, but can also be used as a guideline to protect coronary perfusion as well. The coronaries fill during diastole and MAP is much closer to diastolic pressure than to systolic pressure.

$$\text{MAP} = \frac{\text{syst} - \text{diast}}{3} + \text{diast}$$

To actually measure coronary perfusion pressure, subtract either RAP or PAWP from the aortic diastolic pressure.

$$\text{coronary perfusion pressure} = \text{aortic diastolic} - \text{PAWP}$$

$$70 \text{ mm Hg} = 80 - 10$$

Normal coronary perfusion pressure is 70–75 mm Hg. In Mr. Hall, coronary perfusion pressure (60 − 25) was only 35 mm Hg! Using afterload reduction and positive inotropes would result in a decrease in PAWP, as forward flow from the left ventricle would be enhanced, causing an increase in coronary perfusion pressure.

11. Both cardiac tamponade and myocardial dysfunction may present as:

  Tachycardia
  Hypotension
  Narrowed pulse pressure
  Increased CVP

How can the differential diagnosis be made using common assessment and hemodynamic monitoring techniques?

The incidence of cardiac tamponade after cardiac surgery is 3.4–7%; however, it is a potentially lethal complication requiring prompt diagnosis and treatment. The classic signs and symptoms of cardiac tamponade include:

    a. Resistance to right heart filling
       i. Increased CVP
      ii. Neck vein distention
     iii. Kussmaul's sign
    b. Reduction in CO
       i. Hypotension
      ii. Narrowed pulse pressure
     iii. Pulsus paradoxus
     iv. Tachycardia
    c. Fluid accumulation around heart
       i. Widened mediastinum on chest x-ray
      ii. Muffled heart sounds
     iii. Decreased ECG voltage

However, these signs and symptoms are less reliable after cardiac surgery. The mediastinum often appears widened as the result of the distortion in the AP view. Heart sound muffling and decreased ECG voltage may be a function of opening the pericardium.

More reliable signs and symptoms of cardiac tamponade in the postoperative cardiac surgical patient include:

Serum Creatinine (>1.6 mg%). Serum creatinine level is a sensitive, although nonspecific, indicator of inadequate renal perfusion secondary to decreased CO.

Pressure Plateau (LAP-RAP 0–2 mm Hg) Sustained. Normally left heart pressures exceed right heart pressures. In tamponade, RAP, RVEDP, PADP, PAWP, LAP, and LVEDP equalize (pressure plateau), so in cardiac tamponade RAP = or > LAP/PAWP. The RA and LA waveforms would demonstrate elevated a and v waves with an exaggerated x descent with brief or absent y descent (Fig. 7.1).

Chest Tube Drainage (>1400 ml Postoperatively Cumulative). Bleeding into the chest cavity can predispose a patient to development of tamponade and increased bleeding can be predictive of increased risk of tamponade.

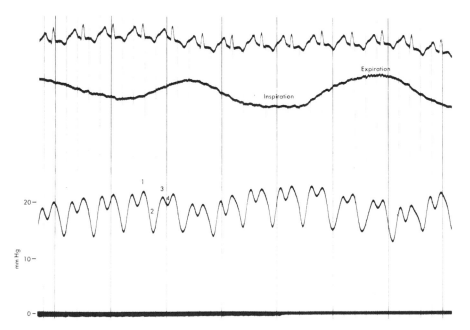

Figure 7.1. Right atrial waveform in cardiac tamponade. Note: elevated a and v waves with exaggerated X descent. (Reproduced by permission from Daily EK, Schroeder JS. Hemodynamic waveforms. St. Louis, 1983, The C.V. Mosby Co.)

12.   Should chest tubes be stripped postoperatively?

Chest tubes are customarily placed in the mediastinum and/or pleural space following cardiac surgery to measure the amount of drainage and to prevent possible cardiac tamponade. Routine nursing orders usually call for periodic stripping of chest tubes; however, concern has been raised about possible injury to intrathoracic structures adjacent to the chest tube openings from the negative pressure generated by the stripping procedure. Some manufacturers of disposable chest drainage units have added a manual filtered vent for controlled entry of air to lower residual negative pressure to the desired level. Others use a vented sump drain in which a stream of air is drawn continuously from the atmosphere through the tubing to move drainage along. Sump tubes are contraindicated for drainage of the pleural space because air entry required for sump action would bring normal intrapleural negative pressure toward ambient level and promote collapse of lung tissue; in contrast, entry of atmospheric air into the mediastinum and a change in ambient pressure does not disrupt cardiac function. Further study is needed, however, before nursing policy on this issue is finalized.

As mentioned previously, mediastinal chest tubes should be stripped carefully, if at all, after a LIMA graft, because of the proximity of the tip of the tube to the graft.

13.   What is the effect of increasing temperature in the open heart patient?

Patients characteristically overwarm following hypothermia. The warming device should be removed when the rectal temperature reaches 98.4°F (36.9°C). Even so, slight to moderate hyperthermia is often present in the first 24 hr postoperatively. As body temperature rises, the tissue oxygen demands increase. The body's initial response to meet this need is to increase the cardiac output, followed by increased extraction of oxygen or use of the venous oxygen reserve. In addition, an increase in body temperature shifts the oxyhemoglobin dissociation curve to the right, thereby decreasing hemoglobin's affinity for oxygen and facilitating oxygen unloading at the tissue level.

It is not advisable to wean the patient or consider extubation until the patient is normothermic. Frequently, the patient wakes up, appears alert, but falls back asleep during the warming process. This occurs because as vessels dilate upon rewarming, blood flows to areas previously vasoconstricted due to hypothermia. As blood flows through previously underperfused tissues, it picks up residual anesthetic and essentially reanesthetizes the patient.

14. Why is it necessary to keep the patient normotensive?

Hypertension may cause rupture of the suture lines at the site of the graft anastomosis. Hypotension, on the other hand, will decrease the blood flow through the graft and could cause the graft to clot off. Brisk antegrade flow and good distal runoff are the most important flow factors in maintaining graft patency.

15. How is the heart protected during open heart surgery?

Periods of induced ischemia are necessary to provide a motionless field and may be accomplished by intermittent aortic occlusion. The aorta is cross-clamped and ventricular fibrillation is induced, allowing the coronary anastomosis to be performed. The clamp is then removed and the heart defibrillated. The proximal aortic anastomosis is then done while the heart is being perfused.

Often, the "safe" ischemic period is prolonged by the use of hypothermia, which reduces myocardial oxygen consumption and tissue metabolism. Systemic hypothermia may be accomplished through a heat exhanger in the extracorporeal circuit. Cold solutions also can be poured over the heart to provide topical cooling. It is important to provide uniform cooling because the subendocardium is especially vulnerable to ischemia owing to its high energy requirements and its terminal position in the coronary artery distribution. Usually, hypothermic perfusion of the coronary arteries is performed for rapid, thorough and reliable cooling. Direct coronary perfusion is generally a reliable method except in the presence of coronary stenosis, which impedes flow to the distal bed. Cold solution may be infused through bypass grafts or via the coronary sinus in such instances.

In addition to reducing the myocardial oxygen demands, perfusion of the coronary arteries with solutions colder than 10°C will eventually cause electromechanical arrest and thus a still operative field. However, immediate diastolic arrest, termed "cardioplegia" can be produced by adding potassium to the cold solution. At present, hypothermic potassium arrest is the most widely used method to protect the myocardium during cardiac surgery.

16. What are the relevant nursing diagnoses?

Decreased CO related to CAD

Impaired gas exchange related to atelectasis and intrapulmonary shunting

Altered body temperature (hypo- and hyperthermia)

Potential for infection related to invasive monitoring lines

Pain related to sternal splitting and extensive dissection of LIMA

Sleep pattern disturbance related to environmental stimuli

SUGGESTED READINGS

Bland RD, Shoemaker WC. Common physiologic patterns in general surgical patients: Hemodynamic and oxygen transport changes during and after operation in patients with and without associated medical problems. Surg Clin 1985;65(4):793–799.

Daily EK, Schroeder JS. Hemodynamic waveforms. St. Louis: CV Mosby, 1983.

Duncan CR, Erickson RS, Weigel RM. Effect of chest tube management on drainage after cardiac surgery. Heart Lung 1987; 16(1):1–9.

Jansen KJ, McFadden PM. Postoperative nursing management in patients undergoing myocardial revascularizations with the internal mammary artery bypass. Heart Lung 1986;15(1):48–54.

Kern LS. Advances in the surgical treatment of coronary artery disease. J Cardiovasc Nurs 1986;1(1):1–14.

Sarabu MR, McClung JA, Fass A, et al. Early postoperative spasm in left internal mammary artery bypass grafts. Ann Thorac Surg 1987;44:199–200.

Seifert PC. Protection of the myocardium during cardiac surgery. Heart Lung 1983; 12(2):135–142.

Sider L. Interpretation of the postoperative chest radiograph. Crit Care Q 1986; 9(3):71–83.

Vitello-Cicciu J, Stewart SL, Griffin EL. Coronary artery disease. In: Kinney MR, Packa DR, Dunbar SB, eds. AACN's clinical reference for critical-care nursing. 2nd ed. New York: McGraw-Hill, 1988:571–658.

White KM. Completing the hemodynamic picture: SVO_2. Heart Lung 1985;14(3): 272–280.

Wiland AP, Walker WE. Physiologic principles and clinical sequellae of cardiopulmonary bypass. Heart Lung 1986;15(1): 34–39.

CHAPTER 8

Femoral Popliteal Bypass

Virginia Byrn Huddleston, RN, MSN, CCRN

Ethel Jordan is a 78-year-old woman admitted to the ICU following femoral popliteal bypass on her left lower extremity. She was admitted to the hospital with a complaint of severe ischemic rest pain and several small gangrenous areas on the toes of her left foot. She has insulin-dependent diabetes mellitus, hypertension, coronary artery disease, and a 50-year history of smoking. She underwent coronary artery bypass grafting for triple vessel disease 10 years prior to this admission; therefore, her saphenous veins were unavailable for use, and a prosthetic graft was placed.

On arrival in the unit, Ms. Jordan was awake and following commands. She was in normal sinus rhythm with occasional PACs and PVCs. She was receiving crystalloids via the proximal port of the pulmonary artery catheter. She had a radial arterial line that showed a pressure of 150/90. Her temperature was 97°F. She was placed on 40% face mask, and auscultation of her chest revealed coarse crackles bilaterally. Her nasogastric tube was clamped, and assessment of her abdomen revealed a soft, round belly with hypoactive bowel sounds. A Foley catheter was draining adequate amounts of pale, yellow urine. The patient was placed on a warming blanket and given intravenous morphine sulfate in attempts to decrease her blood pressure.

Vital Signs		Hemodynamic Parameters	
BP	150/90	CVP	10
HR	94	PAP	32/15
		PAWP	10
		CO	4.6

QUESTIONS AND ANSWERS

1. **What is a femoral popliteal bypass?**

   Vascular bypass procedures are titled by the site of graft attachment; therefore, a femoral popliteal bypass involves a graft anastomosed proximally to the femoral artery and distally to the popliteal artery. The blockage may exist at any point between the anastomoses. The distal anastomosis to the popliteal artery may be above or below the knee, depending on the site of the occlusive lesion.

2. **What factors contributed to Ms. Jordan's development of infraingui-
nal atherosclerosis?**

>   Age
>   Diabetes mellitus
>   Hypertension
>   Smoking

3. **What complications is Ms. Jordan at risk for following her femoral
popliteal bypass?**

>   Graft thrombosis
>   Hemorrhage
>   Edema
>   Lymphatic leakage
>   Infection

4. **Describe important assessment parameters and nursing interventions
for the first 48 hr postoperatively.**

   The major goal of care in the first 48 hr is the maintenance of
hemodynamic stability and graft patency. The majority of patients
undergoing a femoral poplitcal bypass have preexisting cardiac or
pulmonary disease, and the stress of surgery could potentiate dysrhythmias, myocardial ischemia, MI, CHF, or pulmonary edema.
Hourly measurements should include PAP, PAWP, CVP, BP, heart
rate, urine output, and cardiac output if inotropic drips are being
titrated.

   Aggressive pulmonary toilet is indicated, because Ms. Jordan is on
bedrest, has a history of smoking, and has received a fluid load in the
Operating Room. Special care must be taken to monitor fluid shifts
occurring at 48–72 hr. Third-spaced fluid is sequestered back into the
circulation during this time, so the patient should be assessed for
evidence of pulmonary edema or myocardial infarction. Lasix may
be given to assist the patient in unloading the excess fluid as it moves
back into the vasculature.

   The patient is maintained on bedrest with knees straight to prevent
additional stress to the graft site, especially if the bypass extends
below the knee. Kinking with subsequent occlusion could lead to
thrombosis, ischemia, and limb loss. Neurovascular checks are performed every 1–2 hr to monitor for graft patency, embolic phenomena, and compartment syndrome, especially if reoperation was necessary.

5. **Why is it necessary to maintain Ms. Jordan's blood pressure within a narrow range?**

    In order to maintain graft patency and integrity, the blood pressure must be controlled. If the patient becomes hypotensive, the risk of graft thrombosis increases greatly. Vasopressors may be used judiciously to maintain a systolic blood pressure slightly above normal, but care must be taken not to markedly increase the pressure because extreme hypertension can cause anastomotic leaks, breakdown, hemorrhage, and loss of the graft.

6. **On day 2, the nurse caring for Ms. Jordan is unable to palpate or auscultate via Doppler a previously present left dorsalis pedis pulse. Ms. Jordan's left foot is cooler and becoming mottled. What is occurring and why?**

    Thrombosis is occurring, most likely at the graft itself. This is considered a surgical emergency, and the physician is notified immediately. There are many contributing factors to the development of this complication. They include:

    > Inadequate arterial inflow
    > Proximal clamp injury leading to impaired flow
    > Disturbance of distal flow by intimal flaps
    > Graft constriction by tissue or nerve fiber bands
    > Twists or kinks in the graft
    > Decreased cardiac output
    > Vasospasm (especially with poor use of vasopressors)
    > Inadequate run-off in the distal vessels
    > Inadequate preparation of the graft
    > Thromboemboli

7. **Following embolectomy, flow is adequately restored, and Ms. Jordan is returned to the ICU. Postoperative laboratory tests reveal a potassium of 5.8 mEq/liter and a pH of 7.29. ABGs are otherwise within normal limits. Describe the pathophysiology and treatment of this complication.**

    Due to the lack of tissue perfusion distal to the occlusion, muscle ischemia and cell death occur, liberating potassium, myoglobin, and lactic acid. Upon reperfusion, these substances are released into the systemic circulation. All three can produce major complications if not treated promptly.

    Myoglobin precipitates in the renal tubules, which can lead to acute tubular necrosis (ATN). Damage can be reduced if sodium bicarbonate is administered to alkalinize the urine and prevent precipitation of the acid hematin. (See Chapter 36, "Rhabdomyolysis.")

Fluid volumes and mannitol are also given to flush the tubules and maintain a urine output of >100 ml/hr.

The lactic acid not only causes acidemia and alterations in enzyme function, but it also potentiates the hyperkalemia. As the pH becomes more acidic, hydrogen ions are driven into the cell, causing potassium ions to move from the cell into the serum in order to maintain electrical neutrality. The administration of sodium bicarbonate also assists in returning the pH and potassium to homeostatic levels.

A combination of hypertonic glucose (D_{50}) and insulin may also be given to lower the potassium level. Potassium is carried into the cell concurrently with the insulin-mediated uptake of glucose. These are short-term measures, so if potassium levels remain increased after pH correction, cation-exchange resins (Kayexalate) may be required to further reduce the potassium concentration and prevent cardiac irregularities.

8. What other complications is Ms. Jordan at risk for following reperfusion?

> Compartment syndrome
> Pulmonary embolus

Along with the by-products of cell lysis, recent research has also implicated oxygen free radicals in reperfusion injury. Following reperfusion, hyperemia, increased capillary permeability, and microhemorrhage often occur. Edema and increased compartmental pressures ensue, resulting in nerve and muscle damage. The lower leg is divided into four compartments by the crural fascia. The compartments are relatively fixed in size; therefore, any increase in compartment contents causes the hydrostatic pressure within the compartment to increase. Interstitial fluid is the most common precipitating factor, but blood and cellular swelling may also contribute to pressure increases. Normal compartment pressure is <20 mm Hg.

Signs and symptoms of compartment syndrome include severe pain, muscle weakness, paresthesias, pain on passive stretch, and compartment tenseness. Compartment pressures >40–45 mm Hg require a fasciotomy to relieve compartment pressure. The presence of pedal pulses is not indicative of safe, physiologic compartment pressures, so other parameters must be assessed, including color, temperature, and capillary refill. Compartment pressures may also be measured directly using a needle and pressure transducer setup.

During the time of occlusion and ischemia, venous pooling may occur in the affected extremity with sluggish venous return. If venous thrombosis develops, multiple emboli may be released following restoration of arterial circulation. A pulmonary embolic event or ARDS could then result.

9. **Why is graft infection such a devastating complication of arterial bypass surgery?**

Graft infection is much more common in prosthetic grafts, because the artificial material represents a foreign body. Graft infection can lead to false aneurysm, anastomotic breakdown, hemorrhage, sepsis, thromboemboli, DIC, amputation, and organ dysfunction. The graft usually must be removed. Flow is restored by either replacing the graft or performing other procedures, such as extraanatomic bypass.

10. **Describe the etiology and pathophysiology of a graft infection.**

Graft infections occur primarily in the groin area secondary to invasion by staphylococcus organisms. This area's proximity to the perineum, chronic colonization of skin folds, and extensive lymphatic network all promote the development of graft infection. Also, the graft is relatively superficial at this position and more prone to infiltration.

The placement of the graft in the body initiates a foreign body response. Phagocytes, complement, and the coagulation cascade may all be activated with a concomitant release of cytotoxic enzymes. Abscesses and the knitted graft itself can sequester bacteria in areas inaccessible to host defenses.

Contamination may occur during actual operative placement of the graft, especially if skin contact is made. If distal infections are present, the lymph may be contaminated. During femoral dissection, lymph fluid may spill into the field and cause direct infection of the graft at that time. Lymph leaks in the postoperative period may also infect the graft. Bacteria from other systemic sources such as pneumonia, urinary tract infection, and catheter sepsis may also predispose the graft to bacterial colonization.

Meticulous hemostasis, ligation of lymph vessels, and soft tissue coverage are necessary to protect the graft at the femoral site. Promotion of wound healing by strict aseptic technique, gentle handling of tissues, adequate nutrition, and oxygenation all aid in reducing the risk of graft infection.

11. List the signs and symptoms of graft infection.

Incisional swelling
Local tenderness
Drainage-purulent or serous (lymph leak)
Pulsatile mass (false aneurysm)
Diminished distal pulses
Leukocytosis
Fever

12. What nursing diagnoses apply in this case?

Alteration in peripheral tissue perfusion related to atherosclerosis and thromboembolic events
Potential for impaired skin integrity secondary to immobility, decreased tissue perfusion, and diabetes mellitus
Anxiety related to ICU environment
Pain related to operative procedure and decreased tissue perfusion
Potential for infection secondary to groin incision, distal necrosis, and diabetes mellitus
Ineffective airway clearance related to immobility, sedation, and pulmonary dysfunction secondary to long smoking history

SUGGESTED READINGS

Appleton D. Vascular disease and postoperative nursing management. Crit Care Nurs 1985;5(5):34–42.

Bernhard VM, Towne JB, eds. Complications in vascular surgery. 2nd ed. New York: McGraw-Hill, 1985.

Foreman MD. Arterial prosthetic graft infections: The pathophysiologic basis of nursing care. Focus Crit Care 1985;12(5):22–28.

Guzetta CE, Dossey BM. Cardiovascular nursing: Bodymind tapestry. St. Louis: CV Mosby, 1984.

Hallett JW. Trends in revascularization of the lower extremity. Mayo Clin Proc 1986;61:369–76.

Hallett JW, Brewster DC, Darling RC. Manual of patient care in vascular surgery. Boston: Little, Brown & Co, 1982.

Wagner MM. Pathophysiology related to peripheral vascular disease. Nurs Clin North Am 1986;21(2):195–206.

Wilson SE, Veith FJ, Johnson RW, Williams RA, eds. Vascular surgery: Principles and practice. New York: McGraw-Hill, 1987.

CHAPTER 9

Hypertensive Crisis

Jacquelyne V. Prince, RN, MSN

Hattie Goodman is a 58-year-old cafeteria worker who was diagnosed as having essential hypertension 5 years ago. She has a history of poor compliance with her antihypertensive therapy plan. Ms. Goodman presented to the Emergency Department with severe headache, nausea, blurred vision, and weakness. Her past medical history was significant for "forgetting" to take her clonidine and smoking two packs of cigarettes/day for the past 40 years.

Ms. Goodman's physical examination showed an obese (240 pound) woman sitting up in a chair, holding her head, and crying. Her vital signs were:

BP	188/130 (both arms)
HR	120
Resp	18
Temp	98.7°F

The cardiac monitor showed sinus tachycardia with occasional PACs. Funduscopic examination revealed retinopathy with exudates, hemorrhage, and papilledema. The radial and femoral pulses were bounding bilaterally, but the pedal pulses were obtainable only via Doppler. She had 2+ pedal edema. Auscultation of the heart revealed an S_4 and a soft S_3. No abdominal bruits were audible. Breath sounds were essentially clear. Chest x-ray demonstrated left ventricular predominance with mild pulmonary venous engorgement.

Initial laboratory values were as follows:

Electrolytes		CBC	
Na	140	Hgb	15.3
K	3.6	Hct	48
Cl	102		
CO_2	18		
Gluc	162		

Renal Values		ABGs (Room Air)	
Creat	2.8	pH	7.34
BUN	34	$PaCO_2$	31
Uric acid	7.0	PaO_2	85
		SaO_2	95%
		HCO_3	19

Ms. Goodman was transferred from the Emergency Department to the ICU. Upon arriving in the unit, she complained that her head ached so badly that she "couldn't stand it any more." Her blood pressure at that time was 230/142 in both arms. She began to have projectile vomiting, and her neurological examination revealed nystagmus and mental confusion. An arterial line was inserted in the right radial artery. Her blood pressure was 245/145 by monitor and 230/150 by cuff. A sodium nitroprusside (Nipride) drip was started at 0.5 μg/kg/min and titrated to bring the diastolic pressure down to 115–120 mm Hg. Ms. Goodman's blood pressure was checked by monitor before and after each adjustment of the Nipride drip and at least every 5–10 min. Nursing documentation during this time included blood pressure, heart rate, Nipride infusion rate, and level of consciousness. A Foley catheter was placed and urine output was measured hourly. Over the next 12 hr, the Nipride was titrated and the diastolic pressure brought down to 90–100 mm Hg.

On the second hospital day, Ms. Goodman was started on captopril, 12.5 mg PO BID. The Nipride infusion was tapered and then discontinued. The patient remained on hourly vital signs and neurological checks. Patient teaching regarding hypertension and compliance was begun.

The arterial line was discontinued on the morning of the third hospital day. Ms. Goodman's blood pressure was 152/98. Her captopril was increased to 25 mg PO TID and she was transferred to the floor. Patient teaching regarding hypertension and compliance was continued.

QUESTIONS AND ANSWERS

1. **What is a hypertensive crisis?**

   Hypertensive crisis is a loosely defined clinical event marked by significant blood pressure elevation and characteristic clinical findings. While the absolute blood pressure criterion for hypertensive crisis is not universally agreed upon, a diastolic blood pressure of >140 mm Hg is considered to be serious, warranting immediate treatment. In addition, the patient with malignant hypertension or hypertensive encephalopathy generally demonstrates papilledema with retinal hemorrhages and exudates. Other clinical manifestations may include severe headache, projectile vomiting, visual disturbances, transient paralysis, convulsions, stupor, and coma. Cardiac decompensation and declining renal function are not uncommon in these patients.

2. **Hypertensive crisis can be divided into two categories, hypertensive emergency and hypertensive urgency. Distinguish between the two and give examples of each.**

   Hypertensive emergencies pose a significant and immediate threat to the patient's life by threatening the cardiovascular, neurologic, and/or renal systems. Immediate blood pressure reduction, within hours, is essential. The following are examples of hypertensive emergencies:

Hypertensive encephalopathy
Acute aortic dissection
Pulmonary edema
Pheochromocytoma crisis
Monoamine oxidase (MAO) inhibitor + tyramine interaction
Intracranial hemorrhage
Eclampsia

Hypertensive urgencies are situations where the patient's elevated blood pressure poses a serious risk to the patient if it is not treated aggressively. Patients generally do not require invasive monitoring or IV medication. Blood pressure should be lowered within 24 hr. The following are identified as hypertensive urgencies:

Hypertension associated with coronary artery disease
Severe hypertension in the kidney transplant patient
Postoperative hypertension
Uncontrolled hypertension in the patient requiring surgery
Moderate rise of blood pressure (diastolic >120) without evidence of end organ damage

3. **Ms. Goodman demonstrated papilledema, nystagmus, and mental confusion, which are symptoms of hypertensive encephalopathy. What is the mechanism responsible for this?**

When the cerebral blood vessels are subjected to a sustained, extreme elevation of blood pressure, they lose the ability to autoregulate. Autoregulation is the brain's ability to maintain a constant rate of blood flow despite changes in arterial blood pressure or intracranial pressure. An increase in arterial pressure causes vasoconstriction of the cerebral vessels, while a decrease in arterial pressure causes vasodilatation. Autoregulation keeps cerebral blood flow essentially constant for a range of mean arterial pressures (MAP) from approximately 50 to 170 mm Hg. With sustained elevations in arterial blood pressure, the autoregulatory mechanism may be impaired. When cerebral blood vessels dilate, cerebral blood flow increases, and the excessive pressure drives the fluid out of the vessel into the cerebral tissue, causing cerebral edema.

4. **What heart sounds are likely to be present during a hypertensive crisis?**

S_4
S_3
Murmur of aortic regurgitation

5. **Which organs are most likely to be damaged with sustained severe elevations in blood pressure?**

    Prolonged severe hypertension causes fibrinoid necrosis of the intima and media of the arteriole. Blood vessels are constricted and blood flow to major organs is restricted, which eventually causes ischemia and/or infarction of target organs. The organs that are most susceptible to damage are the kidneys, eyes, heart, and brain.

    Complications of hypertension include:

    Blindness
    Renal failure
    Stroke
    Coronary artery disease
    Aortic dissection
    Peripheral vascular disease

6. **How does a hypertensive crisis place the patient with atherosclerotic heart disease at risk for myocardial infarction?**

    When a hypertensive crisis occurs, the afterload is dramatically elevated. The left ventricle has to pump against increased resistance, which increases the myocardial oxygen demand. If the patient is tachycardic, myocardial oxygen demands are increased even more. Because the atherosclerotic changes in the coronary arteries diminish coronary artery blood flow, an imbalance between myocardial oxygen supply and demand may occur. If severe, this may precipitate a myocardial infarction. Patients with ischemic heart disease must be taught the importance of controlling their blood pressure with medication and should be advised of the complications of uncontrolled hypertension.

7. **Ms. Goodman's creatinine was 2.8 mg/dl and her BUN was 34 mg/dl. What is the significance of these values?**

    The kidney is one of the first organs damaged by prolonged hypertension. It is likely that Ms. Goodman has sustained renal parenchymal damage secondary to hypertension.

8. **Ms. Goodman had "forgotten" to take her clonidine for the past week. This led to an event known as "clonidine withdrawal syndrome." Briefly describe this phenomenon.**

    When clonidine is abruptly discontinued or sometimes rapidly tapered, a syndrome has been noted that is evidenced by palpitations, nausea, anxiety, sweating, headache, and nervousness as well as marked elevation of blood pressure. In some patients, blood pressure increases beyond the pretreatment level. The occurrence of rebound hypertension has been noted with use of this drug.

9. **Ms. Goodman's hypertensive crisis was precipitated by failure to take her antihypertensive medication. What are some other potential causes of hypertensive crisis?**

   Untreated or inadequately treated essential hypertension
   Renal disease (glomerulonephritis, collagen vascular disease, renal vascular disease)
   Adrenal dysfunction (Cushing's syndrome)
   Coarctation of the aorta
   Drug interactions with MAO inhibitors
   Pheochromocytoma
   Drug abuse

10. **Ms. Goodman was initially treated with intravenous Nipride. How does this drug work, and what are the nursing considerations during the administration of Nipride?**

    Nipride is the drug of choice in hypertensive crisis, as it is a potent vasodilator with almost immediate effects. Nipride is supplied in 50-mg vials, which must be reconstituted with D_5W. A common preparation of a Nipride drip consists of 50 mg of Nipride in 250 ml of D_5W. This drug must be administered via infusion pump and should be piggybacked into another line of D_5W so that it can be stopped if hypotension occurs. The maintenance dose is 0.25–8.0 $\mu g/kg/min$, with the average dose being 3 $\mu g/kg/min$. Nipride is unstable in solution and deteriorates rapidly when exposed to light, so the bag should be wrapped in protective foil. The tubing should not be wrapped, so that the solution can be observed for color changes. If the solution changes from its characteristic brown to blue, green, or red, it should be discarded and replaced. A fresh solution should be hung every 24 hr due to decomposition of the mixture. Nipride is metabolized to thiocyanate. Thiocyanate toxicity may occur with prolonged (>48 hr) or high dose infusion (>15 $\mu g/kg/min$) or when renal insufficiency exists. Symptoms of thiocyanate toxicity include fatigue, nausea, tinnitus, blurred vision, and delirium. Serum thiocyanate levels should be checked after 48 hr of administration. Levels <10 mg/dl are considered safe.

    Before a Nipride infusion is started, an arterial line should be placed for direct arterial monitoring. Nipride is a potent drug and precipitous drops in blood pressure can occur. The duration of action of Nipride is only 3–5 min; so if hypotension is detected immediately, the drug can be turned off and the pressure brought back to normal before disastrous consequences occur.

11. **Ms. Goodman's blood pressure was 230/150 by cuff and 245/145 by arterial line. Is this a normal discrepancy, or was it likely that the monitor blood pressures were inaccurate?**

    The arterial line blood pressure was accurate. An arterial line is said to correlate with the cuff pressure if the systolic pressure is 0–20 mm Hg higher by monitor and the diastolic pressure is 0–10 mm Hg lower by monitor. In order to ensure accurate readings, the air fluid interface on the transducer should be leveled with the right atrium (fourth intercostal space, midaxillary line). The monitor should be calibrated every 4 hr. No air bubbles should be allowed in the transducer dome or the pressure tubing. The cuff pressure should be checked at least once every 4 hr. As long as the arterial line and cuff pressures correlate, pressures should be taken by monitor.

12. **What steps can be taken to ensure accurate cuff blood pressures in a patient who does not have an arterial line?**

    The bladder of the cuff should fit completely around the arm and cover two-thirds of the length of the upper arm. The arm should be supported at heart level on the bed or overbed table. The cuff should be rapidly inflated until the pulse disappears, and then inflated an additional 30 mm Hg. The cuff should then be deflated at 2–3 mm Hg/sec.

    In the patient recovering from hypertensive crisis, standing BP should be monitored with a cuff to assess for orthostasis.

13. **What other drugs may be used in hypertensive emergencies?**

    See Table 9.1.

14. **Describe the role of nifedipine in treatment of hypertensive crisis.**

    Nifedipine is a calcium blocker which lowers the blood pressure by decreasing the total peripheral resistance. Nifedipine has the advantage that its use does not require invasive monitoring. It is useful while waiting for arterial line insertion and IV administration of an antihypertensive agent. Ten to 20 mg of nifedipine given sublingually or orally can lower the blood pressure within 5–15 min. The duration of treatment effect is 3–5 hr.

15. **Aortic dissection is a dreaded complication of uncontrolled hypertension. What is aortic dissection and what symptoms are indicative of its occurrence?**

    Aortic dissection is a longitudinal tear in the aortic wall caused by the driving pressure of a column of blood. The most common causes

Table 9.1. Drugs for hypertensive emergencies[a]

Drug	Route and Dose	Onset	Duration	Comments
Parental therapy				
Nitroprusside	IV, 0.25–8 µg/kg/min	Seconds	3–5 min	Thiocyanate toxicity may occur with prolonged (>48 hours) or high dose infusion (>15 µg/kg/min), particularly in renal insufficiency
Diazoxide	IV, 50–150 mg every 5 min or as infusion of 7.5–30 mg/min	1–5 min	4–24 h	Should not be used for patients with angina pectoris, myocardial infarction, dissecting aneurysm
Trimethaphan	IV infusion pump, 0.5–5 mg/min	1–5 min	10 min	Drug of choice for treatment of aortic dissection
Labetalol	IV, 2 mg/min or 20 mg every 10 min (can go to 80-mg doses); maximum cumulative dose, 300 mg	5 min or less	3–6 h	Prompt response; can be followed by same drug taken orally
Hydralazine	IM or IV, 10–20 mg	10–30 min	2–4 h	May precipitate angina, myocardial infarction
Acute oral therapy				
Nifedipine	10–20 mg orally or sublingually	5–15 min	3–5 h	Generally good response; short duration of action; optimal dosage not standardized
Clonidine	0.2 mg orally initially, then 0.1 mg/hr, up to 0.8 mg	½–2 hrs	6–8 h	Prominent sedation
Captopril	6.5–25 mg orally	15 min	4–6 h	Generally good, sometimes excessive response
Minoxidil	5–10 mg orally	½–1 h	12–16 h	Tachycardia, fluid retention

[a] From Ram CV, Hyman D. Hypertensive crises. J Intensive Care Med 1987;2(3):151–162.

of aortic dissection include trauma and hypertension. The classic symptom of aortic dissection is sudden, severe chest pain that is not associated with respiration and not relieved by changes in position. The pain may radiate to the back or the neck. A difference in blood pressure between the two arms or between upper and lower extremities is indicative of aortic dissection. Diminished femoral pulses and bruits over the chest's posterior interspaces may also occur. There may be a lag between the radial and femoral pulse. Other symptoms include pale, cool skin, sluggish capillary refill, apprehension, nausea, vomiting, confusion, lethargy, oliguria, and signs of congestive heart failure.

16. Ms. Goodman's ECG demonstrated left ventricular hypertrophy. Why does this occur in hypertension, and what are the ECG criteria?

Left ventricular hypertrophy (LVH) results from the left ventricle having to pump against a chronically increased afterload. Criteria for diagnosing LVH vary considerably in the literature. The most widely accepted system is the Estes' Scoring System, which follows. A score of ≥ 5 indicates LVH; 4 indicates probable LVH.

Estes' Scoring System for LVH

1.	R or S in limb lead:	20 mm or more	
	S in V_1, V_2, or V_3:	25 mm or more	3
	R in V_4, V_5, or V_6:	25 mm or more	
2.	Any ST shift (without digitalis)		3
	Typical "strain" ST-T (with digitalis)		1
3.	LAD: $-15°$ or more		2
4.	QRS interval: 0.09 sec or more		1
5.	I.D. in V_{5-6}: 0.04 sec or more		1
	Total		10

17. Captopril (Capoten) has also been used to lower blood pressure in urgent situations. Identify considerations when this drug is used.

Captopril is an oral angiotensin-converting enzyme inhibitor. In patients previously treated with diuretics and in patients with renal artery stenosis, the response to the drug is variable and severe hypotension can occur.

18. Identify the nursing diagnoses associated with the care of the patient in hypertensive crisis.

Potential for infection related to presence of invasive lines
Sleep pattern disturbance related to environmental stimuli

Knowledge deficit related to disease management procedures, practices, and/or self-care health care management
Anxiety related to unfamiliar environment
Potential or actual noncompliance with medical regime
Alteration in comfort related to pain, nausea, and vomiting

REFERENCES

Alspach JG, Williams SM. Core curriculum for critical care nursing. 3rd ed. Philadelpha: WB Saunders, 1985.

Baker KG, Doyle JE, Ekers MA, et al. Controlling hypertension. In: Hamilton HK, ed. Nurses clinical library: Cardiovascular disorders. Springhouse, PA: Springhouse Corp., 1984:56–73.

Bursztyn M, et al. Hypertensive crisis associated with nifedipine withdrawal. Arch Intern Med 1986;146:397.

Cunningham SG. Nonpharmacologic management of high blood pressure. Cardiovasc Nursing 1987;23(4):18–22.

Ferguson RK, Houston MC, Jackson JE, Liebson PR. Hypertensive emergency. Patient Care 1987;21(13):124–139.

Gonzalez DG, Ram VS. New approaches for the treatment of hypertensive urgencies and emergencies. Chest 1988;93(1):193–195.

Levy DB. The nifedipine effect. Emergency 1988;20(5):18–19.

Linton AL. Hypertensive crisis. In: Sibbald WJ, ed. Synopsis of critical care. Baltimore: Williams & Wilkins, 1988:28–30.

Trounson L. Hypertensive crisis. Post Anesthesia Nursing 1988;3(2):102–106.

CHAPTER 10

Hypovolemic Shock

Mary K. Roberts, RN, MSN, CCRN

Andrew Jones is a 34-year-old convenience store clerk who sustained a gunshot wound to the right chest during a robbery. When the paramedics arrived, his BP was barely palpable at 50 mm Hg, his heart rate was 130, and his respiratory rate was 35. His skin was pale, cold, and clammy with delayed capillary refill, his radial pulse was weak and thready, and he was unresponsive. His respirations were deep and rapid and supplemental oxygen was administered via 100% nonrebreathing mask. Two 14-gauge peripheral IV lines were inserted, and Ringer's lactate was infused at a wide open rate.

Upon arrival in the Emergency Department, Mr. Jones' BP was 90 mm Hg systolic, heart rate 120, and respiratory rate 26. He was restless and responded only to pain. His skin was pale and cool, and his capillary refill had a defined delay. His chest expansion was unequal and his breath sounds were grossly diminished on the right side.

A 36F chest tube was inserted in the right 8th intercostal space in the midaxillary line. Fifteen hundred ml of blood were immediately evacuated, with bleeding continuing up to 2500 ml in 30 min.

Mr. Jones' admission ABG and CBC results were as follows:

ABGs (100% nonrebreathing mask)		CBC	
pH	7.21	Hgb	8.2
$PaCO_2$	45	Hct	24.1
PaO_2	91	Plat	263
SaO_2	95%	RBC	2.17
HCO_3	15	WBC	5.8

A Foley catheter was inserted and 100 ml of clear, yellow urine was obtained. Fluid replacement continued, with 6 liters of Ringer's lactate and 4 units of type O-Rh-negative blood infused over the 30-min period prior to surgery.

In the Operating Room, a right thoracotomy with right pneumonectomy was performed, with repair of the right axillary artery. Mr. Jones received 14 liters of crystalloid, 20 units of packed red blood cells, 6 units of fresh frozen plasma, and 10 units of platelets. He was transferred to the Cardiovascular Thoracic ICU (CVTICU).

Upon admission, Mr. Jones is still anesthetized. He is hemodynamically stable with a heart rate of 96, BP 110/70 and CVP of 10. He is being mechanically ventilated at an assist control rate of 12 and is not assisting at this time. His skin is warm and dry, pulses are palpable, and capillary refill is normal. The nurse notes that his thoracotomy dressing is blood-soaked and diffuse oozing is apparent from all insertion sites. Significant clinical data are as follows:

Coagulation		CBC	
PT	18.7	Hgb	10.1
PTT	71.9	Hct	32
Fibrinogen	78	WBC	5.3
		Plat	108
		RBC	4.6

QUESTIONS AND ANSWERS

1. **Define hypovolemic shock.**

    Hypovolemia is defined as a diminished circulatory fluid volume. Shock is defined as a low flow state with poor tissue perfusion. The term hypovolemic shock implies a condition in which there is a decrease in intravascular volume resulting in inadequate tissue perfusion and insufficient cellular oxygenation.

2. **Was Mr. Jones in hypovolemic shock when the paramedics arrived? What clinical manifestations of hypovolemic shock did he exhibit?**

    Yes, Mr. Jones was in hypovolemic shock when the paramedics arrived. The clinical indicators included:

    > Tachycardia
    > Weak, thready pulse
    > Hypotension
    > Pale, cold, clammy skin
    > Defined delay in capillary refill
    > Deep, rapid respirations
    > Altered level of consciousness

    Clinical evaluation of hypovolemic shock focuses on assessment of tissue perfusion. Parameters to consider include neurological status, heart rate, blood pressure, pulse pressure, quality of respirations and respiratory rate, urine output, and capillary blanch test.

3. **Why was Ringer's lactate the fluid of choice for Mr. Jones' initial fluid resuscitation?**

    Ringer's lactate is a crystalloid solution (salt solution that contains electrolytes). In addition to providing intravascular volume replacement, crystalloids replenish extracellular stores of sodium, chloride, and water. Ringer's lactate most closely approximates the plasma electrolyte composition. It is a balanced electrolyte solution of sodium chloride, potassium chloride, calcium chloride, and sodium lactate in water. Normal saline may also be used to replace fluid volume. Normal saline contains greater amounts of sodium and chloride than Ringer's lactate but lacks calcium and potassium. In massive amounts, it can cause hypokalemia and hypernatremia. In addition, normal saline can lead to a hyperchloremic acidosis, thus worsening the acidotic state present in hypovolemic shock. This occurs because the high concentration of chloride in normal saline causes bicarbonate ions to be released in the kidney tubules, thus lowering the bicarbonate level in the extracellular fluid.

4. What other fluids might be considered in initial resuscitation of hypovolemic shock?

Data exist that support the use of colloids in resuscitation of the hypovolemic shock patient. Colloids include normal human serum albumin, plasma protein fraction, dextran, and hetastarch. Colloids increase the osmotic pressure gradient within the vascular compartment and augment intravascular volume by osmosis. The side effects associated with some colloids as well as the much greater expense involved in colloid resuscitation are contributing factors to the wider use of crystalloids. Crystalloids have the additional advantage of restoring the electrolyte balance.

5. What is the preferred route of vascular access for fluid resuscitation in hypovolemic shock?

Prompt restoration of intravascular volume with maintenance of adequate tissue perfusion is the primary treatment goal in hypovolemic shock. Short large-bore intravenous catheters are preferred. Such catheters will allow for rapid, massive infusion of fluid and blood, without the risks involved in central line placement. If percutaneous intravenous access is unobtainable, the second choice would be a cut-down of the saphenous vein. Placement of central lines is reserved for the period following initial resuscitation. A CVP line is most helpful in evaluating volume status.

6. A CVP line is inserted in Mr. Jones' right subclavian vein during surgery. What are the potential complications of CVP insertion?

Pneumothorax is the most common complication, so a follow-up chest x-ray must be obtained as soon as possible. If the catheter is out of normal position, infiltration of fluid into the pleural cavity may cause a hydrothorax. Bleeding from an injured vein or an adjacent artery may lead to hemothorax. Air embolism may occur during insertion, or it may occur if the IV administration set becomes disconnected from the catheter hub. Cardiac dysrhythmias may also be induced if the catheter tip is in the right ventricle.

Four hours after admission to the CVTICU, Mr. Jones' BP dropped to 72/50, his heart rate rose to 120, and his CVP was 3 mm Hg. He received 2 liters of Ringer's lactate over the next hour, at which time his BP was 86/60, heart rate 112, and CVP 5 mm Hg. His urine output for the last hour was 25 ml. A pulmonary artery catheter was inserted.

7. **Placement of a pulmonary artery catheter allows for accurate and detailed cardiopulmonary assessment. What hemodynamic alterations would be expected in hypovolemic shock?**

   CVP decreased due to decreased right heart filling pressure
   PAWP decreased due to decreased left ventricular filling pressure
   CO decreased due to decreased preload, increased afterload
   SVR increased due to intense peripheral vasoconstriction

   Mr. Jones' initial hemodynamic profile revealed the following:

CVP	2
PAP	20/10
PAWP	2
CO	4.0
CI	1.8
SVR	1420
BP	88/66

8. **What therapy would be appropriate at this point?**
   Mr. Jones' profile indicates volume depletion. Therefore, fluid therapy is the appropriate treatment. Replacement therapy may be with either a crystalloid or a colloid solution.
   Hemodynamic values that reflect adequate resuscitation are:

CVP	>5
MAP	>70
PAWP	>8
CI	>2.5

9. **During the initial resuscitative period, Mr. Jones received 4 units of packed red blood cells. Why?**
   Mr. Jones presented with a gunshot wound to the chest and progressive shock. In such cases, it is highly likely that blood replacement will be necessary in order to restore adequate oxygen-carrying capacity. Blood component therapy is considered after the patient's response to the initial resuscitative fluids has been evaluated. Although Mr. Jones' clinical presentation improved with initial

fluid therapy, he continued to be hypotensive. The massive continuing hemorrhage displayed by Mr. Jones also indicates a loss of at least 30% of total blood volume, which is a primary indication for blood component therapy.

Mr. Jones' hematocrit of 24.1 and hemoglobin of 8.2 are also low. However, because of hemoconcentration, reported values may be misleading after acute hemorrhage. As volume is replaced, the hematocrit drops as a result of hemodilution. Because of these fluctuations, the degree of blood loss may not be reflected in these values for 4–6 hr. Therefore, all clinical indicators of volume and oxygenation adequacy, not just hematocrit and hemoglobin, require evaluation. These include:

> Mean arterial pressure, >70
> Heart rate, 60–100 beats per minute
> Respiratory rate, 10–20 breaths per minute
> Mental status, alert, oriented, and following commands
> Skin, warm and dry
> Capillary blanch test, <2 sec
> Urine output, >0.5 ml/kg/hr

10. What is autotransfusion? Would it be useful in this case?

Autotransfusion is the collection and transfusion of a patient's own blood. Autotransfusion may be performed using blood collected from the pleural cavity or mediastinal area, or from the abdomen if no colon or small bowel injury exists. Because Mr. Jones' hypovolemic shock has been precipitated by a massive hemothorax, autotransfusion could be useful in replacing the patient's blood loss. Salvaged blood must be reinfused within 4 hr of collection.

Autologous blood provides the safest source of red blood cells by eliminating the risk of posttransfusion hepatitis and other infections or immunologic complications of homologous blood. The platelet count in salvaged blood is low, and those platelets present may be dysfunctional. Therefore, this blood is a reliable source only of red blood cells.

11. What factors in Mr. Jones' case indicate a coagulopathy?

An elevated prothrombin and partial thromboplastin time, decreased platelet count and fibrinogen level, and diffuse oozing of blood indicate a coagulopathy. This coagulopathy may be a complication of massive blood transfusion. This is attributed to resuscitation with fluid and blood deficient in both coagulation factors and platelets. To prevent further blood loss and consequently a volume deficit, this coagulopathy must be resolved. Hypothermia has also been implicated in contributing to coagulopathies.

Treatment includes administration of fresh frozen plasma and platelets. Cryoprecipitate may also be transfused if fresh frozen plasma does not correct the fibrinogen level.

12. **What are other complications of massive blood transfusions?**
The major complications include hypothermia, hypocalcemia, hypomagnesemia, shifts in potassium level, and acid-base alterations.
Hypothermia is caused by transfusion of refrigerated stored blood. The clinical effects of hypothermia include increased affinity of hemoglobin for oxygen, impaired tissue oxygenation, and defective clotting.
The citrate present in stored blood binds with the transfused patient's calcium and magnesium. This causes decreased ionized calcium levels and hypomagnesemia.
The majority of patients receiving blood transfusions do not need calcium supplements. The average adult who is not hypothermic and has adequate hepatic function is able to metabolize citrate at a quantity equal to the amount present in up to 20 units of whole blood every hour. Identifying those patients who need calcium supplementation during transfusion is difficult. Measuring the ionized calcium and monitoring the QT interval for prolongation are of some value and are recommended during the rapid infusion of citrated blood.
Potassium tends to leak out of the red blood cells in stored blood. Therefore, when multiple units of blood are transfused, hyperkalemia is theoretically possible. However, in the hypoperfused, acidotic patient, its occurrence with massive transfusion is rare, because the actual load of extracellular potassium in blood is low. Hypokalemia is a more common occurrence, due to metabolic alkalosis from the metabolism of citrate to bicarbonate. Because both hypokalemia and hyperkalemia are detrimental to myocardial function, plasma potassium levels should be carefully monitored in these patients.

13. **When Mr. Jones arrived in the Emergency Department, his pH was 7.21, $PaCO_2$ 45, PaO_2 91, and HCO_3 15. What was his acid-base status? What was the etiology of this acid-base imbalance?**
Mr. Jones was in a metabolic acidosis. Oxygen transport is decreased in hypovolemic shock because of the reduction in cardiac output. Tissue oxygen demands exceed supply. Anaerobic metabolism occurs, and lactic acid is produced. The buffer systems are depleted, and metabolic acidosis is the result.
The patient in hypovolemic shock might present with a low $PaCO_2$. This is the result of hyperventilation as a compensatory mechanism for the metabolic acidosis.

14. **List the major compensatory mechanisms in hypovolemic shock and briefly explain each:**

    Sympathetic Response

    The sympathetic response, including the baroreceptor reflex, is activated within 30 sec after hemorrhage. This response initiates vasoconstriction in the arterioles and veins and causes β-adrenergic stimulation to increase heart rate, contractility, and speed of conduction.

    Renin-Angiotensin-Aldosterone System

    Angiotensin formation causes potent vasoconstriction, which supports the falling blood pressure. Aldosterone causes increased conservation of water and salt by the kidneys, which augments intravascular fluid volume.

    Synthesis of Antidiuretic Hormona (ADH)

    ADH creates constriction of arteries and veins and promotes water retention by the kidneys.

    Body Fluid Shifts from Interstitial Spaces into the Intravascular Space

    This includes absorption of large quantities of fluid from the interstitial spaces and the intestinal tract to return the blood volume back to normal.

    Reverse Stress-Relaxation of the Circulatory System

    In an attempt to restore adequate circulation, the blood vessels decrease in size to constrict the blood volume that remains. These mechanisms all work to return cardiac output and arterial pressure to normal levels.

15. **Mr. Jones' hypovolemic shock resulted from hemorrhage. What are the common causes of hypovolemic shock?**

    Loss of blood volume
      Trauma
      Hemorrhage
      Hemothorax
      Hemoperitoneum
    Loss of plasma volume
      Burns
      Bowel obstruction
      Peritonitis
      Pancreatitis
      Ascites
    Water loss: dehydration
      Diuretic therapy
      Uncontrolled diabetes mellitus
      Diabetes insipidus
      Severe vomiting or diarrhea

16. What are the possible renal complications of hypovolemic shock?

The renal complication most frequently seen is acute tubular necrosis due to reduced renal perfusion during shock. The degree of renal damage is related to the severity and duration of shock. The serum creatinine level should be closely monitored as an estimate of the functional capacity of the kidney.

17. What nursing diagnoses apply in this case?

Altered peripheral tissue perfusion related to decreased circulating blood volume

Fluid volume deficit related to blood loss secondary to posttraumatic hemorrhage

Potential for fluid volume deficit related to blood loss secondary to posttransfusion coagulopathy

Anxiety related to the disruption in the individual's physiological and psychological integrity

Potential for infection secondary to presence of invasive catheters and lines

SUGGESTED READINGS

American College of Surgeons, Committee on Trauma. Advanced trauma life support course (student manual). Chicago: American College of Surgeons, 1985.

Casey MF. Hypovolemic shock. In: Sommers MS, ed. Difficult diagnoses in critical care nursing. Rockville, MD: Aspen Systems, 1989:1–25.

Guyton AC. Textbook of medical physiology. 2nd ed. Philadelphia: WB Saunders, 1986.

Kruskall MS, Mintz PD, Bergin JJ, Johnston MF, Klein HG, Miller JD, Rutman R, Silberstein L. Transfusion therapy in emergency medicine. Ann Emerg Med 1988;17(4):55–63.

McQuillan KA, Wiles CE. Initial management of traumatic shock. In: Cardona, VC, Hurn PD, Mason PJ, Scanlon-Schilpp AM, Veise-Berry SW, eds. Trauma nursing: From resuscitation through rehabilitation. Philadelphia: WB Saunders, 1988:160–173.

Meyers K, Hickey M. Hypovolemic shock. Crit Care Nurse Q 1988;11(1):57–67.

Roberts MK. Fluid resuscitation in the adult trauma patient. Orthopaedic Nursing 1989;8(6):41–47.

Rutledge R, Sheldon G, Collins M. Massive transfusion. Crit Care Clin 1986;2(4):791–804.

Traverso LW, Lee WP, Langford MJ. Fluid resuscitation after an otherwise fatal hemorrhage: I. Crystalloid solutions. J Trauma 1986;26(2):168–175.

CHAPTER 11

Inferior Myocardial Infarction with Right Ventricular Infarction

Kathleen H. Toto, RN, MSN, CCRN

Kenneth Jackson is a 37-year-old automobile mechanic. While working on a car, he experienced a 10-min episode of substernal chest pain accompanied by shortness of breath, which subsided with rest. While eating lunch an hour later, he again experienced the sudden onset of severe substernal chest pain which he described as "feeling like I was being kicked in the chest." The pain was accompanied by dyspnea, diaphoresis, and nausea. This time the pain was not relieved by rest, and 10 min later he sought help at a nearby fire station. At the fire station, it was suggested that he was merely hyperventilating and attempts were made to calm him. He experienced worsening dyspnea and diaphoresis and began having radiation of pain to his left scapula. He was brought to the hospital by ambulance at his request. In the ambulance, Mr. Jackson was placed on a cardiac monitor and was noted to be in the rhythm shown in Figure 11.1 with a stable blood pressure. He converted back to normal sinus rhythm (NSR) before reaching the hospital.

Mr. Jackson arrived in the Emergency Department at 12:30 PM, approximately 30 min after the onset of pain. He continued to complain of severe chest pain and shortness of breath.

Physical examination revealed the following vital signs:

BP	110/86
HR	68
Resp	22
Temp	98.8

He was alert and oriented but anxious. He had an S_1, S_2 without S_3, S_4 or murmur. He was in NSR without evidence of heart block. No jugular venous distention was noted. His breath sounds were clear to auscultation. Gastrointestinal and genitourinary examinations were normal. A 12-lead electrocardiogram was obtained (Fig. 11.2).

Mr. Jackson had never been hospitalized, but had received outpatient treatment in an alcoholic treatment center. While undergoing treatment, he was told that he had hypertension, but no medications were prescribed. Relevant family history included: father diabetic, hypertensive, died of MI at age 48; grandmother had several MIs, died of CVA at age 66; and male cousin on father's side died of an MI at age 35.

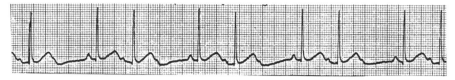

Figure 11.1. Wenckebach (second degree heart block, Type I).

Mr. Jackson admitted to smoking one package of cigarettes a day for the past 15 years. His cholesterol and triglyceride levels on admission were normal. He had no history of diabetes and his serum glucose level on admission was 132 mg/dl.

After review of the initial 12-lead electrocardiogram, a dextrocardiogram was obtained (Fig. 11.3).

Mr. Jackson was given oxygen via nasal cannula at 2 liters/min. Morphine sulfate, 2 mg, was given by IV push every 5 min for relief of chest pain. Hydrocortisone, 100 mg, was given by IV push, and the streptokinase protocol was initiated at 1:15 PM. Mr. Jackson received streptokinase 1.5 mg, in 50 ml of D_5W over 1 hr via infusion pump into a peripheral IV. He was also given a bolus of lidocaine, 100 mg, and a lidocaine drip was started at 2 mg/min via infusion pump.

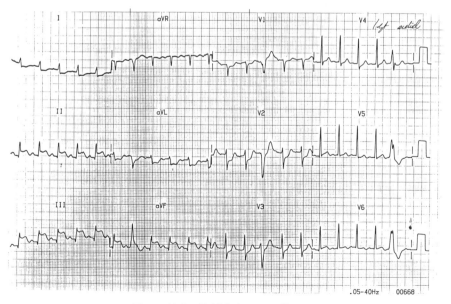

Figure 11.2. Initial electrocardiogram.

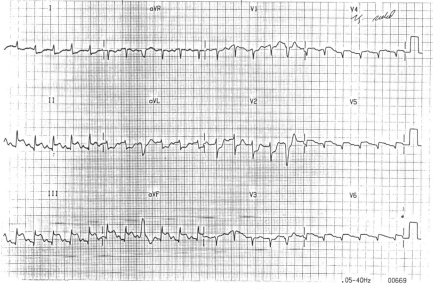

Figure 11.3. Dextrocardiogram.

At 1:30 PM, after 12 mg of morphine, Mr. Jackson denied chest pain and shortness of breath. Vital signs were:

BP   110/84
HR   72
Resp   20

Cardiac monitoring showed the rhythm depicted in Figure 11.4.

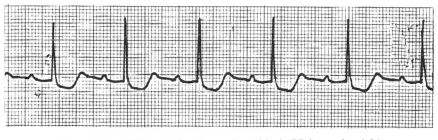

Figure 11.4. NSR with first degree heart block. PR interval = 0.26.

At approximately 2:00 PM, Mr. Jackson was given heparin, 5000 units, by IV push and started on a heparin drip at 1000 units/hr via infusion pump.

At 3:10 PM, he was still in the Emergency Department waiting for a bed in the CCU. Cardiac monitoring showed the rhythm depicted in Figure 11.5.

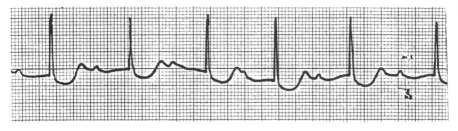

Figure 11.5. NSR with worsening first degree heart block. PR interval = 0.40.

Another 12-lead ECG was done and shortly thereafter the patient's heart rate dropped to 54 with a BP of 70/42. Atropine, 0.5 mg, was given by IV push for the rhythm shown in Figure 11.6.

Mr. Jackson continued to receive atropine up to a total dose of 2 mg with only transient increases in heart rate. He was then started on an isoproterenol (Isuprel) drip to keep his HR above 80. The drip was continued until external pacing could be initiated. At 4:30 PM, Mr. Jackson was transported to the CCU on a portable monitor showing an underlying rhythm of 2 : 1 heart block with a ventricular rate of 54.

Several hours later, Mr. Jackson converted to NSR and the external pacemaker was discontinued; however, he remained hypotensive and required intravenous normal saline (NS) infusions to raise his BP. At 6:00 PM, his BP was stable at 102/74 with continued NS infusions. He remained in NSR rate of 88/min with 2–3 PVCs/min.

Throughout the night Mr. Jackson continued to have intermittent ventricular dysrhythmias (PVCs, 4–5 beat runs of ventricular tachycardia). He was loaded with 1 gm of procainamide (Pronestyl) and started on an intravenous infusion at 1 mg/min. The lidocaine drip was discontinued. By the following morning, Mr. Jackson had received a total of 7500 ml of intravenous NS to maintain his blood pressure. His lungs remained clear to auscultation but marked jugular venous distention was noted. He also developed an S_3. His extremities were warm and well perfused. Serial 12-lead ECGs, cardiac enzymes, and coagulation studies were done.

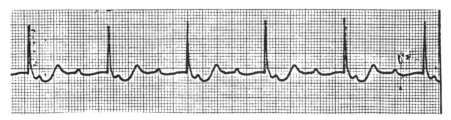

Figure 11.6. Fixed ratio 2 : 1 AV block (second degree).

By the next day, Mr. Jackson's condition had improved. He was in NSR with 1–2 PVCs/min on 1 mg/min Pronestyl infusion. His blood pressure was elevated at 130/100 and treatment with captopril was initiated at 12.5 mg PO TID.

He remained on the heparin infusion titrated to keep his PTT 2–2½ times normal. At 6:00 AM the morning after admission, his PTT was 60.7 sec. He had no evidence of bleeding and his hematocrit was stable at 46%.

Cardiac enzyme series revealed a creatine kinase peak to 2157 units/liter at 6:00 AM the morning after admission with CK-MB of 419 units/liter. The 12-lead ECG at this time showed small Q waves in leads II, III and AVF without ST elevation.

Mr. Jackson was discharged 13 days after admission on aspirin, 325 mg PO q am, and captopril, 25 mg PO TID.

QUESTIONS AND ANSWERS

1. **What are the components of the patient history in a patient with suspected myocardial infarction?**

   The patient history is by far the most important source of information contributing to the diagnosis of MI. Besides providing information relating to symptoms, a careful history will also allow the nurse to identify and evaluate the impact of the disease on the patient and family, likelihood of compliance with past and future therapeutic regimens, as well as the patient's emotional stability, fears, and threshold of discomfort. The general history should include past medical history, personal habits such as alcohol intake and cigarette smoking, family history, and the exact nature of the patient's work, as this will provide valuable information to facilitate discharge planning. A history for the risk factors of ischemic heart disease must also be pursued. These include family history, hypertension, cigarette smoking, diabetes mellitus, and long-term use of birth control pills.

   Next, the patient should be questioned regarding the symptoms of heart disease, including chest pain, dyspnea, syncope, palpitations, edema, cough, and fatigue. Many of the symptoms can be caused by conditions other than heart disease. A complete history is the most helpful method of determining the etiology of these symptoms.

   A history of the symptom of chest pain should include the location and character of chest pain, radiation, what precipitates and relieves the pain, duration, frequency, pattern of recurrence, and associated symptoms. Observing the patient's gestures during this part of the history may be helpful. If the patient clenches his or her fist over the chest while describing the pain (Levine's sign), this is a strong indication that it is ischemic in origin. Angina pectoris may be described as discomfort rather than pain. The patient may complain of pressure, burning, squeezing, or strangling. The discomfort can radiate to the neck, shoulders, extremities, jaw, or teeth.

The discomfort of myocardial ischemia usually cannot be localized or reproduced by external pressure. If a patient can point to a particular site of discomfort, it is not likely angina.

In some instances, the patient may not experience any discomfort in the chest. Myocardial ischemia may manifest as dyspnea, indigestion, gas, dizziness, diaphoresis, nausea, and pain in the arms, jaw, teeth, neck, or shoulders. This would be the patient's "anginal equivalent." The anginal equivalent is extremely important to document and communicate between shifts so that episodes of myocardial ischemia are not misinterpreted and appropriate treatment can be initiated. It is interesting to note that anginal equivalents above the mandible and below the umbilicus are very uncommon.

Chest discomfort associated with angina is generally short in duration, 2–10 min, whereas chest discomfort associated with myocardial infarction may last for several hours. Angina is often brought on by exertion but may also occur at rest. Rest and/or nitroglycerin commonly relieve anginal pain but will not relieve chest pain due to myocardial infarction.

Dyspnea is often associated with myocardial infarction but can also occur due to a variety of other pulmonary and cardiac disorders. Dyspnea is an abnormal symptom when it occurs at rest or at a low level of physical activity. Dyspnea often accompanies the chest pain of myocardial infarction but may occur exclusive of chest pain as the patient's anginal equivalent. Dyspnea occurring with acute MI or with myocardial ischemia is due to pulmonary congestion.

The nurse should also question the patient about other symptoms accompanying chest pain, in particular diaphoresis and palpitations. Symptoms of myocardial ischemia are often associated with autonomic symptoms such as diaphoresis and nausea or vomiting. Chest pain associated with palpitations may be due to acute MI with tachyarrhythmias.

2. Identify the risk factors Mr. Jackson has for myocardial infarction.

> Hypertension
> Cigarette smoking
> Strong family history

3. Discuss the ECG recognition of acute myocardial infarction and right ventricular infarction (RVI).

The standard 12-lead ECG is used to aid in the diagnosis of left ventricular (LV) injury, infarct, and ischemia. Specific areas of the left ventricle can be evaluated by looking at representative leads as follows:

Inferior wall—II, III, AVF
Lateral wall—I, AVL, V_5, V_6
Anterior wall—V_1, V_2, V_3, V_4
Posterior wall—V_1, V_2, V_3 (reciprocal changes)

In acute transmural myocardial infarction, ST segment elevation will occur within 1 min of the onset of injury. ST segment elevation will occur in the leads representing the injured area of the myocardium. If no further injury or extension of the MI occurs, the ST segment elevation will begin to resolve over a period of hours to days.

Q waves are the next ECG change that will be seen in transmural infarction. A pathologic Q wave is the component of the QRS complex that has an initial negative deflection from the isoelectric line, is at least 0.04 sec wide, and usually >4 mm in depth. See Figure 11.7.

Small, nonpathologic Q waves are normally present in leads I, III, AVL, V_5, and V_6. Pathologic Q waves represent infarction and develop over a period of hours to days after the onset of myocardial infarction. As the ECG evolves, the Q waves get deeper and the R waves disappear. Hence the term, "loss of R wave" is used in interpreting the evolutionary ECG changes in acute MI. Q waves may take years to disappear and often never do resolve. It is important to remember that the electrocardiographic diagnosis of MI in a patient with a left bundle branch block (LBBB) will be extremely difficult. A LBBB will produce Q waves in several leads that are unrelated to infarction.

ST depression and T wave inversion are ECG changes that accompany ischemia. Transient ST depression is the ECG change that occurs with ischemia associated with angina. T wave inversion is the electrocardiographic manifestation of ischemia, which may be seen with angina or as an evolutionary change associated with acute myo-

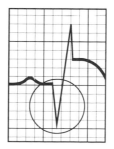

Figure 11.7. Q wave.

cardial infarction. With acute MI, T wave inversion usually develops 6–24 hr after the initial injury and takes months to years to resolve. Transient T wave inversion can also be seen in classical angina and unstable angina with the occurrence of chest pain. It is important to remember that the 12-lead ECG has limited sensitivity and specificity for diagnosis of MI. Many of the ECG changes discussed above can occur in settings other than myocardial infarction, such as pericarditis and hyperkalemia (ST elevation), and digitalis administration (ST depression).

In Mr. Jackson's case, the initial 12-lead ECG demonstrated ST elevation and small Q waves in leads II, III, and AVF indicative of acute inferior myocardial infarction. Eventually, Mr. Jackson's ECG evolved, as evidenced by the progressive change of the small Q waves to pathologic Q waves in the inferior leads. The ST depression present in leads V_1 through V_3, I, and AVL is representative of either reciprocal changes of an acute inferior infarction or anterior and lateral ischemia. Reciprocal changes (ST depression) occur in leads that are opposite the infarcted area (see below):

Transmural Infarction	Reciprocal Changes
Inferior	I, AVL, V_1, V_2, V_3
Anterior	II, III, AVF
Lateral	V_1, V_2, V_3

The reciprocal changes will resolve as the ST elevation in the infarcted area subsides.

RVI cannot be diagnosed from the standard 12-lead ECG. However, a dextrocardiogram, using right precordial leads, can be extremely useful. The positioning of the right precordial leads is a mirror image of the positioning of the left precordial leads in a standard 12-lead ECG as follows:

Lead	Placement
V_1R	4th intercostal space, left sternal border
V_2R	4th intercostal space, right sternal border
V_4R	5th intercostal space, midclavicular line
V_3R	Between V_2R and V_4R
V_6R	Right midaxillary line, horizontal to V_4R
V_5R	Between V_4R and V_6R

Mr. Jackson's dextrocardiogram was consistent with RVI as evidenced by ST segment elevation in V_4R, V_5R, and V_6R. See dextrocardiogram (Fig. 11.3).

A dextrocardiogram should be obtained in all patients with acute inferior infarction, as 37–52% of all acute inferior MIs are also associated with acute RVI. Occlusion of the right coronary artery (RCA) is usually associated with inferior MI. In addition to supplying the inferior surface of the left ventricle, the RCA also supplies the right ventricle in most people. Additionally, the RCA supplies blood flow to the sinoatrial (SA) node in 60% of the population and the atrioventricular (AV) node in 90% of the population. Therefore, considering coronary blood flow, inferior MIs are commonly associated with right ventricular infarctions and dysrhythmias arising from ischemia to the SA and AV nodes (bradyarrhythmias and heart blocks).

4. Differentiate the forms of atrioventricular heart block and discuss their pathogenesis.

The conduction of an impulse can be slowed or completely blocked at various sites along the conduction pathway. AV block is an abnormality of conduction between the atria and ventricles and can occur in either the AV node or the specialized conduction system below the AV node (infranodal). There are three degrees of AV block. In first degree AV block, there is a conduction delay at the AV node. The ECG manifestation of a first degree AV block is a PR interval >0.20 sec (normal is 0.12–0.20 sec). Causes of a first degree AV block include vagal stimulation, pharmacologic agents (digitalis, β-adrenergic blocking agents, some calcium channel blockers), and several cardiac disorders including acute myocardial infarction. A first degree heart block occurring in a patient receiving the pharmacologic agents listed above would not necessarily mandate an alteration in dosage or discontinuation of the drug. First degree heart block occurring with acute MI is usually seen with inferior MIs and requires no specific therapy. However, the patient should be monitored for the development of more serious forms of heart block.

Second degree heart block is divided into two subclassifications: Mobitz I or Wenckebach, and Mobitz II. Mobitz I is characterized by progressive lengthening of the PR interval until a P wave is not followed by a QRS. The PR interval following the nonconducted P wave will return to the initial baseline PR interval. In most patients, Mobitz I is located at the AV node, but it can occur in the bundle branches. Usually the QRS is narrow (0.04–0.10 sec), as there is no intraventricular conduction delay. Mobitz I can be caused by digitalis excess, intense vagal stimulation, and cardiac disorders such as acute MI. When occurring due to MI, Mobitz I is most frequently seen in acute inferior infarctions. If the patient's BP is adequate and he or she is otherwise asymptomatic (no shortness of breath, syncope, PVCs, or chest pain), Mobitz I usually does not require treatment. If symptomatic, the patient may be treated with atropine, Isuprel, or a temporary pacemaker. In the setting of acute inferior MI, Mobitz I usually resolves within 5–6 days and does not require permanent pacing.

Unlike Mobitz I, Mobitz II is due to a block in intraventricular conduction and therefore is associated with QRS prolongation. In Mobitz II, the PR interval is constant and QRS complexes are dropped intermittently. See the example shown in Figure 11.8.

Mobitz II rarely occurs due to digitalis excess. Mobitz II may be seen with acute MI, but is usually seen with anterior MI rather than inferior. Predictably, Mr. Jackson did not develop Mobitz II heart block. Mobitz II is much more likely to progress to third degree heart block. Treatment requires prompt insertion of a temporary pacemaker, and subsequent implantation of a permanent pacemaker is frequently required.

Fixed ratio 2 : 1 AV block is another form of second degree heart block. It is characterized by a fixed PR interval and two P waves to each QRS. Every other QRS is dropped, and the atrial rate is two times the ventricular rate. If the block is in the AV node, the QRS will be narrow. This is treated similar to Mobitz I. If the block is infranodal, the QRS will be wide and this will be treated like Mobitz II.

In third degree, or complete AV block, the atria and ventricles are controlled by independent pacemakers, which are not in synchrony with each other. The block can be in the AV node, the bundle of His, or the bundle branches. If the block is high (AV node) the ventricular rate will usually be 40–60/min and the QRS narrow. This is seen more typically when it occurs with acute inferior MI.

If the block is below the AV node, the ventricular rate is more likely to be 15–40 and the QRS wide (>0.10 sec). This is typically seen with acute anterior MI. In third degree heart block, the atrial rate is faster than the ventricular rate. Third degree AV block can also be caused by digitalis intoxication, hyperkalemia, cardiac disorders, or as a complication of surgical procedures such as mitral valve replacement. When third degree heart block develops as a complication of inferior MI, it is usually temporary. If the patient is symptomatic, treatment might include atropine, Isuprel, and temporary pacing. However, when third degree heart block occurs as a complication of anterior MI, it is usually permanent, necessitating implantation of a permanent pacemaker.

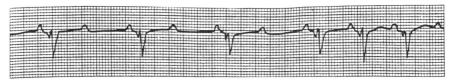

Figure 11.8. Mobitz II.

Mr. Jackson developed all of the heart blocks discussed above except Mobitz II and third degree. At 12:20 PM, (in the ambulance), he was noted to be in a Wenckebach (Mobitz I) rhythm (see Fig. 11.1) with a stable blood pressure. Note the lengthening of the PR interval from 0.16 to 0.20 sec and then a P wave that is not followed by a QRS. Mr. Jackson was in this form of second degree heart block for only a short time before converting back to NSR. He then developed a first degree heart block in the Emergency Department at 1:30 PM (see Fig. 11.4.) This ECG tracing shows normal sinus rhythm at a rate of 72/min with a PR interval of 0.26 sec, a first degree AV block. Several hours later, at 3:10 PM, Mr. Jackson's PR interval lengthened to 0.40 sec, as his first degree AV block worsened (see Fig. 11.5). About one-half hour later, he progressed to second degree heart block, 2:1, with a ventricular rate of 54/min, an atrial rate of 108/min, and a blood pressure of 70/42 (see Fig. 11.6). The QRS complex was narrow, signifying the impulse pacing the ventricles was originating from a location above the bundle branches, most likely the AV node or bundle of His. Because he was hypotensive, Mr. Jackson required treatment of his second degree heart block consisting of atropine 0.5-mg doses by IV push every 5 min up to a total dose of 2 mg. He did not respond well to the atropine and an Isuprel drip was then initiated. Because Isuprel is a β-adrenergic stimulator, it increases heart rate and myocardial contractility. This results in increased myocardial oxygen consumption and can potentially extend an acute myocardial infarction. Therefore, this drug must be given with extreme caution to the acute MI patient and temporary pacing should be initiated as soon as possible.

5. **Describe the clinical presentation of a patient with a RVI.**

Clinical features of RVI include hypotension, jugular venous distention, and clear lungs. These clinical findings may also be present with other forms of right ventricular dysfunction, such as pulmonary hypertension. Many patients with RVI do not have any of the clinical signs listed above. In fact, the clinical syndrome associated with RVI is thought to occur in only 3–8% of all cases of acute MI. Clinical recognition of RVI is often seen only in patients with extensive RV involvement. Because of the low incidence of symptomatology with RVI, many times it goes unrecognized and misdiagnosed.

Jugular venous distention (JVD) is a sign of elevated central venous pressure as the jugular veins communicate almost directly with the right atrium. RVI can cause an elevation in right ventricular end-diastolic pressure, which in turn increases right atrial pressure and results in JVD. Upon auscultation of the lungs in a patient with acute inferior myocardial infarction (IMI) and RVI, breath sounds are often clear. This is unlike other hypotensive acute MI patients in which pulmonary edema may be present due to left ventricular pump failure. In acute IMI with RVI, the patient is hypotensive because of RV failure rather than LV failure. In RVI the RV acts as a passive conduit between the right atrium and the pulmonary circulation and ultimately the left heart. Right ventricular contractility is impaired and this results in inadequate left ventricular preload. The following illustrates the hemodynamic profile of a patient with RVI:

> Elevated RA pressure
> Normal or low PAWP pressure
> RA pressure equal to or greater than PAWP
> Hypotension

Mr. Jackson did not have a pulmonary artery catheter in place so clinical findings were relied upon to interpret both right and left ventricular function. Right ventricular dysfunction was signified by JVD and hypotension. Indicators of left ventricular dysfunction (rales, S_3) were notably absent.

The treatment of a patient with RVI who is hypotensive or hypoperfusing includes intravenous fluid administration to raise LV filling pressures and restore forward cardiac output. Intravenous NS is usually given. Rapid infusion of NS will increase RV output and subsequently LV preload and cardiac output. During this treatment, it is important to assess the patient's breath sounds, as rales would signify LV failure. This is most likely to occur in patients who have sustained significant LV myocardial damage. Once volume loading has been accomplished, if the cardiac output remains low, positive inotropes such as dobutamine may be useful. Besides its positive inotropic effect, dobutamine decreases pulmonary vascular resistance (PVR). Lowering PVR will reduce impedence to RV ejection and result in improved RV cardiac output as well.

Mr. Jackson required only volume loading to stabilize his blood pressure. He received a total of 7500 ml of NS and did not require pharmacologic support for his cardiac output. His blood pressure stabilized after volume loading and his lungs remained clear, suggesting hemodynamic stability.

In treating the patient with acute IMI and RVI, it is important to remember that these patients are very sensitive to preload reduction, as this would further reduce LV filling. Diuretics should not be given unless LV failure is present. Furthermore, venodilators such as nitroglycerin should be administered very cautiously, as they may cause a profound fall in cardiac output and blood pressure in these patients.

6. Discuss the indications, methods, and side effects of intravenous streptokinase administration.

Streptokinase is a thrombolytic agent given to reestablish coronary artery blood flow in the patient with acute myocardial infarction in an attempt to preserve functional myocardium. When given intravenously, streptokinase is administered as a 1.5 million unit dose, diluted in D_5W or NS, and given over 30–60 min. To be effective, streptokinase must be administered within 6 hr of the onset of chest pain. The greatest benefit is thought to occur in patients who receive streptokinase within the first 3–4 hr after the onset of chest pain. Once the streptokinase infusion is complete, the patient is bolused with 5000 units of IV heparin and then started on an infusion of 1000 units/hr. This infusion rate is adjusted after 4 hr to maintain the activated partial thromboplastin time (PTT) 2–2½ times normal. The patient must be watched closely for bleeding from puncture sites and the gastrointestinal tract, including guaiac testing of all stools.

Side effects of streptokinase administration include bleeding, allergic reactions (5% of patients), and hypotension. The most common allergic reaction is fever and rash; anaphylaxis is rare. Allergic reactions can be avoided by administering steroids and antihistamines prior to treatment. Aside from bleeding, another major side effect of streptokinase is sudden hypotension occurring during administration of the drug. This occurs in approximately 15% of patients and may necessitate vasopressors for support. The incidence of hypotension can be reduced by slow, controlled infusion of the drug and decreased dosage in patients with lower body weights.

For a more detailed discussion of streptokinase and other thrombolytic agents, see Chapter 15, "Thrombolytic Therapy for Acute Myocardial Infarction."

Mr. Jackson arrived in the Emergency Department 30 min after the onset of chest pain and received streptokinase 45 min later. Prior to receiving streptokinase, he was given hydrocortisone, 100 mg IV to prevent an allergic reaction. The streptokinase was infused slowly and did not cause hypotension in Mr. Jackson's case. A heparin bolus and infusion was then initiated and a PTT checked every 4 hr. His PTT was maintained between 90 and 110 sec during the infusion. In Mr. Jackson's case, it was not clear that reperfusion occurred. He did exhibit some signs of reperfusion such as ventricular ectopy. However, at 4 hr after streptokinase administration, his ST segments remained elevated and pathologic Q waves did develop. A radionuclide ventriculogram (MUGA) scan 8 days after admission revealed a right ventricular ejection fraction of 50% (lower limit of normal) with free wall hypokinesis and a left ventricular ejection fraction of 60% with a defect in segmental wall motion consistent with a small inferoseptal MI. Although it did not appear that streptokinase prevented Mr. Jackson from having a myocardial infarction, it may have helped to limit the extent of the infarction.

7. **What are the nursing implications of caring for a patient receiving transcutaneous pacing (external pacemaker)?**

Transcutaneous pacing is a noninvasive form of cardiac pacing. The heart is paced using two large electrodes placed in the anterior position (over ECG V_3 position) and in the posterior position (in the left subscapular region). The electrodes are then attached to an external pulse generator by pacing cables. The pulse generator has a dial to set the milliamperes (mA), which ranges from 50 to 210 mA. The pacing rate is set on another dial. Rates of up to 300/min may be selected. Temporary transcutaneous pacing may be initiated to treat the following:

> Symptomatic bradydysrhythmias
> Mobitz II
> Back-up for permanent pacemaker malfunction
> Overdrive for tachydysrhythmias

Nursing management of the patient receiving transcutaneous pacing is directed at reducing the patient discomfort associated with electrical stimulation of the chest wall. Each time the pacemaker fires, it is equivalent to moderately pounding on the chest with a closed fist.

Administration of diazepam (Valium) will usually make the patient more comfortable. If pain continues, it could be due to improper electrode placement and usually can be relieved by moving the electrode further away from the large pectoralis muscle. If failure to capture occurs, this may be resolved by moving the electrode to the ECG V_6 position. Should the patient require defibrillation, the pacing cables should be disconnected from the generator during defibrillation to prevent electrical damage to the pulse generator.

In order to minimize pacemaker malfunction, it is important that the electrodes maintain good contact with the skin. Cleansing and abrading the skin prior to electrode placement will facilitate good contact. Prior to application, check the electrode for sufficient gel. When external pacing is discontinued, check the patient for skin burns. It is also very important to teach both the patient and the family about external pacing, it's purpose, discomfort involved, and side effects (skin burns) prior to the initiation of pacing.

8. What are the pertinent nursing diagnoses in this patient with acute inferior MI and right ventricular infarction?

Alteration in comfort related to chest pain (myocardial ischemia)

Decreased cardiac output related to impaired right ventricular performance

Decreased cardiac output related to dysrhythmias

Potential for fluid volume excess related to therapeutic volume expansion

Potential for discomfort and skin burns related to transcutaneous pacing

SUGGESTED READINGS

Braunwald E, ed. Heart disease. A textbook of cardiovascular medicine. 3rd ed. Philadelphia: WB Saunders, 1988.

Hillis LD, Firth BG, Winniford MD, Willerson JT. Manual of clinical problems in cardiology. 3rd ed. Boston: Little, Brown & Co, 1988.

Kapoor AS. How to recognize right ventricular infarction. J Crit Care Illness 1987; 2(2):15–19.

Kapoor AS. Stepwise approach to managing right ventricular infarction. J Crit Care Illness 1987;2(5):27–34.

Kleven MR. Comparison of thrombolytic agents: Mechanism of action, efficacy, and safety. Heart Lung 1988;17(6), (part 2):750–755.

Persons CB. Transcutaneous pacing: Meeting the challenge. Focus Crit Care 1987; 14(1):13–19.

Robinson JS. Acute right ventricular infarction: Recognition, evaluation, and treatment. Crit Care Nurse 1987;7(4):42–53.

White HD, Rivers JT, Maslowski AH, et. al. Effect of intravenous streptokinase as compared with that of tissue plasminogen activator on left ventricular function after first myocardial infarction. N Engl J Med 1989;320(13):817–821.

CHAPTER 12

Mitral Valve Replacement

Marsha Halfman-Franey, RN, MSN

Edith Fry is a 50-year-old woman who presents with complaints of fatigue and SOB when climbing stairs or walking briskly. She had documented rheumatic heart disease, stemming from a bout of rheumatic fever at age 12. She began experiencing progressive SOB in high school, which led to a cardiac catheterization and mitral commissurotomy 10 years ago. Penicillin prophylaxis was initiated in adolescence, and she has continued it to the present. She is now admitted for further evaluation and possible mitral valve replacement.

ECG. Normal sinus rhythm with 1st degree AV block (PR 0.23 sec).

Chest X-ray. Cardiomegaly with prominent left atrium, left atrial appendage, and right ventricle, with minimal cephalization of flow.

Myocardial Scan. Normal resting left ventricular ejection fraction (LVEF) of 68%, with exercise LVEF of 71%; normal wall motion.

Echocardiogram. Decreased E to F slope; mild left atrial enlargement; calcified and thickened mitral valve leaflets with doming of anterior leaflet and parallel motion of posterior leaflet; calculated mitral valve area of 0.9 cm². This is "critical" stenosis and surgery is definitely indicated in this case.

Cardiac Catheterization. Normal coronary arteries; modest decrease in rate of left ventricular filling; mitral valve is thickened in appearance.

Pulmonary Artery Wedge Pressure		**Right Ventricular Pressure**	
v wave	29	Systolic	44
a wave	27	Diastolic	8
Mean	20		

Pulmonary Artery Pressure		**Right Atrial Pressure**	
	44	Mean	7
Diastolic	25		
Mean	30		

Oxygen Saturation Data		Left ventricle	94%
Pulmonary artery wedge	96%		
Pulmonary artery	74%	Superior vena cava	72%

Mean cardiac
output   4.2 liters
             /min
Cardiac index   2.36
Gradient   12 mm Hg
   at rest for mitral valve
Mitral valve
   area   1.1 cm^2
Pulmonary vascular
   resistance   190

Ms. Fry underwent a mitral valve replacement with a St. Jude prosthesis. When median sternotomy was performed, the right ventricle was inadvertently entered and she was immediately placed on cardiopulmonary bypass via the usual cannulation sites. Her operative course was plagued with constant oozing and she subsequently left the operating room with a Hgb of 4 gm/dl.

In anticipation of a rocky postoperative course, a pulmonary artery oximetry catheter was inserted. She had an arterial line in place and was on a Servo ventilator with acceptable blood gases on an FIO$_2$ of 0.40. She had a brief run of a paroxysmal supraventricular tachycardia, which converted spontaneously. Generally, though, her postoperative course was remarkably uneventful and she was discharged 10 days postoperatively.

QUESTIONS AND ANSWERS

1. **What is the role of rheumatic fever in acquired valvular heart disease?**
   Rheumatic fever remains the primary cause of acquired valvular heart disease, especially involving the mitral valve. Rheumatic fever is quite rare in developed countries due to antibiotics, and most people think we no longer have rheumatic fever in the United States. However, a new type of rheumatic fever seems to be occurring. Outbreaks have recently been observed almost simultaneously in Utah, Ohio, Pennsylvania, and Hawaii. These outbreaks were not associated with higher rates of group A β-hemolytic streptococcal pharyngitis as was the case previously. Additionally, a much higher incidence of carditis was found among suburban or rural white children, reversing the traditional pattern in which black children were the chief victims.

   Rheumatic fever causes long-term pathologic changes that include:

   Fusion of commissures
   Fibrosis and thickening of valve leaflets
   Shortening, fibrosis, and fusion of the chordae tendinae and/or papillary muscles
   Calcification of the valve leaflets

It takes approximately 10–20 years for these changes to develop, and the patient is usually female. The mitral valve is most frequently affected, although combined mitral/aortic valve disease is common. The predilection for left-sided heart valves seems to be related to the increased pressure and turbulence associated with the left side of the heart.

The incidence of valvular problems is related to hemodynamic stress. The mitral valve is more frequently involved than the aortic valve. This is because the closed mitral valve is subjected to higher hemodynamic stress than the closed aortic valve. The explanation for this is that the closed mitral valve is subjected to systemic arterial systolic pressure because the aortic valve is open during systole. The closed aortic valve is subjected only to systemic diastolic pressure because it is open during systole.

2. **What other conditions may lead to surgical replacement of the mitral valve?**

Mitral valve prolapse, the most commonly diagnosed valvular disorder in the United States, is the most frequent cause of pure mitral regurgitation requiring mitral valve replacement. In this condition, one leaflet (usually the posterior) protrudes into the left atrium during systole. This occurs secondary to an increase in the spongiosa layer of the valve leaflet, and stretching of the chordae tendinae.

Mitral annular calcification, a degenerative process commonly seen in elderly patients, is probably the result of the stress of the mitral apparatus opening and closing 2.5–3 billion times during a lifetime. This lesion produces a clinical picture that may be very similar to that of rheumatic heart disease and may necessitate mitral valve replacement.

In the medical setting, rupture or dysfunction of the papillary muscles or chordae tendinae may occur secondary to myocardial infarction. In its most benign manifestation, "functional" regurgitation may result due to left ventricular dilatation distorting the geometry of the valve apparatus relative to the chamber size. When profound mitral regurgitation occurs on an acute basis, there is not time for compensatory mechanisms to be activated and the patient goes into acute failure with increased v waves in the left atrial pressure or pulmonary artery wedge tracing (Fig. 12.1). Immediate afterload reduction and mitral valve replacement are indicated.

Less frequent etiologies include:

Tumor
Left atrial myxoma
Bacterial vegetations

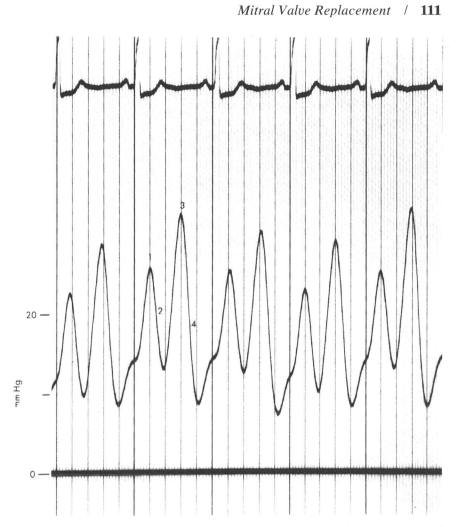

Figure 12.1. PAW trace with elevated v waves due to mitral regurgitation. *1*, a wave of 26 mm Hg; *2*, *x* descent *3*, v wave of 32 mm Hg; *4*, *y* descent. (Reproduced with permission from Daily EK, Schroeder JS. Hemodynamic waveforms. St. Louis, 1983, the C.V. Mosby Co., p. 79.)

Dysfunction of mitral valve prostheses
Trauma

3. How does mitral valve disease affect waveform components and validity of data obtained from hemodynamic monitoring?

The essential relationship in pulmonary artery pressure monitoring is:

$$
\text{PAD} = \begin{matrix} (\text{LAP}) \\ \text{PAWP} \end{matrix} = \text{LVEDP}
$$

This relationship is valid because there are no valves in the pulmonary vasculature and the mitral valve is open during diastole, allowing the catheter positioned in the pulmonary artery (PA) to accurately reflect left ventricular filling pressure. However, disease in the mitral valve disrupts that relationship so PAWP/LAP ≠ LVEDP. Therefore, assessment of LVEDP using the pulmonary artery catheter is invalid in cases of mitral valve disease.

In mitral stenosis, the left atrium needs to contract with greater force to push blood through the stenotic valve orifice. The a wave reflects atrial systole and therefore is usually increased in the presence of mitral stenosis (Fig. 12.2).

The mean wedge pressure usually is around 20–30 mm Hg in mitral stenosis; however, LVEDP is usually low because blood flow into the left ventricle is restricted.

Mitral regurgitation, on the other hand, is manifested by an elevated v wave. The v wave represents the atrial events that occur during ventricular systole. Blood refluxes across the incompetent valve and causes the v wave to be much higher than the a wave. In this instance, the value of the a wave is a better indicator of LVEDP than mean PAW.

4. **Describe the hemodynamic consequences of mitral stenosis, including presenting symptoms. How is this valvular defect different from the others?**

   Before hemodynamic consequences develop from mitral stenosis, the cross-section of the mitral valve must be reduced from 4–6 to 2.5 cm^2 or less. Because of the stenotic opening between the left atrium and left ventricle, the left atrial pressure must increase to maintain normal left ventricular filling. The left atrium hypertrophies and dilates, often leading to atrial fibrillation (with possible systemic emboli), hoarseness (due to compression of the left recurrent laryngeal nerve), and dysphagia. The increased left atrial pressure leads to elevated pulmonary pressures, resulting in dyspnea, which is worsened by exercise. Severe, long-standing mitral stenosis may present as pulmonary edema, hemoptysis, and possibly right heart failure.

   Mitral stenosis is the only valvular defect that spares the left ventricle. Because less blood passes through the tight mitral valve, the left ventricular cavity and aorta are often small. Cardiac output and blood pressure may be reduced, leading to increased fatigability.

Hemodynamic Consequences of Mitral Stenosis

Forward	Backward
Decreased LVEDP	Increased LAP
Decreased CO	Increased a wave
Decreased BP	Increased pulmonary pressures

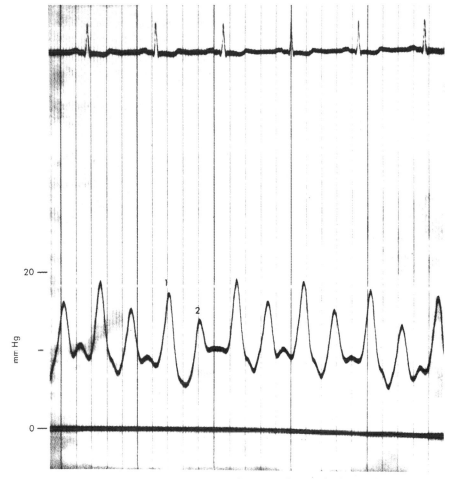

Figure 12.2. PAW trace with exaggerated a and v waves due to mitral stenosis. Note that a wave (*1*, 18 mm Hg) is higher than v wave. (Reproduced with permission from Daily EK, Schroeder JS. Hemodynamic waveforms. St. Louis, 1983, The C.V. Mosby Co., p. 78.)

5. Considering the pathophysiology of mitral stenosis, what heart sounds might you expect?

The classic auscultatory findings in mitral stenosis include:

Loud apical first sound due to closure of the stenotic mitral valve

Opening snap caused by the snapping of the stenotic valve into the ventricle during early diastole in response to rapidly changing pressure gradients

Rumbling apical diastolic murmur (intensity of murmur changes with flow and may actually disappear in end-stage disease)

Increased pulmonic second sound if pulmonary hypertension is present

An S_3 or S_4 gallop is rare because the left ventricle is protected from failure. An S_3 is caused by blood turbulence in the rapid ventricular filling period of early diastole. (This finding may be normal in young athletes but is abnormal in the adult patient population.) Stenosis inhibits rapid ventricular filling, and slow ventricular filling occurs all through diastole—hence, no S_3 on the left side. A left ventricular S_4 is never heard.

If the patient has progressed to right ventricular failure, right-sided S_3 and S_4 might be heard. S_4 is common because atrial contraction results in increased turbulence in an already full right ventricle. S_3 may be present due to increased turbulence during rapid filling of an already full right ventricle.

6. **What are the physiologic differences in the patient receiving a mitral valve replacement for mitral stenosis as opposed to mitral regurgitation?**

In mitral regurgitation, the output of the left ventricle is divided into systemic (forward) and regurgitant (backward) flow. The amount of flow in each direction depends on the severity of the insufficiency and the resistance to outflow through the aortic valve, which is primarily determined by the systemic vascular resistance. Regurgitant flow increases as the degree of insufficiency increases and/or as systemic vascular resistance increases. Once the incompetent valve is replaced, the only outlet from the left ventricle is forward into the systemic circulation. The left ventricle must now eject blood against full systemic vascular resistance. If the left ventricle is already compromised, valvular replacement and elimination of regurgitation can result in left ventricular failure. Whereas the ejection fraction preoperatively is often in the 70–85% range, this reflects the hyperdynamic state of the ventricle and the two outlets with differing resistances and is not useful in predicting left ventricular function postoperatively.

Mitral stenosis, on the other hand, spares the left ventricle. However, its effects on the pulmonary circulation may well determine surgical success. Long-standing mitral stenosis may result in actual changes in the pulmonary arteries, resulting in pulmonary hypertension and right heart failure. In most cases, pulmonary hypertension is usually reversible following surgical correction of the stenosis.

As in all cases of valvular heart disease, the New York Heart Association classification is the best predictor of success. Operation should be recommended before cardiac decompensation occurs.

7. **Did Ms. Fry have pulmonary hypertension?**

According to the cardiac catheterization report, Ms. Fry's pulmonary artery pressures were 44/25 mm Hg, with normal PAP being 20–30/8–15 mm Hg. The pulmonary circuit is a very compliant one, however, and in this case, pulmonary vascular resistance was not elevated. Ms. Fry's PVR = 190 dyn/sec/cm^{-5}; normal is 200–250 dyn/sec/cm^{-5}. It was expected that her pulmonary artery pressures would decrease postoperatively, and that is exactly what happened.

Initially, increased blood volume in the pulmonary circuit is well tolerated because the pulmonary circuit is very compliant. (Blood flow to the lungs may increase 3–4-fold before PAP rises appreciably.) If the pulmonary vessels are subjected to sustained, increased pressures, they begin to hypertrophy and pulmonary vascular resistance may rise rapidly. Once vessel morphology changes, pulmonary hypertension may not be reversible. Often, the ratio of SVR to PVR is calculated. Normally,

$$\frac{250 \text{ PVR}}{1000 \text{ SVR}} = 0.25$$

As the pulmonary vascular resistance increases, the ratio changes

$$\frac{500 \text{ PVR}}{1000 \text{ SVR}} = 0.50$$

and surgery may not be beneficial to the patient because of irreversible pulmonary changes.

If Ms. Fry had had significant pulmonary hypertension, it would have been essential to closely monitor her right heart function (CVP, pulmonary artery systolic). The right ventricle is very sensitive to afterload and will fail in the face of increased pulmonary vascular resistance. Her right ventricular pressures were a little elevated but the right ventricular diastolic and right atrial pressures were very near normal values. Increases in pulmonary vascular resistance occur as a response to hypoxia, so maintenance of oxygenation postoperatively was a priority in Ms. Fry's case.

8. **What ECG findings are characteristic of mitral stenosis?**

ECG. The ECG is not specific for mitral stenosis and often is not a good indicator of the severity of the disease. However, the following changes may occur:

a. P mitrale may be seen in lead II if atrial enlargement has occurred.

The normal P wave, usually measured in lead II, does not exceed 3 mm in height or 0.11 sec in duration. Since the P wave represents atrial depolarization, atrial hypertrophy is often manifested on ECG by either an abnormally tall, peaked P wave (P pulmonale, secondary to cor pulmonale; right atrial (RA) hypertrophy) or by an abnormally wide P wave (P mitrale, secondary to mitral stenosis; left atrial (LA) hypertrophy) in lead II (Fig. 12.3). The characteristic M shape of P mitrale in this lead is due to LA depolarization being delayed by the increase in left atrial muscle mass. In the same vein, left atrial enlargement is also exhibited by a diphasic P wave in V_1 in which the negative deflection exceeds the positive deflection. The V_1 electrode placement is used because it sits right over the atria.

b. If atrial fibrillation is present, large fibrillatory waves in V_1 may indicate right heart involvement. A flat fibrillatory baseline may indicate irreversible atrial fibrillation.

c. Right ventricular hypertrophy. The right ventricle is not usually affected unless pulmonary hypertension is present. In mitral stenosis, right ventricular hypertrophy on ECG almost always indicates a pulmonary artery systolic pressure of >35 mm Hg.

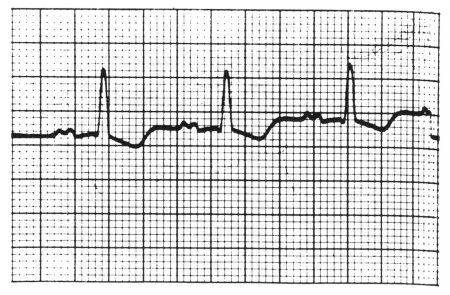

Figure 12.3. P mitrale in lead II from a patient with mitral stenosis. (From Vitello-Cicciu J, Lapsley DP. Valvular heart disease. In: Kinney MR, Packa DR, Dunbar SB, eds. AACN's Clinical Reference for Critical-Care Nursing. 2nd ed. New York: McGraw-Hill, 1988, 702.)

Right ventricular hypertrophy (RVH) might go unnoticed on ECG unless the thickness of the right ventricle exceeds left ventricular thickness. In RVH, a large R wave is recorded in V_1 as the mean wave of depolarization moves toward the electrode, and a large S wave is inscribed in V_6 as the mean wave of depolarization moves away from it. Voltage is one of the two criteria used for recognition of RVH:

$$R \text{ wave} \geq S \text{ wave in } V_1$$

or

$$R \text{ wave in } V_1 + S \text{ wave in } V_6 \geq 11 \text{ mm}$$

Ms. Fry's ECG was essentially normal. She did, however, have an increased PR interval (0.23 sec). In patients with abnormal P wave duration, it is helpful to measure the PR segment rather than the PR interval so that the influence of the P wave width is eliminated (Fig. 12.4).

The PR interval includes the P wave and ends with the beginning of the QRS complex. This interval represents depolarization of the atria and the spread of the depolarization wave up to and including the AV node. In instances in which the P wave is abnormally widened, the PR interval might exceed 0.20 sec. Ms. Fry's P waves were not abnormal, however, and she may have been experiencing a conduction defect due to atrial dilatation and hypertrophy.

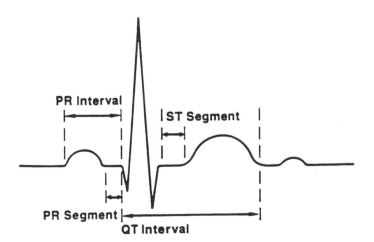

Figure 12.4. Identification of normal intervals and segments on surface ECG.

9. **What are the typical cardiac catheterization findings in mitral stenosis?**

The most important finding on cardiac catheterization in mitral stenosis is the pressure gradient across the mitral valve with elevated LAP/PAWP (Fig. 12.5). In mitral stenosis, left atrial pressure no longer mirrors left ventricular pressure during diastole. Instead, LAP reflects the pressure required for the left atrium to push blood across the stenotic valve and is not representative of the actual filling pressure in the left ventricle. Left ventricular filling pressure is much lower due to the restriction of blood flow across the mitral valve.

The gradient across the valve depends on the severity of the stenosis, the duration of diastole, and the stroke volume. It is possible that there will be little or no gradient at rest in a patient with a small stroke volume, slow heart rate, and mild stenosis. Exercise testing is usually done in an attempt to accentuate the stenosis by increasing the cardiac output. Ms. Fry's diastolic gradient was only 12 mm Hg, but it should be noted that this was at rest.

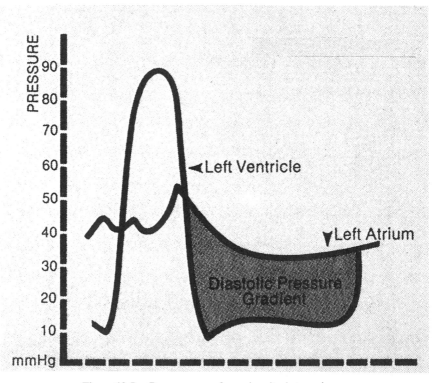

Figure 12.5. Pressure waveforms in mitral stenosis.

Ms. Fry's cardiac output was within normal limits but her cardiac index was a little low. Indexing of cardiac output allows the variable of body weight to be eliminated and is a much more precise indicator of left ventricular function than cardiac output.

10. On Ms. Fry's oximetry run, oxygen saturation fell from 96% in the pulmonary artery wedge position to 94% in the left ventricle. Did she have some other problem?

It is perfectly normal to see a slight decrease in oxygen saturation from the pulmonary circuit to the left heart. This "shunt" is due to the venous drainage from the thebesian, bronchial, and pleural circulation which enter into the left heart chambers. A saturation of 96% in the pulmonary artery wedge position is a little low and indicates a pulmonary problem due to slight amount of fluid in the lungs (increased PAP).

11. What surgical options exist for patients with mitral valve disease?

Mitral commissurotomy of stenotic and fused rheumatic leaflets was the first successful reparative surgery and continues to be performed in patients without significant mitral regurgitation, valvular calcification, or loss of audible opening snap. The fused leaflets of the mitral valve are manually defused under direct visualization (heart open). This enlarges the valve orifice and allows the patient to retain his or her natural valve, which is more desirable than mitral valve replacement. This procedure is more likely to restore normal function when performed early in the course of the disease, before the valve is irreparably damaged.

In mitral insufficiency, repair or reconstruction of the valve (valvuloplasty) is gaining popularity. Valvuloplasty may include:

Leaflet reconstruction
Chordal repair
Annulus remodelling

These procedures have a lower operative mortality than valve replacement and are often performed early in the course of the disease. In addition, a patient's own valve that is adequately repaired is preferable to the prosthetic valves in use today.

When valve replacement is indicated, there is a wide choice of mechanical or biologic valves available. However, all prosthetic valves are inherently stenotic as placement of the sewing ring within the valve annulus decreases the valve orifice. The use of supraannular prostheses is being considered to alleviate this problem. In essence, prosthetic valves do not provide a cure, but rather impose a different form of valvular disease.

12. **Ms. Fry had had previous cardiac surgery. What increased risks did she face?**

The median sternotomy incision for cardiac surgery has been used since the early 1970s. Advantages of this approach include:

Ease of access to most areas of the heart
Avoidance of the lungs
Ease of closure

Generally, the pericardium is not closed postoperatively. This facilitates drainage through the chest tubes, thereby decreasing the potential for cardiac tamponade.

Unfortunately, these two techniques pose risks for patients facing reoperation, as adhesions frequently form following the initial surgery. Reentering the chest through a median sternotomy can result in catastrophic hemorrhage due to injury to:

Anterior cardiac chambers (right atrium or ventricle)
Anterior great vessels (vena cavae, pulmonary artery, aorta)
Anterior saphenous vein bypass grafts or left internal mammary grafts to left anterior descending or right coronary artery

Additionally, division of the adhesions is time consuming, and cardiac and coronary anatomy may be obscured. Postoperative mortality and morbidity are slightly higher than for the initial operation, and bleeding is more of a problem, resulting in an increased need for blood replacement.

Ms. Fry suffered an inadvertent incision in her right ventricle, which had adhered to the posterior aspect of her sternum following her previous surgery. Catastrophic hemorrhage resulted and the surgical team moved quickly to place her on bypass to ensure perfusion while the laceration was repaired. It is now customary to have a lateral chest film taken on all patients scheduled for reoperation to ascertain whether or not cardiac structures have adhered to the sternum. In addition, both groins are prepared so that the patient can be placed on cardiopulmonary bypass via femoral cannulation either prior to sternal reentry or in case of problems.

13. **Ms. Fry received several units of blood upon her return to CVTICU. She was still hypothermic (temperature, 96.2°F via bladder probe). What potential impact do these factors have on oxygen delivery in the postoperative period? What does her $S_{\bar{v}}O_2$ tell you about the balance between O_2 supply and demand?**

Ms. Fry might well have had some oxygen transport problems postoperatively. Her hemoglobin level was critically low, and hemoglobin is required to carry oxygen to the systemic capillary bed.

While blood transfusion will increase the hemoglobin level, banked blood is deficient in 2,3-diphosphoglycerate (2,3-DPG). Decreased serum levels of 2,3-DPG shift the oxyhemoglobin dissociation curve to the left, impairing oxygen unloading at the tissue level. Hypothermia also shifts the oxyhemoglobin dissociation curve to the left, impairing oxygen unloading and threatening tissue oxygenation. Fortunately, Ms. Fry's tissue oxygen demands were reduced in the immediate postoperative period, as she was still partially anesthetized, paralyzed, and on controlled ventilation. The balance between her oxygen supply and demand was normal, as reflected by her $S_{\bar{v}}O_2$ of 80%.

14. **Within the hour, Ms. Fry's $S_{\bar{v}}O_2$ readings dropped from 80 to 60%. What actions should the nurse take?**
   Because ABGs and Hgb levels were recently checked and found to be adequate, a reduced cardiac output or increased tissue oxygen demand is the most likely cause of a reduced $S_{\bar{v}}O_2$. This is a distinct possibility, because the ability of Ms. Fry's left ventricle to handle the increased blood volume presented through the new mitral valve is not known. The patient could also have a primary right heart problem because she did have some right ventricular involvement preoperatively. The best way to determine what the problem is is to measure her cardiac output and look at the total cardiopulmonary profile. Her CO was 6 liters/min and her PA readings were as follows:

PAP	30/15	SaO₂	97%
PAWP 12		S$_{\bar{v}}$O₂	60%
SVR	1500	Hgb	13

Because PAD and PAWP are essentially equal (normal gradient of 1–4 mm Hg), there does not seem to be a problem between the right and left heart. PAWP is a little low, and Ms. Fry might benefit from some volume to maximize the Starling forces. However, her CO is good and her oxygen delivery is over 1000 ml of O_2/min. ($13 \times 1.39 \times 0.97 \times 6 \times 10 = 1052$ ml of O_2/min). When her venous oxygen transport is calculated ($13 \times 1.39 \times 0.60 \times 6 \times 10 = 650$ ml of O_2/min), it is obvious that she is consuming more than the usual 200–250 ml of O_2/min. Her ability to compensate for the increased demand by increasing her cardiac output is entirely appropriate and attention should be directed toward discovering the reason for her increased tissue oxygen demand. Ms. Fry was found to be waking up, shivering, anxious, and in pain. Nursing interventions included covering her with warm blankets and administering morphine sulfate, 5 mg IV push.

15. **Ms. Fry chose to have a mechanical valve inserted as opposed to a tissue valve because she did not want to ever require another open heart procedure. What are the advantages and disadvantages of each type of valve?**

    The mechanical valves require anticoagulation while tissue valves do not. Ms. Fry felt she could handle the anticoagulation routine as she worked in a health care facility. Her past history demonstrated a high rate of compliance with therapy.

    The mechanical valves last longer than do tissue valves. It seems apparent that porcine valves last about 10 years. Ms. Fry did not want to have this valve replaced again. (Porcine valves in children show a surprisingly high rate of calcification and are generally not considered for children under the age of 15 years.)

    The tissue valves have better hemodynamics, in that the blood flow through them closely resembles normal. However, the bileaflet design of the St. Jude valve does allow central flow as opposed to the caged ball or tilting disc valves. In addition, the low profile design is particularly suited for small left ventricular chambers.

    Mrs. Fry was not prepared for the audible sound of the valve. She was initially very upset and actually unable to sleep because of this.

16. **What is a perivalvular leak? How would it be manifested in this patient?**

    A perivalvular leak is a leak around the valve annulus secondary to suture line disruption. Perivalvular leak is the most common abnormality of implanted valve function, whether with tissue or mechanical valves. Periprosthetic leaks resulting from detachment of part of the sewing ring from the annulus are suggested by the presence of new murmurs and signs of hemolysis (RBCs in urine, jaundice, and anemia) secondary to blood trauma between the prosthesis and the valve annulus.

    In the mitral position, a pansystolic murmur best heard at the apex or a systolic ejection murmur may herald the appearance of a leak. However, almost all mitral valve prostheses (even tissue ones) are associated with a short systolic murmur.

17. **What other postoperative complications may result from mitral valve replacement?**

    There have been various reports in the literature dealing with rupture of the left ventricular free wall and left ventricular outflow tract obstruction following mitral valve replacement. Left ventricular outflow tract obstruction may complicate mitral valve replacement in an abnormally small or hypertrophied nondilated heart.

18. Ms. Fry will need to be anticoagulated for the rest of her life. Why?

Thromboembolism is a risk with all mechanical valves. Although the St. Jude valve has a lower rate of thromboembolism (1.0%/patient/year) of any currently available mechanical prosthesis, thromboembolic events are twice as common in mitral valve as compared to aortic valve replacement and result from thrombotic material on the prosthesis as well as an accelerated platelet consumption. Conditions that increase the risk of thromboembolism include:

Large left atrium
Enlarged heart
Low cardiac output
Atrial fibrillation
Endocarditis

Those at highest risk of thromboembolism are also at highest risk of complications from antithrombotic therapy. Additionally, although a patient with a mechanical aortic valve can probably be off anticoagulation for 3–5 days without much added risk of thrombosis or thromboembolism, these risks increase significantly in the first 24 hr with a mitral valve prosthesis. The loss of a previously audible prosthetic click is an abnormal finding that may represent thrombosis of the prosthesis.

19. Is prophylactic antibiotic therapy required following mitral valve replacement?

Yes. Prosthetic valve endocarditis (PVE) occurs in 4–5% of patients following valve replacement. "Early" PVE occurs in the first 60 days postoperatively and is usually due to staphylococcus or a Gram-negative bacillus. Aggressive early valve replacement may be required, as these organisms are frequently resistant to antibiotic therapy. The mortality rate is 60–90%.

"Late" PVE occurs after 2 months postoperatively, is usually caused by staphylococcal or streptococcal infection, and is usually precipitated by dental procedures, genitourinary manipulation, or GI procedures.

Clinical manifestations of PVE include fever, a new murmur, perivalvular leak, or embolic symptoms.

Mechanical valves are more likely to become infected beneath the site of attachment, leading to ring abscess. The infection with tissue valves is usually limited to the cusps, which allows greater contact between the infecting organisms and antibiotic agents. Thus, antibiotic therapy is usually more effective in infections occurring in tissue valves as compared to mechanical valves.

20. What are the appropriate nursing diagnoses?

Alteration in fluid balance related to hemorrhage
Impaired gas exchange related to atelectasis
Alteration in peripheral tissue perfusion related to decreased cardiac output
Potential for infection related to presence of invasive lines
Alteration in comfort related to incisional pain
Sleep pattern disturbance related to environmental stimuli
Anxiety related to audible sound of prosthetic valve

SUGGESTED READINGS

Baas L, Kretten C. Valvular heart disease: Its causes, symptoms and consequences. RN 1987;Nov.:30–35.

Baas L, Kretten C. Valvular heart disease: Surgery and postop care. RN 1987; Dec: 38–44.

Gotsman MS. Rheumatic fever in the 80's. Cardiovasc Rev Rep 1985;6(8):935–957.

Husebye DG, Pluth JR, Piehler JR, et al. Reoperation on prosthetic heart valves. J Thorac Cardiovasc Surg 1983;86:543–552.

Johnson J. Valvular heart disease in the elderly. J Cardiovasc Nurs 1987;1(2):72–81.

Schakenbach LH. Physiologic dynamics of acquired valvular heart disease. J Cardiovasc Nurs 1987;1(3):1–17.

Siefert PG. Surgery for acquired valvular heart disease. J Cardiovasc Nurs 1987; 1(3):26–40.

Whitman GR. Prosthetic cardiac valves. Prog Cardiovasc Nurs 1987;2:116–124.

CHAPTER 13

Non-Q Wave Myocardial Infarction

Laura E. Luecke, RN, BSN, CCRN

Maria Garcia is a 64-year-old widow who was in her usual state of health until 1 month prior to admission, when she began having chest pain. This pain became a daily event, occurring at rest or with exertion, often lasting several hours every day. She described the pain as a "gripping" feeling over her left chest area, sometimes radiating to both arms and to her neck. On the evening of admission, while at rest at home, she had a sudden onset of chest pain, also a "gripping" feeling over her left chest which radiated to both arms. She became nauseated and vomited three times. She was diaphoretic but denied SOB. She called her son, who drove her to a neighborhood clinic. When her chest pain was not relieved after 3 nitroglycerin, she was sent to the county hospital Emergency Department, arriving at 4 AM. Risk factors for coronary artery disease included a history of hypertension and obesity.

Ms. Garcia was placed on a cardiac monitor, which showed sinus tachycardia. Her vital signs were:

BP	210/116
HR	112
Resp	20
Temp	98.6°F

O$_2$ via 2 liters per nasal cannula was started.

Physical examination revealed an anxious, obese, diaphoretic female. She was alert and oriented. No JVD was noted, and normal S$_1$, S$_2$ were auscultated. Her lungs were clear to auscultation, and her extremities were warm and well perfused without edema. A 12-lead ECG was done, which showed ST depression in I, II, AVL, AVF and V$_3$–V$_6$, compatible with inferolateral ischemia. The physician was notified. Nifedipine and propranolol were given, and the patient was transferred to the CCU.

Ms. Garcia's admitting diagnosis was unstable angina (USA), rule out myocardial infarction (ROMI). She was felt to have a good "story" for USA and her ECG changes were compatible with ischemia. Upon arrival in the CCU, she denied chest pain, and her cardiac monitor showed NSR.

Vital signs

BP	142/80
HR	84
Resp	24
Temp	98.4° F

125

She was placed on Isordil, nifedipine, propranolol, and aspirin. Serial cardiac enzymes, isoenzymes, and ECGs were ordered.

Cardiac enzymes and isoenzymes were as follows:

	Day 1			Day 2
	5 AM	2 PM	6 PM	4 AM
CK	156	653	583	375
LDH	155	324	290	307
AST	56	137	133	99
CK-MB	0	12%	9%	6%
LDH$_1$/LDH	8%	31%	42%	39%

ECG on day 2 showed ST depression V$_3$–V$_6$, T wave inversion II, III, AVF.

Based on her history, ECG changes, and increased CK and CK-MB, a non-Q wave myocardial infarction in the inferolateral region was suspected. An echocardiogram showed a normal sized left ventricle with lateral hypokinesis. Her medical regimen was continued, except her nifedipine was discontinued and she was placed on diltiazem. The nurse monitored Ms. Garcia closely for recurrence of chest pain, ischemic ECG changes, or a second rise in cardiac enzymes. Ms. Garcia remained stable and was transferred to the cardiac rehabilitation unit on day 4. Results of a lipoprotein analysis, showing hyperlipidemia, were as follows:

Total cholesterol	241
Triglycerides	134
VLDL	22
LDL	177
HDL	42

The dietitian was called to initiate intensive dietary instruction for a 30% fat, low caloric diet. Prior to discharge, a 24-hr Holter monitoring study was done and showed rare, unifocal, ventricular ectopic beats with an average rate of <1/hr. No ST changes were noted. A radionuclide scan showed a left ventricular ejection fraction of 60%, and a right ventricular ejection fraction of 70% with no wall motion abnormalities. A submaximal exercise test was attempted, but the patient could not ride a bicycle. She ambulated in the hospital without difficulty. Ms. Garcia was discharged on day 12, to be followed closely for any recurrent chest pain and hyperlipidemia.

QUESTIONS AND ANSWERS

1. **Define the terms Q wave and non-Q wave MI.**

Previously, an MI was classified clinically as transmural or nontransmural, also called subendocardial, based on the presence or absence of new Q waves on the ECG. Patients who developed Q waves were thought to have had a transmural myocardial infarction, involving the full thickness of the myocardial wall. Patients who displayed only ST, T wave changes were thought to have had a nontransmural or subendocardial MI. Studies have shown that the ECG does not always correlate with the pathology. Nontransmural MIs may produce Q waves and transmural MIs may not always produce Q waves. Some have suggested that the terms Q wave and non-Q wave infarct should be used, and these terms are gaining recognition in cardiology literature. More important than the nomenclature, reports indicate differences in the pathology, clinical course, and mortality of non-Q wave MIs versus Q wave MIs.

2. **How does the pathology of a non-Q wave MI compare with a Q wave MI?**

   A thrombus completely occluding the coronary artery is present in the majority of Q wave infarctions. An incomplete or transient thrombus that spontaneously reperfuses is present in the majority of non-Q wave infarctions. This may leave a stenosed coronary artery supplying an area of the myocardium at risk for future ischemic events.

3. **What is the incidence of non-Q wave MIs?**

   Approximately 1 of 4 MIs are non-Q wave MIs. Some studies have shown that non-Q wave MIs affect a slightly older population and slightly more women.

4. **How is a Q wave MI and a non-Q wave MI diagnosed?**

   Q Wave MI.   Serial ECGs for the first 36 hr post-MI show early ST elevation followed by development of new pathological Q waves.

   Non-Q Wave MI.   Changes on the ECG are restricted to persistent ST and/or T wave changes. Changes most commonly include ST depression and or T wave inversion; however, studies have shown up to 30–40% may display ST segment elevation. ST and T wave changes are not specific for only MI, but can indicate other conditions such as ischemia, digoxin toxicity, or strain. Thus, diagnosis can be made only with the presence of history and positive isoenzyme studies. In addition, more non-Q wave MI patients have a history of previous angina than do patients with Q wave MIs.

5. **Ms. Garcia had a history of typical ischemic chest pain associated with nausea and vomiting unrelieved by nitroglycerin. She had angina 1 month prior to admission. She had risk factors of hypertension, obesity, and hyperlipidemia. Her ECG showed persistent ST depression. How did her isoenzyme studies corroborate the diagnosis of non-Q wave MI?**

The use of cardiac enzymes to diagnose MI is discussed in Chapter 16, "Unstable Angina and Percutaneous Transluminal Coronary Angioplasty." Creatinine kinase (CK) found in the heart, brain, and skeletal muscles, is the most sensitive enzyme for diagnosing MI. However, elevations of CK also occur in patients with other conditions, such as seizures, alcohol intoxication, diabetes mellitus, muscular diseases, muscular trauma, and pulmonary embolus, and in patients who are defibrillated or have received intramuscular injections.

CK can be broken down into isoenzymes that are more organ-specific and more reliable in diagnosing MI. CK-MM is found in the skeletal muscle and heart. CK-BB is found in the brain and kidney. CK-MB is found primarily in the cardiac muscle. CK-MB increases in all cases of MI. If the serum level is less than 2%, a diagnosis of MI can be ruled out. One exception is post-open heart surgery, or cardiac trauma, which elevates the CK-MB.

If an MI is suspected, CK and CK-MB should be measured on admission and a minimum of 12 and 24 hr later. Many institutions send CK and CK-MB samples every 6–8 hr for 24 hr and then every day for 3 days. CK-MB rises 4–6 hr after the onset of pain, peaks 12–20 hr later, and returns to normal in 2–3 days.

Lactic dehydrogenase (LDH) is found in many tissues including the brain, heart, liver, kidneys, red blood cells, and skeletal muscles. LDH rises 8–12 hr after the onset of pain, peaks in 24–48 hr, and returns to normal in 10–14 days. If a patient delays coming to the hospital, the longer elevation time of LDH makes it useful in detecting an MI. LDH alone is not a sensitive indicator of MI because it is present in many tissues, but the LDH_1 isoenzyme is present only in the heart. LDH_2 is found primarily in the blood, LDH_3 in the heart and skeletal muscle, and LDH_4 and LDH_5 in the liver and skeletal muscle. LDH_1 rises in 4 hr after an MI, peaks in 48 hr, and returns to normal in 10 days. If the LDH_1 rises above 36% of the total LDH, it is suggestive of an MI.

Ms. Garcia's CK-MB and LDH_1 rose above normal. In patients with a non-Q wave MI, cardiac enzymes often show a lower peak CK and an earlier peak CK than patients with a Q wave MI. One study showed an average peak CK of 1334 in a Q wave MI, and 520 in a non-Q wave MI. Time to peak averaged 22.5 hr in a Q wave MI, and 16.9 hr in a non-Q wave MI. The higher peak CK in a Q wave MI is consistent with a larger area of myocardial necrosis as compared with a non-Q wave MI. The earlier peak seen in a non-Q wave MI is due to spontaneous reperfusion of the ischemic myocardium, creating an earlier "washout" of enzymes from the ischemic area.

6. **Why might it be important to differentiate between a Q wave MI and non-Q wave MI when planning the patient's care?**

   Differences in the clinical course and prognosis have been observed. Q wave infarcts are associated with a higher mortality in the acute hospital phase. They are usually larger infarcts and are associated with a higher incidence of complications such as shock, myocardial rupture, and late phase ventricular tachycardia. Overall, non-Q wave MIs have a lower complication rate in the acute phase, but a higher incidence of reinfarction and recurrent angina later. Data indicate that in-hospital mortality is lower in non-Q wave MI, but the long-term prognosis is similar to that of a Q wave MI. Although a non-Q wave MI appears to have a smaller area of necrosis, there is a large area of myocardium in jeopardy for future ischemic events. Although the infarct-related coronary artery is not totally occluded, it is usually severely stenotic, leaving myocardium at risk for reinfarction. Some state that a non-Q wave MI is a "noncompleted" MI, to be considered unstable due to a risk of reinfarction and residual angina in the myocardial area in jeopardy. Ms. Garcia was monitored carefully for complaints of chest pain, ischemic ECG changes, and elevations of CK-MB isoenzymes. Up to 23% of patients with non-Q wave MI reinfarct, with an average time of 10 days after the initial infarct. Some studies have found recurrent chest pain, female sex, and obesity to be statistically significant predictors for future ischemic events.

7. **Discuss the treatment of the patient with a non-Q wave MI.**

   The patient with a non-Q wave MI has myocardium perfused by a stenosed coronary artery still at risk for reinfarction and ischemia. Aspirin is given to prevent platelet aggregation. Calcium channel blockers and nitrates may help prevent vasoconstriction of the coronary artery. Studies have found diltiazem to be effective in reducing the incidence of reinfarction. If a patient displays signs of ongoing ischemia, coronary angiography is usually done and percutaneous transluminal coronary angioplasty or revascularization may be indicated.

8. **How is the patient assessed for risk of future ischemic events?**

   As stated, the patient is monitored for clinical signs and symptoms of ischemia. Risk after an acute myocardial infarction is related primarily to the amount of left ventricular dysfunction, the presence of postinfarction ischemia, and ventricular dysrhythmias. Left ventricular function should be measured. Exercise testing should be done before discharge if the patient is without angina, preferably with radionuclide studies. Presence of ventricular dysrhythmias and ischemic ST-T wave changes can be assessed with 24-hr Holter monitoring. Left ventricular function is usually well preserved in the non-Q wave MI patient. Residual ischemia and ventricular dysrhythmias are the main risks. If the Holter monitoring or exercise testing reveal significant ischemia, coronary angiography is needed. If significant ventricular dysrhythmias are present, antiarrythmic therapy may be given, although it is not known if antiarrythmic therapy improves survival.

9. What about risk factor control in Ms. Garcia?

Risk factor control is fundamental in the long-term control of coronary artery disease. Ms. Garcia's hypertension was under control with β-blockers and calcium channel blockers.

Treating hyperlipidemia has been shown to slow the progression of coronary artery disease. The National Cholesterol Education Program recommends that anyone with a serum cholesterol level of >200 mg/dl with coronary artery disease or two other risk factors should have a lipoprotein profile checked including triglycerides, high density lipoprotein cholesterol (HDL), and low density lipoprotein cholesterol (LDL).

Ms. Garcia's lipoprotein analysis reveals an elevated total cholesterol, elevated LDL, decreased HDL, and normal triglycerides for her age and sex. The goal of treatment should be to decrease the LDL cholesterol and increase the HDL cholesterol to the 50% range for her age and sex. She is at increased risk due to her known coronary artery disease, obesity, and hypertension. She needs intensive dietary instruction for a 30% fat, low caloric diet. Weight loss will lower her LDL cholesterol and she may be able to achieve a normal level at her optimum weight. If her LDL cholesterol remains elevated after 3–6 months of diet, drugs will be considered.

It is important to remember that total cholesterol and triglycerides are useful for screening, but a lipoprotein analysis is needed to evaluate the patient for appropriate treatment. If Ms. Garcia's LDLs had been lower and her HDLs higher, at the appropriate level for her age and sex, she would not need to be treated for hyperlipidemia.

10. What nursing diagnoses apply in this case?

Potential for alteration in peripheral tissue perfusion related to acute myocardial infarction

Potential for further alteration in myocardial tissue perfusion related to high incidence of future ischemic events in non-Q wave MIs

Alteration in comfort related to myocardial ischemia

Knowledge deficit related to health risks associated with obesity
Knowledge deficit regarding the relationship between diet and hyperlipidemia
Potential for alteration in cardiac output and tissue perfusion related to dysrhythmias

SUGGESTED READINGS

André-Fouet A, Pillot M, Leizorovicz A, et al. "Non-Q wave," alias "nontransmural" myocardial infarction: A specific entity. Am Heart J 1989;117:892–902.

Cheitlin MD. Non-Q wave infarction: Diagnosis, prognosis, and treatment. Adv Intern Med 1988;33:267–294.

DeWood M. Clinical implications of coronary arteriographic findings soon after non-Q wave acute myocardial infarction. Am J Cardiol 1988;61:36F–38F.

Frye RL, Gibbons RJ, Schaff HV, et al. Treatment of coronary artery disease. J Am Coll Cardiol 1989;13:957–968.

Gibson RS. Non-Q wave myocardial infarction: Diagnosis, prognosis, management. Curr Probl Cardiol 1988;XIII:1–72.

Maisel AS, Scott N, Gilpin E, et al. Complex ventricular arrythmias in patients with Q wave versus non-Q wave myocardial infarction. Circulation 1985;72:963–970.

Nicod P, Gilpin E, Dittrich H, et al. Short and long-term clinical outcome after Q wave and non-Q wave myocardial infarction in a large patient population. Circulation 1989;79:528–536.

Nixon JV. Non-Q wave myocardial infarction. Am J Med Sci 1986;292:173–181.

Stone PH, Raabe DS, Jaffe AS, et al. Prognostic significance of location and type of myocardial infarction: Independent adverse outcome associated with anterior location. J Am Coll Cardiol 1988;11:453–463.

CHAPTER 14

Ruptured Aorta

Wendy L. Baker, RN, MS, CCRN

Marsha Gellin is a 43-year-old factory worker who was the driver of a car struck broadside by a pickup truck. She was found 10 feet from her car. On presentation to the Emergency Department, she complained of pain in her right chest, right leg, and left shoulder. Further evaluation revealed fractures of right ribs 4 through 6, a fractured right femur, and a right patellar fracture. Her past medical history was significant for an exploratory laparotomy 12 years ago with a tubal ligation. Ms. Gellin smokes 1 pack of cigarettes/day but denies any alcohol use.

Physical Examination. The patient is in moderate distress with multiple abrasions on her face. Blood pressure is 120/50, heart rate 118, respirations 24, and temperature 99°F. There is a 2 × 3 cm avulsion laceration lateral to her left eye. Pupils are equal and reactive to light. Heart rate and rhythm are regular and no murmurs, gallops, or rubs are present. Her lungs are clear, and moderate right rib and sternal tenderness are present. The abdomen is soft and nontender with bowel sounds present. Rectal tone is normal and stool is guaiac positive. Her right leg is in an air splint and she is tender over the right midthigh and right knee. Although there is ecchymosis over her left shoulder, there is a good range of motion. Cranial nerves II–XII are intact. Motor and sensory examination findings are within normal limits and distal pulses are present and equal in all extremities.

X-ray Findings. X-rays demonstrated a right midshaft, displaced femur fracture, a right patellar fracture, and a question of mediastinal widening. An arch aortogram revealed an intimal injury at the level of the ligamentum arteriosum, without extravasation.

Relevant laboratory data included:

Electrolytes		CBC		ABG (Room Air)	
Na	140	Hgb	11.8	pH	7.51
K	3.4	Hct	31.5	PaCO$_2$	31
Cl	106	WBC	10.5	PaO$_2$	42
CO$_2$	22	Plat	245,000	SaO$_2$	76%
Gluc	134			HCO$_3$	22
BUN	12				

Hospital Course. The patient was taken immediately to the Operating Room and the aorta was repaired using a Dacron graft interposition. A shunt bypass was used during the 46-min procedure. The patient received pentobarbital, a nitroprusside (Nipride) infusion, 2 units of packed red blood cells, 2 units of whole blood, 1 liter of Plasma-lyte, and 4900 ml of electrolyte solution intraoperatively. The fractured left femur was also fixed during this same operative period, which took approximately 6 hr.

Approximately 10 hr postoperatively, the assessment demonstrated the following:

Vital Signs		Ventilator Settings	
BP	142/80	Mode	SIMV
HR	104	Rate	10
Resp	10	FIO_2	0.60
Temp	101.6° F	Tidal volume	750
CVP	9	PEEP	7.5

ABG			
pH	7.43	Urine Output	80 ml/hr
$PaCo_2$	35	Creat	1.0
PaO_2	53		
SaO_2	82%		
HCO_3	22		

Peripheral pulses were present and equal in all extremities. The patient followed simple commands, and muscle strength was 5/5 in all extremities. On auscultation of the lungs, crackles were audible throughout, and breath sounds were diminished on the left side and in both bases.

QUESTIONS AND ANSWERS

1. **What is the likelihood that someone with traumatic rupture of the aorta will be alive on arrival at a hospital?**

    Eighty to ninety percent die at the scene. Of those who arrive at the hospital and do not receive definitive treatment, most will die within 1 week. One-third of the patients who suffer blunt chest trauma will have a traumatic tear of the thoracic aorta. Sixteen percent of automobile accident fatalities are due to aortic rupture. Patients thrown from the car, as this patient was, have twice the likelihood of presenting with a ruptured aorta as those who remain in the car.

2. **Why would you expect a favorable outcome in this patient with an aortic rupture?**

    She did not have extensive dissection of the aorta, which would have made operative repair and hemostasis more difficult. In addition, this patient was hemodynamically stable on arrival in the Operating Room, and she had little preinjury disease.

3. **Does Ms. Gellin's injury history make you suspicious that she is at high risk for an aortic injury? Why/Why not?**

    Yes. In the United States, traumatic aortic injury most often occurs as a result of high speed deceleration injury (especially when the occupant is wearing a shoulder harness), usually due to motor vehicle accidents (MVA). However, these injuries may also occur after falls from heights, airplane accidents, kicks by animals, sudden burial by landslide, and penetrating injuries to the mediastinum. Information should always be obtained about damage to the vehicle, death or injuries of other victims, the severity of the patient's associated injuries, and the mechanism of those injuries. Other injuries that would arouse suspicion of aortic rupture include fracture of the first and second ribs, left clavicular fractures near the sternal border, high sternal fractures, and penetrating parasternal chest wounds.

4. **Is the anatomical location of Ms. Gellin's injury consistent with the three most common locations of thoracic aorta rupture?**

Yes. Her injury was at the level of the ligamentum arteriosum. Because the thoracic aorta is relatively mobile, tears most often occur at points of anatomical fixation. Although the aorta may be torn anywhere along its length, the site of 90% of ruptures is at the aortic isthmus, just distal to the origin of the left subclavian artery where the vessel is attached to the chest wall by the ligamentum arteriosum. Besides injury to the aortic isthmus, other potential areas of injury include: the supravalvular portion of the ascending aorta; the innominate artery, which may be avulsed from the aorta; the aortic arch; other portions of the descending thoracic aorta; the abdominal aorta; and combinations of these (Fig. 14.1).

5. **How does deceleration cause injury to the aorta?**

With the enormous shearing forces acting maximally on the aorta, which is fixed at the ligamentum arteriosum, deceleration from impact causes the inner layers of the vessel (intima and media) to tear. The adventitia (outer layer) may be the only layer to remain intact. It then balloons out into a pseudoaneurysm. If the aorta is partially transected and the patient survives, surrounding tissue may form a partial circumferential hematoma and tamponade the aneurysm. Pseudoaneurysms may also form between the two ends of a totally transected aorta.

6. **Why do the history and physical examination provide valuable information but not necessarily provide diagnostic information?**

Although the aorta may have been damaged at the time of a high speed MVA, causing tearing of the intima and media, there may not be rupture when the patient arrives at the hospital. Clinical signs and symptoms are present in less than one-half, and up to one-third have no evidence of external trauma. Thus, the strongest argument for

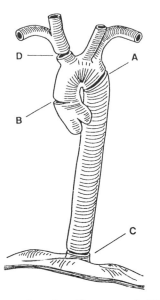

Figure 14.1. Sites of aortic rupture in order of frequency. **A,** Distal to left subclavian artery at the level of the ligamentum arteriosium. **B,** Ascending aorta. **C,** Lower thoracic aorta above diaphragm. **D,** Avulsion of innominate artery from aortic arch. (From Frey C. Initial management of the trauma patient. Philadelphia: Lea & Febiger, 1976: 321.)

such an injury is the accident history and vague symptoms such as retrosternal chest pain.

7. Were Ms. Gellin's symptoms consistent with those frequently seen after aortic rupture?

Although the only real symptom Ms. Gellin experienced was her left shoulder pain, this picture is quite common in injury to the thoracic aorta. Symptoms often will not become apparent until rupture occurs. The most frequent symptom is retrosternal chest pain or intercapsular pain. Pressure from a localized hematoma can cause dyspnea and stridor from tracheal or bronchial compression, dysphagia from esophageal compression, or superior vena caval syndrome from caval compression. (This is rare but results from rupture of the ascending aorta and is evidenced by prominence of superficial veins, facial edema, dyspnea, and complaints of fullness of the head and neck.) The most common physical finding is hypotension (systolic BP, <100 mm Hg). If bleeding has progressed to shock, look for restlessness, confusion, hypotension, tachycardia, tachypnea, decreased urinary output, and cool, moist, clammy skin. Localized aneurysms developing in the aortic isthmus late after trauma may cause hoarseness, cough, and dysphagia from compression of the adjacent recurrent laryngeal nerve, bronchus, and esophagus. Auscultation of the heart may reveal a systolic murmur, which radiates to the back medially and to the left scapula in 25% of patients with aortic rupture.

8. **What are common roentgenographic findings suggestive of aortic injury?**

   Common roentgenographic findings suggesting aortic injury are multiple rib fractures, an obscured aortic knob, widened mediastinum, left pleural effusion, rightward shift of the trachea, and depression of the left mainstem bronchus. Although other injuries common in multiple trauma can cause a widened mediastinum, i.e., pneumothorax or hemothorax, this is also classic for a ruptured aorta. Only one of five chest x-rays with widened mediastinum represent a ruptured aorta.

9. **What is the best way to position a patient for the anterior-posterior chest film?**

   A truly erect anteroposterior chest film is best, with the patient tilted a few degrees forward from the vertical axis to facilitate recognition of a widened mediastinum. This may be very difficult, or impossible, in the trauma patient who does not yet have the spine cleared of fracture.

10. **Do the associated injuries Ms. Gellin suffered commonly occur with aortic rupture?**

    Yes. Force severe enough to result in an aortic tear also often causes severe associated injuries, with femoral fracture being very common. Aortic rupture is often difficult to diagnose because of other serious injuries, such as: hip fractures, closed head injuries, and ruptured spleens. Thus, when hypovolemic hypotension is present, bleeding may be from either the aortic injury or exsanguinating intra-abdominal hemorrhage. About two-thirds of patients with aortic rupture have clear-cut evidence of other thoracic trauma. The remaining one-third are surprisingly free of symptoms of chest wall injury.

11. **Did Ms. Gellin exhibit the triad of findings that can be helpful in identifying aortic injury (but that are often not present?)**

    This is unclear because we don't have blood pressures from several extremities. (Often this is difficult if multiple extremities are fractured.) However, when possible, it is always a good idea to check for the following: (*a*) difference in pulse amplitude between upper and lower extremities, (*b*) hypertension in the upper extremities, and (*c*) widening of the mediastinum shown on the chest x-ray.

12. Why is spinal cord injury a complication of aortic rupture or its surgical repair?

Infarction of the spinal cord is caused by ischemia. The principal blood supply to the spinal cord arises between the tenth thoracic and second lumbar vertebra. Thus, if the injury is of the proximal thoracic aorta, the filling pressure near the origin of the spinal arteries is low and ischemia is likely. With severe ischemia, infarction can occur within 20–30 min, depending on the systemic blood pressure and the collateral circulation. Therefore, the goal during surgical correction of a ruptured thoracic aorta is to keep cross-clamp time to <20 min or use a shunt that provides sufficient blood flow to keep distal aortic pressure above 60 mm Hg.

13. How should you prepare to take Ms. Gellin from the Emergency Department or ICU to the arteriograph suite?

Be prepared for full cardiopulmonary arrest. Although a patient with a thoracic aortic injury may present with stable vital signs, exsanguinating hemorrhage is a constant threat. Make sure the patient is transported on a monitor. Have patent, large bore, intravenous access, plenty of IV fluid, a box of arrest drugs, and a manual resuscitator bag.

14. Why is it important for you to know the length of time the patient's aorta was cross-clamped during surgery?

Cross-clamping times longer than 20–30 min can result in severe ischemia, which is believed to cause spinal cord injury. The patient should be carefully assessed for neuromuscular dysfunction postoperatively. Cross-clamping the aorta for longer periods of time can be more safely done if the patient is placed on a bypass machine. However, this requires heparinization, which is unsafe if the patient also has a closed head injury.

15. What is the most likely reason that this patient received Nipride intraoperatively?

Ms. Gellin received Nipride for blood pressure control intraoperatively to regulate mean and systolic pressure. By keeping blood pressure relatively low, vessel and graft anastomosis stress are minimized. The goal preoperatively and intraoperatively is usually to keep the systolic blood pressure between 90 and 100 mm Hg.

16. **What pathophysiology underlies the nursing assessment of the patient after aortic rupture repair?**

    Hypoperfusion below the level of the graft is the major concern, as it may cause ischemia and multisystem organ failure.

17. **In what type of aortic injuries is postoperative hypertension most likely to be a problem?**

    Aortic isthmus repairs often require antihypertensive drugs (usually Nipride) to keep the systolic, diastolic, and mean blood pressure within acceptable limits.

18. **What other systems are likely to reflect ischemia after aortic surgery and require close monitoring?**

    The gastrointestinal and the renal system are at greatest risk for ischemia. Gastrointestinal assessment should include return of bowel function and presence of abdominal distention, fever, or abdominal pain. Hypoperfusion of the kidneys can result in renal impairment or failure. The urine output, urine electrolytes, creatinine, and BUN should be followed closely.

19. **Why should chest tube drainage be monitored closely after surgery for repair of a ruptured thoracic aorta?**

    Because there is little permanent bonding of the graft to the aorta, graft leaks or blow-outs can occur. Careful monitoring of chest drainage for dramatic increases or decreases in volume provides information about graft leakage.

20. **What other factors, besides cross-clamp time, are likely to influence the outcome from surgical repair of aortic rupture?**

    The patient's age, previous cardiovascular status, and additional injuries to other body systems each have prognostic significance.

21. **Besides bleeding from the new graft site, what is another major concern with any new graft and what would you assess for related to this problem?**

    Infection is always a threat when grafts are implanted. Detection of infection at graft sites is difficult, as symptoms are nonspecific: malaise, elevated white blood cell count, and fever. Occasionally a graft will clot if infected, causing symptoms of ischemia below the level of the graft.

22. **What is the probable reason for the patient's postoperative oxygenation problem? What could improve her oxygenation?**

When the posterior lateral thoracotomy incision was made to repair the aorta, the left lung was allowed to deflate to expose the isthmus of the aorta. This intraoperative deflation, in addition to the quantity of fluids received intraoperatively, probably impaired oxygenation. The patient should be positioned with her "good" (right) lung down to maximize blood flow to the good lung and improve oxygenation. The physician should be notified of Ms. Gellin's hypoxemia and might consider placing a pulmonary artery catheter to assist in determining the etiology of the low PaO_2. Another reasonable intervention would be to obtain an order to increase the PEEP to 10, with an ABG checked 30 min later.

23. **What are the major nursing diagnoses most often seen in the patient with a ruptured thoracic aorta?**

Altered renal tissue perfusion related to cross-clamping of aorta
Altered gastrointestinal tissue perfusion related to cross-clamping of aorta
Potential for infection related to graft placement
Decreased cardiac output related to increased afterload
Potential impaired physical mobility related to spinal cord ischemia
Impaired gas exchange related to atelectasis.

SUGGESTED READINGS

Hurn PD. Thoracic injuries. In: Cardona VC, Hurn PD, Mason PJ, Scanlon-Schilpp AM, Veise-Berry SW, eds. Trauma nursing: From resuscitation through rehabilitation. Philadelphia: WB Saunders, 1988: 478–482.

Kite JH. Cardiac and great vessel trauma: Assessment, pathophysiology, and intervention. J Emerg Nurs 1987;13(6):346–351.

Merrill WH, Lee RB, Hammon JW, et al. Surgical treatment of the acute traumatic tear of the thoracic aorta. Ann Surg 1988;207(6):699–706.

Pate JW. Traumatic rupture of the aorta: Emergency operation. Ann Thorac Surg 1985;39(6):531–537.

Schorr RM, Critenden M, Indeck M, et al. Blunt thoracic trauma: Analysis of 515 patients. Ann Surg 1987;206:200–209.

Sommers, MS. Nursing care of patients with blunt cardiac trauma. Crit Care Nurse 1987;5(6):58–66.

CHAPTER 15

Thrombolytic Therapy for Acute Myocardial Infarction

Laura E. Luecke, RN, BSN, CCRN

Frank Rossetti, a 43-year-old male caterer, awakened at 3:30 AM with substernal pain, which he described as a tightness radiating into his neck and left arm. This sensation was associated with diaphoresis and mild nausea. He had no vomiting or shortness of breath. He immediately came to the Emergency Department, arriving at 4:30 AM. Mr. Rossetti was placed on a cardiac monitor, vital signs were taken, and oxygen therapy per nasal cannula was initiated.

Mr. Rossetti's physical examination revealed an anxious, morbidly obese male (estimated weight 350 pounds). He was alert and oriented. His BP was 130/90, heart rate 88, and respiratory rate 20. S_4, S_1, and S_2 were auscultated. Breath sounds were equal with bibasilar rales and a few scattered wheezes. His extremities were warm and well perfused. Mr. Rossetti's past medical history was unremarkable. Risk factors for heart disease included:

> Cigarette abuse of 1½ packs/day for 30 years
> Father had first myocardial infarction at age 40, died of myocardial infarction at age 60
> Morbid obesity

Mr. Rossetti was asked to "rate" the severity of his chest pain on a scale of 1 to 10, with 10 being the most severe. He rated his chest pain an "8."

At 4:40 AM, a 12-lead ECG was done. The nurse noted ST elevation in leads II, III, AVF, V_1–V_6, indicative of an acute extensive anterolateral and inferior myocardial infarction. The physician was called immediately. Mr. Rossetti received one nitroglycerin (NTG) 1/150 sublingually without relief. The NTG was repeated at 4:45 AM without relief. At 4:50 AM, the 12-lead ECG was repeated and the results were unchanged. One inch of nitropaste was applied without relief. At 4:55 AM, morphine, 2 mg, was given slow IV push. The cardiologist was called to evaluate the patient for thrombolytic therapy with recombinant tissue plasminogen activator (rt-PA). Mr. Rossetti met all the screening criteria. A careful history and examination were performed to assess for potential bleeding problems. None were identified. At 5:30 AM, a second IV line was started. A heparin lock was also inserted for blood specimen collection. He received a 100-mg bolus of lidocaine and a drip was started at 2 mg/min. At 5:35 AM, 6 mg of rt-PA were given IV push, followed by an infusion. Over the first hour, 54 mg were to be infused, followed by 20 mg over the second hour and 20 mg over the third hour. At 5:37 AM, Mr. Rossetti was bolused with 5000 units of heparin followed by a continuous IV infusion of 1000 units/hr. He received one child's aspirin, 81 mg. At 5:45 AM, Mr. Rossetti was transferred to the CCU. At 6:45 AM, he experienced a dramatic relief of his chest pain. A 12-lead ECG was done and revealed less ST segment elevation. At 8:00 AM, the nurse noted ventricular bigeminy, trigeminy, and quadrigeminy. The patient's vital signs were stable. He remained on lidocaine at 2 mg/min and was monitored for signs of residual ischemia. He had no complaints of chest pain. His ECG and cardiac enzymes were done every 4 hr.

The CK results for the first 24 hr were as follows:

Day 1		Day 2	
5:30 AM	58	1:30 AM	496
9:30 AM	320	5:30 AM	399
1:30 PM	587		
5:30 PM	634		
9:30 PM	588		

Mr. Rossetti was continued on aspirin, one 81-mg tablet every day. His heparin infusion was titrated to keep his PTT 45–60 sec. He was carefully monitored for signs of bleeding. Eleven hours after rt-PA administration, the nurse noted a hematoma, approximately 15 × 10 cm, on his right groin. Upon investigation, she learned that Mr. Rossetti had blood drawn from both femoral veins in the Emergency Department prior to rt-PA administration. A pressure dressing was applied. On day 2, a hematoma, approximately 4 × 4 cm, was noted on his left groin. Right groin bruising had extended around his flank. By day 3, the hematomas had expanded further and Mr. Rossetti's hematocrit had dropped from 40 to 25%. His heparin infusion was stopped. He was transfused with 2 units of packed red blood cells, and his hematocrit rose to 35%. His aspirin dose was increased to 325 mg q day. He experienced no further problems and was transferred to the cardiac rehabilitation unit. Twenty-four hour ECG monitoring showed no ST changes and no ectopy. An exercise radionuclide ventriculogram showed a left ventricular ejection fraction (LVEF) of 57%, increasing to 64% with exercise. Because the patient weighed 350 pounds and the fluoroscopy table weight limit was 300 pounds, cardiac catheterization was not performed. The decision was made to treat him medically and monitor him closely. He was discharged on day 9.

QUESTIONS AND ANSWERS

1. **What is the rationale for using thrombolytic therapy in the patient with an acute myocardial infarction?**

   Eighty to 90% of patients with acute Q wave infarcts have a coronary artery thrombus obstructing the infarct-related coronary artery in the first few hours after the event (1). The cause of the thrombus is not well established. Thrombus formation almost always occurs at the site of a coronary atherosclerotic plaque. Thrombosis usually results from plaque rupture or endothelial injury with resultant hemorrhage, platelet aggregation, and release of vasoactive substances.

   Blood clots are formed in the body as a result of platelet aggregation at the site of endothelial injury with the formation of fibrin threads. Prothrombin activator catalyzes prothrombin into thrombin. Thrombin converts fibrinogen into fibrin threads. Studies have shown that lysis of the coronary thrombosis and reperfusion can be achieved by giving intracoronary or intravenous thrombolytic agents aimed at interrupting the formation of the fibrin threads.

   A second rationale for the use of thrombolytic therapy related to the finding that myocardial infarction is not a static but a dynamic event. Dogs with coronary artery occlusion followed by reperfusion showed predictable degrees of necrosis depending on the length of coronary artery occlusion (2). Forty minutes of coronary artery occlusion followed by reperfusion resulted in the necrosis of 45% of the myocardial wall thickness supplied by the occluded coronary artery. Three hours of occlusion resulted in necrosis of ⅔ of the supplied wall thickness. Six hours of occlusion resulted in necrosis of 80–85% of the supplied wall thickness. By 6–24 hr, the necrosis was almost transmural. Therefore, necrosis proceeded from the subendocardium to the epicardium in a "wave front" that was time related. Prompt thrombolysis and reperfusion were found to decrease infarct size, salvage myocardium, and decrease mortality by limiting the duration of total coronary artery occlusion.

2. **Compare streptokinase, urokinase, and tissue plasminogen activator.**

   Streptokinase is derived from streptococci bacteria. Streptokinase binds to free and fibrin-bound plasminogen and activates plasminogen to form plasmin. Plasmin acts to dissolve clots in the body by digesting fibrin threads, fibrinogen, and clotting factors V, VIII, and XIII. A systemic lytic state is produced until clotting factors and fibrinogen are resynthesized, which is usually in 24–36 hr. Because streptokinase is derived from a bacteria, it is a foreign protein and may stimulate antibody production. If antibodies develop, the thrombolytic effect may decrease, and allergic reactions including hypotension and anaphylaxis may occur. Up to 5% of patients have antibodies to streptokinase.

If a patient has received streptokinase previously or has had a recent streptococcal infection, another thrombolytic agent must be used. Streptokinase has a half-life of 18 min but the systemic lytic state lasts up to 24–36 hr. Streptokinase may not be the preferred choice if the patient becomes unstable or needs coronary angiography or surgery. Studies indicate that intravenous streptokinase achieves coronary artery patency in 50% of patients.

Urokinase is derived from cultured kidney cells. Urokinase, like streptokinase, acts directly on plasminogen to form plasmin and produces a systemic lytic state. However, it has less effect on fibrinogen depletion and is not antigenic, and thus it may be better tolerated than streptokinase with lower incidence of resistance. Urokinase has a half-life of 10–16 min and given intravenously achieves coronary artery patency in 60% of patients.

Tissue plasminogen activator was isolated in 1979 from a melanoma cell line and is now produced using recombinant DNA technology. rt-PA has a weak affinity for free plasminogen and a strong affinity for fibrin-bound plasminogen. Thus, rt-PA activates plasminogen to form plasmin within the thrombus, with less of a systemic lytic effect. rt-PA is nonantigenic and does not produce an antibody response. The half-life of rt-PA is only 5–7 min. Comparative studies of intravenous thrombolytic agents have reported rt-PA to have a patency rate of 70–75%.

The issue of whether one agent is superior to others is still being debated.

Efficacy

Streptokinase and rt-PA have demonstrated similar results in relation to left ventricular function and mortality but studies differ concerning patency rates. Some feel that streptokinase and rt-PA have a similar patency rate if used early after onset of symptoms, but that rt-PA has a higher patency rate than streptokinase after 4–5 hr. Other studies reported that even early after symptom onset, rt-PA achieved higher patency rate than streptokinase (3).

Side Effects

Bleeding is the primary side effect of thrombolytic therapy. Streptokinase and rt-PA have a similar frequency of bleeding episodes, but rt-PA is clot specific and has a shorter half-life, with more rapid restoration of coagulation. rt-PA and urokinase are nonantigenic. Allergic reactions, resistance, and hypotension are not associated with their use.

Cost

An average dose of rt-PA costs about $2000, urokinase costs about $1300, and streptokinase costs only about $150.

3. **List the indications for thrombolytic therapy in a patient with suspected myocardial infarction.**

The patient should show clinical and ECG evidence of an acute transmural MI, with onset of symptoms within the last 6 hr. Clinical evidence of an MI should include chest pain of at least 30 min in duration that does not respond to nitroglycerin. The onset, location, duration, quality, associated signs and symptoms, and aggravating and alleviating factors of the chest pain must be identified to assess the etiology of the chest pain. Presence of risk factors for coronary artery disease should also be assessed to help determine the etiology of the chest pain. Administration of rt-PA to a patient with chest pain due to active peptic ulcer disease, aortic dissection, pericarditis, or cardiac tamponade could cause devastating hemorrhagic complications.

Mr. Rossetti complained of pain suspicious for myocardial infarction—substernal tightness radiating into his neck and left arm, onset at rest 1 hr ago, unrelieved by nitroglycerin. He experienced nausea, which occurs in up to 50% of patients with an MI, especially inferior. Mr. Rossetti's history revealed risk factors for coronary artery disease—smoking, positive family history, and obesity.

If the patient has had at least 30 min of ischemic chest pain and demonstrates ST elevation of at least 0.1 mV in at least two adjacent limb leads or at least two adjacent precordial leads, a transmural MI is probably occurring. Most studies have indicated a decrease in mortality in patients with anterior or multiple location MIs when treated with thrombolytic therapy but no decrease in mortality in patients with inferior or lateral MIs. With conventional treatment, mortality rates are lower in patients with an inferior MI, patients experiencing their first MI, young patients with an MI, and hemodynamically stable patients; therefore, the benefits of thrombolytic therapy may not outweigh the risks. Some conclude that only patients in the following categories should receive thrombolytic therapy: acute anterior MI, acute inferoposterior MI, acute inferior MI with hemodynamic instability, and acute infarction with previous Q wave infarct in a separate area, presenting within 6 hr after the onset of symptoms.

Others feel that thrombolytic therapy should also be used in the patient with a small transmural inferior or lateral MI. Studies have indicated that thrombolytic therapy produced an improvement in left ventricular function as compared to conventional therapy, and this was true for inferior as well as anterior MIs (4). Because patient prognosis following MI is directly related to left ventricular function, many feel that those with evidence of either a large or small transmural MI should receive thrombolytic therapy. A recent review of the TAMI-1 trial (4) suggests that, although thrombolytic therapy is generally thought to be more beneficial in anterior MI's than inferior MI's, inferior MI patients should not be excluded until further mortality data from large studies is available. The role of thrombolytic therapy in the treatment of patients with a non-Q wave infarct manifested by ST depression on the ECG is uncertain at this point and is not routinely recommended unless there is angiographic evidence of a thrombus. Less than 50% of non-Q wave infarctions result from an occlusive coronary thrombus, although a partial thrombus may be involved.

Mr. Rossetti certainly met the ECG criteria. He demonstrated ST elevation in leads II, III, AVF, and V_1-V_6.

The next criteria to consider is duration of pain. Progression of injury can vary with each patient, but the majority of patients have almost complete necrosis by 6 hr after onset of pain (Recall the "wavefront" phenomenon.) Current recommendations advise that duration of chest pain should be >30 min and <6 hr. Patients treated in <3 hr of presentation show the best result. Almost all studies that have shown an improvement in survival and left ventricular function have given the thrombolytic agent within 4 hr. Patients may be treated 3–6 hr after symptom onset, but patency rates of the infarct artery have been shown to be lower, as has preservation of myocardial function. Hence, the risk-benefit ratio must be scrutinized as time passes. At >6 hr, it is widely accepted that the risks may outweigh the benefits unless the patient is experiencing ongoing chest pain and ongoing signs of ischemia. However, some information suggests that late reperfusion may have a beneficial effect on survival even after 4–6 hours, as artery patency is achieved even though it is too late to salvage myocardium. This is currently under investigation (5). Mr. Rossetti arrived at the hospital 1 hr after symptom onset, and received rt-PA approximately 2 hr after symptom onset.

4. **What are contraindications to thrombolytic therapy with rt-PA?**

Because thrombolytic agents dissolve clots both in the coronary artery and any existing protective clots throughout the vascular system, the benefits of thrombolytic therapy must be weighed against the risk of bleeding. A thorough medical and surgical history and physical examination must be done to identify patients at risk for serious bleeding. Examples of absolute contraindications and relative contraindications are given below.

Absolute Contraindications

Active internal bleeding
Aortic dissection
History of cerebral vascular accident
Intracranial or intraspinal surgery within last 2 months
Severe uncontrolled hypertension (systolic BP > 180, diastolic > 110)
Intracranial neoplasm, aneurysm or arteriovenous malformation
Acute pericarditis
Known bleeding diathesis (e.g. hemophilia)
Prolonged CPR

Relative Contraindications

Age > 75 years
Major surgery, organ biopsy, major trauma (particularly cranial) puncture of noncompressible vessel (e.g., jugular) in past 6 months
History of gastrointestinal or genitourinary bleeding
Hepatic dysfunction
Cerebrovascular disease
Subacute bacterial endocarditis
Diabetic retinopathy
Pregnancy
Patients taking anticoagulants

An example of the importance of identifying these risks was discussed by Korsmeyer et al. (6) in their report of a patient who fainted and hit his head during myocardial infarction, but did not report it. The day after he received streptokinase, his mental status changed and a CT scan showed a frontal lobe hematoma. This illustrates the possible risk of thrombolytic therapy and the critical importance of obtaining a thorough patient history.

5. **Invasive assessment by coronary angiography is the only definitive validation of reperfusion, but this procedure is costly and not available 24 hr/day at all hospitals. What noninvasive methods may be utilized at the bedside to assess the likelihood of reperfusion?**

Three noninvasive clinical markers of reperfusion currently available are rapid resolution of chest pain, normalization of ischemic ECG changes, and reperfusion dysrhythmias, but each marker has limitations. Mr. Rossetti displayed all three.

Chest pain in myocardial infarction is due to myocardial ischemia.

If reperfusion occurs, oxygen and nutrients are delivered to the ischemic myocardium and chest pain should be relieved. However, pain is subjective and difficult to quantify. Relief of chest pain may occur in response to narcotics or nitrates rather than reperfusion. Relief of chest pain may also occur when the ischemic myocardium becomes necrotic. Quantifying the pain at the onset of therapy and assessing for changes may help determine if the pain relief is occurring in response to reperfusion.

Normalization of ECG changes, reflected by rapid return of the ST segment elevation to normal, is the most objective sign of reperfusion. ST segment resolution may be delayed because of myocardial "stunning," or depression of myocardial function after an ischemic episode, which may persist for several days.

Reperfusion dysrhythmias have been noted to occur with angiographically documented reestablishment of blood flow to the ischemic myocardium. Reperfusion dysrhythmias result from changes in electrical and chemical gradients caused by the washout of electrolytes and metabolites accumulated in the ischemic myocardium. The most common dysrhythmias associated with reperfusion are ventricular tachycardia, sinus bradycardia, PVCs, accelerated idioventricular rhythm (AIVR), supraventricular tachycardia, ventricular bigeminy, trigeminy, and quadrigeminy, and first, second, and third degree heart blocks. Because dysrhythmias frequently occur due to ischemia and injury in the normal course of an MI, it is difficult to determine if they are due to reperfusion. Therefore, the appearance of reperfusion dysrhythmias is not considered an accurate marker of reperfusion.

If all three markers appear, this is very predictive of reperfusion, but all three appear in only a small percentage of patients. Studies report that complete ST segment resolution is the best predictor of reperfusion, but only 6% of patients display this sign. Partial ST segment resolution occurred in 38% of patients and was a fair predictor. Dramatic relief of chest pain occurred in 29% of patients and was found to be a good predictor of reperfusion (7). As stated previously, the appearance of dysrhythmias is less accurate in predicting reperfusion. Research continues to discover more accurate noninvasive methods to detect reperfusion, including (MM) isoform analysis (a breakdown of the CK-MM isoenzyme), computerized ST segment trend monitoring, signal averaged ECGs, and rapid sequence CT scanning and PET (proton-emission tomography) scanning. Documenting reperfusion may be beneficial so that a back-up strategy to achieve reperfusion, such as PTCA, can be performed if necessary.

6. **Describe how serial analysis of cardiac enzymes may provide evidence of reperfusion.**

    An "early CK peak" is a late indicator of reperfusion. Reperfusion causes a washout of CK from the infarct zone and may accelerate the rate and amount of CK release into the plasma as compared to that occurring with continued occlusion. With reperfusion, an "early peak" may occur in 8–15 hr instead of the 12–24 hr normally seen. Mr. Rossetti's CK peaked in 12 hr. Because CK and CK-MB fractions are late indicators of reperfusion, MM isoforms are being studied that may increase 15–30 min after reperfusion, allowing a more rapid assessment.

7. **Complications associated with thrombolytic therapy include bleeding, coronary artery reocclusion, and reperfusion dysrhythmias. Discuss the prevention, assessment, and management of bleeding complications.**

    Mr. Rossetti had hematomas from groin punctures, which expanded and were associated with a decreased Hct. Surface bleeding, usually from venous and arterial puncture sites and cardiac catheterization access sites, is the most frequently reported bleeding complication (20–40%), with groin hematomas very common. Microscopic hematuria is also seen frequently. Less frequent complications (<10%) include gingival bleeding, epistaxis, hemoptysis, occult blood in stool or emesis, bleeding from abrasions, gross hematuria, and frank GI bleeding. Infrequent complications are retroperitoneal (<1–3%) and intracranial (<0.5%) bleeding.

    Prevention
    a. Identify patients at high risk. In addition to those patients mentioned in question 4, patients at increased risk of bleeding include those undergoing invasive procedures, those of small body size, and those in older age groups.
    b. Establish IV lines prior to rt-PA administration. Three lines are recommended: one for rt-PA, one for lidocaine and heparin, and one for a heparin lock. Maintain IV patency to avoid punctures. Avoid discontinuing access sites for 24 hr. Do not use a noncompressible IV site such as the jugular or subclavian.
    c. Avoid or minimize arterial or venous punctures. Use a heparin lock. Apply pressure to all puncture sites for 30 min or as needed. Cover with a pressure dressing.
    d. Do not give IM injections.
    e. For 24 hr avoid vigorous tooth brushing and use an electric razor for shaving.

f. Avoid unnecessary handling of the patient to minimize bruising, trauma.
g. Post a "bleeding precautions" sign at the bedside.
h. Maintain heparin drip at a level to keep PT/PTT within ordered limits.

Patient Assessment

a. Monitor for bleeding or hematomas from puncture sites.
b. Monitor for bleeding from gingiva, especially in patients with poor dental hygiene. Bleeding from gingiva in a patient with nausea and vomiting may be mistaken for GI bleeding.
c. Monitor vital signs for signs of hypovolemia.
d. Monitor neurological signs frequently for up to 24 hr.
e. Monitor for changes in Hgb, Hct, PT, PTT. The Hct decreases somewhat with rt-PA even without bleeding. Many patients are dehydrated on admission and have a falsely high Hct, which decreases with hydration. PT, PTT should be 1½–2 times normal.
f. Monitor urine and stool for occult blood.
g. Watch for signs/symptoms of retroperitoneal bleeding post-cardiac catheterization, including low back pain, diminished pedal pulses, and muscle weakness.

Management

a. If surface bleeding at an access site occurs, apply direct pressure for at least 20–30 min or until bleeding stops. Cover with a pressure dressing. Continue thrombolytic therapy.
b. If a hematoma develops, mark area with date and time and watch for expansion.
c. If gingival bleeding occurs, aminocaproic acid (Amicar) mouthwash may be used.
d. If major bleeding is noted or if signs of intracranial bleeding occur, discontinue rt-PA and heparin and call the physician immediately.

8. **Discuss the prevention, assessment, and management of coronary artery reocclusion.**

Reocclusion of the infarct-related artery occurs in up to 20% of patients, usually within 24 hr, and may result in reinfarction. Although rt-PA lyses the clot, it does not cure the underlying cause of the clot formation, which is the atherosclerotic plaque. Eighty to 90% of patients have a high grade residual stenosis. Elective PTCA or CABG may be performed to treat the stenosis. The risk of reocclusion increases with severe residual stenosis or with inadequate or interrupted thrombolytic therapy. The ideal regimen to prevent reperfusion is still being debated.

Prevention

a. Maintain rt-PA infusion at ordered rate.
b. Maintain heparin drip as ordered to keep PT, PTT 1½–2 times normal.
c. Administer antiplatelets as ordered—ASA or Dipyridamole may be used.
d. Vasodilators, e.g., nitroglycerin or Isordil may be used.

Assessment

a. Monitor patient for return of signs and symptoms of ischemia: chest pain, nausea, hemodynamic compromise.
b. Monitor ECG for ST segment elevation, T wave inversion, dysrhythmias.
c. Monitor cardiac enzymes for a second rise.

Management

a. Notify physician if any signs of reocclusion are noted.
b. Administer medications for pain/dysrhythmias as ordered.
c. Emergency measures may include cardiac catheterization, repeat thrombolytic therapy, PTCA, or CABG if not eligible for PTCA.

9. **Mr. Rossetti had ventricular bigeminy, trigeminy, and quadrigeminy, a possible consequence of reperfusion. How should reperfusion dysrhythmias be managed?**

   Many thrombolytic therapy protocols initiate prophylactic lidocaine infusions to prevent ventricular dysrhythmias. As in any patient with a myocardial infarction, continuous ECG monitoring should be employed and emergency drugs and equipment should be available. PVCs and accelerated idioventricular rhythm (AIVR), both frequently seen during reperfusion, are usually well tolerated. AIVR is usually a benign rhythm and should not be treated unless there is hemodynamic compromise. Dysrhythmias causing hemodynamic compromise should be treated as dysrhythmias are traditionally treated in the patient with an acute MI.

10. **Identify possible nursing diagnoses for the acute MI patient receiving thrombolytic therapy.**

    Potential for decreased myocardial tissue perfusion related to coronary artery reocclusion
    Potential for cardiac dysrhythmias related to reperfusion
    Potential for decreased blood pressure related to bleeding
    Potential for alteration in comfort related to myocardial ischemia
    Knowledge deficit related to role of risk factors in coronary artery disease

Potential for alteration in peripheral tissue perfusion related to acute myocardial infarction.

REFERENCES

1. Dewood MA, Spores J, Natske R, et al. Prevalence of total coronary occlusion during the early hours of transmural myocardial infarction. N Engl J Med 1980; 303:897–902.
2. Reimer KA, Lower JE, Rasmussen MM, Jennings RB. The wavefront phenomena of ischemic cell death: 1. Myocardial infarct size vs. duration of coronary occlusion in dogs. Circulation 1977;56:786–794.
3. Verstraete M. Thrombolysis after myocardial infarction [Letter]. Lancet 1988; 1:763.
4. Bates ER, Califf RM, Stack RS, et al. Thrombolysis and angioplasty in myocardial (TAMI-1) trial: Influences of infarct location on arterial patency, left ventricular function and mortality. J Am Coll Cardiol 1989;13:12–18.
5. Braunwald E. Thrombolytic reperfusion of acute myocardial infarction: Resolved and unresolved issues. J Am Coll Cardiol 1988;12:85A–92A.
6. Korsmeyer C, Midden AL, Taylor GJ. The nurse's role in thrombolytic therapy for acute MI. Crit Care Nurse 1987; 7(6):22–30.
7. Califf RM, O'Neil W, Stack RS, et al. Failure of simple clinical measurements to predict perfusion status after intravenous thrombolysis. Ann Intern Med 1988;108: 658–662.

SUGGESTED READINGS

Bates ER, Califf RM, Stack RS, et al. Thrombolysis and angioplasty in myocardial (TAMI-1) trial: Influence of infarct location on arterial patency, left ventricular function and mortality. J Am Coll Cardiol 1989;13:12–18.

Braunwald E. Thrombolytic reperfusion of acute myocardial infarction: Resolved and unresolved issues. J Am Coll Cardiol 1988;12:85A–92A.

Brooks-Brunn JA. Thrombolytic intervention and its effect on mortality in acute myocardial infarction: Review of clinical trials. Heart Lung 1988;17(6)(suppl)Part 2:756–761.

Brooks-Brunn JA. Formulating appropriate nursing diagnoses for the patient receiving tissue-type plasminogen activator. Heart Lung 1987;16(6)(suppl)Part 2:787–791.

Cairns JA, Collins R, Fuster V, Passamani E. Coronary thrombolysis. Chest 1989; 95(suppl):735–875.

Califf RM, O'Neil W, Stack RS, et al. Failure of simple clinical measurements to predict perfusion status after intravenous thrombolysis. Ann Intern Med 1988; 108:658–662.

Dewood M, Spores J, Natske R, et al. Prevalence of total coronary occlusion during the early hours of transmural myocardial infarction. N Engl J Med 1980;303:897–902.

Henderson E. Assessment of successful reperfusion after thrombolysis. Heart Lung 1988;17(6)(suppl)Part 2:761–771.

Kennedy JW. Thrombolytic therapy for acute myocardial infarction: A brief review. Heart Lung 1987;16(6)(suppl)Part 2:740–745.

Kleven MR. Comparison of thrombolytic agents: Mechanism of action efficacy, safety. Heart Lung 1988;17(6)(suppl)Part 2:750–755.

Kline E. Management of bleeding in the patient receiving thrombolytic therapy for acute myocardial infarction: A nursing perspective. Heart Lung 1988;17(6) (suppl)Part 2:777–781.

Kline EM. Recombinant tissue-type plasminogen activator in acute myocardial infarction: Role of the critical care nurse. Heart Lung 1987;16(6)(suppl)Part 2:779–786.

Korsmeyer C, Midden AL, Taylor GJ. The nurse's role in thrombolytic therapy for acute MI. Crit Care Nurse 1987;7(6):22–30.

Mark DB, Hlatky MA, O'Connor CM, et al. Administration of thrombolytic therapy in the community hospital: Established principles and unresolved issues. J Am Coll Cardiol 1988;12:32A–43A.

Misinski M. Pathophysiology of acute myocardial infarction: A rationale for thrombolytic therapy. Heart Lung 1988;17(6) (suppl)Part 2:743–750.

Patient selection and care guidelines—
Activase. San Francisco, Genentech,
Inc., 1988.

Ramsden CS. Treatment strategies after successful thrombolysis in acute myocardial infarction. Heart Lung 1988;17(6)
(suppl)Part 2:777–781.

Reimer KA, Lower JE, Rasmussen MM,
Jennings RB. The wavefront phenomena
of ischemic cell death: 1. Myocardial infarct size vs. duration of coronary occlusion in dogs. Circulation 1977;56:786–794.

Sobel BE. Fibrinolysis and activators of
plasminogen. Heart Lung 1987;16(6)
(suppl)Part 2:775–779.

Topol EJ. Clinical use of streptokinase and
urokinase therapy for acute myocardial infarction. Heart Lung 1987;16(6)(suppl)
Part 2:760–774.

Verstraete M. Thrombolysis after myocardial infarction [Letter]. Lancet 1988;
1:763.

CHAPTER 16

Unstable Angina and Percutaneous Transluminal Coronary Angioplasty

Margaret A. Wegner, RN, BSN, CCRN

Carl Harris, a 60-year-old man, presented to the Emergency Department with complaints of exertional chest pain for the past 4 days, culminating in a 15-min episode of chest and jaw pain while watching television on the evening of his arrival. The patient described the pain as a "heavy, deep, burning heartburn" in the center of his chest, which radiated to his left shoulder and the left jaw as an "aching pain." The pain occurred at the end of his daily eight to ten block walk for each of 3 days prior to arrival. Each episode lasted 5 min or less, resolved without intervention other than rest, and was not associated with any other symptoms.

On the morning of arrival, chest and jaw pain were noted at a walking distance of only three blocks, but again resolved spontaneously and occurred without associated symptoms. While watching television that evening, Mr. Harris experienced a 15-min episode of chest and jaw pain accompanied by SOB, diaphoresis, and nausea without vomiting. The episode resolved spontaneously, and Mr. Harris was pain-free on arrival in the Emergency Department.

Mr. Harris stated that he had noticed increasing dyspnea on exertion and fatigue over the past 6 months, which he attributed to his age and relatively sedentary life-style. He denied orthopnea, paroxysmal nocturnal dyspnea, lower extremity edema, family history of cardiac problems, diabetes, hypertension, or coronary artery disease. His history included smoking 2 packs of cigarettes/day for 25 years, but none for the past 13 years. His occupation was noted as retired clerical worker. He had no prior medical history.

On initial examination Mr. Harris did not appear to be in any distress. Normal S_1 and S_2 were auscultated with an intermittent S_4 and no S_3 or murmur. Admission vital signs were:

BP	154/94
HR	66, regular
Resp	16, even and unlabored
Temp	37.1° C

One inch of Nitropaste was applied to his chest wall, resulting in a BP of 128/76 after 30 min.

Laboratory results were significant for normal ABG, CBC, electrolytes, cardiac enzymes, and thyroid function tests. Cholesterol and triglyceride levels were elevated. Admission chest x-ray revealed a normal sized heart. Admission 12-lead ECG showed normal sinus rhythm without ectopy, with normal axis.

Mr. Harris was admitted to the CCU with a diagnosis of new onset unstable angina (USA) and possible myocardial infarction (MI).

QUESTIONS AND ANSWERS

1. What is unstable angina?

Angina pectoris is a syndrome characterized by periods of chest pain or discomfort due to myocardial ischemia. The pain may be described as mild to severe, with gradual to sudden onset. Anginal pain may be located in the sub, mid, or retrosternal area. It frequently radiates to the jaw, neck, shoulder, arm, back, or epigastric area. Descriptions of the quality of this pain range from heavy, pressing, squeezing, crushing, and tightness to a burning or a dull ache. The pain is generally not sharply localized and lasts <15 min. Angina pain is frequently accompanied by nausea, vomiting, diaphoresis, shortness of breath, dyspnea, tachypnea, bradycardia or tachycardia, increase in blood pressure, fear, anxiety, and/or weakness. It is usually precipitated by emotional stress, physical exercise or stress, ingestion of a heavy meal, or exposure to extremes in weather. Relief is generally obtained within 45–90 sec by rest and/or use of sublingual NTG tablets.

USA is also called crescendo or preinfarction angina. In USA, the characteristics of the pain episodes change. Frequency, severity, and/or duration of pain usually increase. The pain may occur with less stimulation, at rest, or while asleep. There may be new associated signs and symptoms or a new pattern of radiation with each anginal attack. Unstable angina may be difficult to distinguish from non-Q wave infarction. (See Chapter 13, "Non-Q Wave Myocardial Infarction.")

2. What factors may precipitate an anginal attack?

Angina is due to myocardial ischemia, resulting from an imbalance between myocardial oxygen supply and demand. This can result from an increase in myocardial oxygen demand, a decrease in myocardial oxygen supply, or a combination of both.

Factors that increase myocardial oxygen demand include:

Dysrhythmias
Hypertension
Hyperthyroidism

Emotional stress (i.e., anxiety)
Physical stress (i.e., exercise)
Structural cardiac abnormalities (i.e., left ventricular aneurysm)

Factors that decrease myocardial oxygen supply include:

Anemia
Atherosclerosis
Dysrhythmias
Embolism
Hypotension
Structural cardiac abnormalities (i.e., aortic valve disease)
Thrombosis (i.e., platelet aggregation)
Vasospasm

The exact events inciting an episode of unstable angina vary from person to person. For most unstable angina attacks, the pathophysiologic mechanism believed to be involved is:

Formation of atherosclerotic plaque(s) in the coronary artery(s).
Disruption or ulceration of the plaque(s), which results in a rough, irregular coronary artery endothelial surface.
Repetitive transient episodes of platelet aggregation, or "plugging," at the site of the plaque(s). These platelets may release substances (i.e., serotonin, thromboxane A_2), which act as coronary artery constrictors.
The decreased blood flow to the myocardium, which is secondary to coronary artery lumen narrowing as a result of the platelet "plug" formation and vasoconstriction, results in an inadequate myocardial oxygen supply to meet the demand. Myocardial ischemia follows.

This process is similar to the process that leads to myocardial infarction. However, in USA, spontaneous lysis occurs before extensive injury develops.

3. **What physiologic changes cause the pain and associated signs and symptoms of USA?**
   Ischemia causes the membranes of the myocardial cells, white blood cells, and platelets to become increasingly permeable. Potassium, serotonin, and histamine are released from these cells into the circulation, where they stimulate the nerve fibers responsible for the sensation of pain. These nerve fibers are also stimulated by lactic acid created by the anaerobic metabolism occurring in the hypoxic myocardial tissues. In the spinal cord, cardiac pain fibers stimulate sensory nerves from other body areas, resulting in the radiation of chest pain to the neck, jaw, shoulders, etc.
   Anginal pain, combined with a decrease in cardiac performance

during pain episodes, stimulates the autonomic nervous system, re-sulting in the associated signs and symptoms.

Admission orders included continuous cardiac monitoring, strict bedrest (to decrease myocardial oxygen demand), and obtaining a 12-lead ECG and cardiac enzyme levels every 6 hr for the first 24 hr. An intravenous line was placed with D_5W infusing at a TKO rate. Mr. Harris was placed on supplemental oxygen at 2 liters/min via nasal cannula. Medication orders included:

heparin	5000 units SC BID
aspirin	one PO q day
Nitropaste (NTP)	1 inch topically q 6 hr
diltiazem	30 mg PO TID (hold for systolic BP <100)

4. What is the goal of medical management in the USA patient?

Ideally, medical management of the USA patient would be aimed at treating the cause of myocardial ischemia in the individual patient. Because it is usually impossible to know the exact cause of ischemia, initial treatment usually includes medications to:

Prevent thrombus formation
Prevent platelet aggregation
Promote vasodilatation
Prevent vasoconstriction
Increase myocardial oxygen supply
Decrease myocardial oxygen demand

5. What are the pharmacological effects of heparin?

Heparin is an anticoagulant that prevents the extension of existing blood clots and inhibits the formation of new blood clots. It does not lyse thrombi already in existence.

Heparin may be administered via the SC or IV route. Administered subcutaneously, the onset of action is within 2–4 hr and the duration of action is 8–12 hr. It is given SC into the fatty layer of the abdomen just above the iliac crest, avoiding the area 2 inches around the umbilicus, using a small gauge needle (26 or 27) of ½–⅝-inch length. A normal SC dose would be 5000 units BID. Whereas subcutaneous heparin at a dose of 5000 units BID is efficacious in preventing deep vein thrombosis, it has minimal effect on systemic clotting.

Heparin given by IV push has its peak within minutes. A normal IV dose would be a 5000-unit IV push bolus, followed by a continuous heparin infusion per infusion pump, titrated to keep the serum partial thromboplastin time (PTT) 1½–2 times the normal value. Heparin administration results in prolonged thrombin time, PT, and PTT. These clotting times usually return to normal 2–6 hr after discontinu-ation of the intravenous heparin infusion.

Side effects of heparin administration include bleeding (i.e., hematuria, hematemesis) and local reactions at the site of injection (i.e., itching, ecchymosis, pain). Protamine sulfate is the antidote used to reverse the effects of heparin. Heparin administration is contraindicated in patients with active bleeding or bleeding tendencies.

While the patient is receiving heparin, all fecal material and emesis should be tested for occult blood. The nurse should assess for bleeding from puncture sites, hematuria, etc. The patient should be instructed to be careful not to bump, bruise, or cut him- or herself while shaving. Coagulation times should be checked every 4–8 hr.

6. **What is the potential benefit of daily aspirin administration in USA?**
    Aspirin, 325–1300 mg PO q day, acts as a platelet aggregation inhibitor, to prevent platelet "plug" formation at the site(s) of coronary artery plaque(s). Major side effects include GI upset and GI bleeding. Taking aspirin with food may decrease the incidence of GI upset without reducing the total amount absorbed. The antiplatelet effects of heparin may last for days.

7. **What are the desired pharmacological effects of nitrates?**
    Nitrates are used to decrease myocardial oxygen demand and increase myocardial oxygen supply simultaneously. This is accomplished by relaxation of vascular smooth muscle cells in both arteries and veins. As blood pools in the dilated peripheral venous system, a decreased amount of blood returns to the heart. This results in a lesser amount of stretch on the myocardial cells at the beginning of each contraction (preload), reducing the myocardial oxygen demand. Myocardial oxygen supply is increased by nitrates, as these medications dilate the coronary arteries, relieve vasospasm, and improve collateral circulation to areas of the myocardium supplied otherwise by diseased coronary arteries.

    Immediate, short-term therapy for chest discomfort due to USA is administration of sublingual NTG tablets (0.3–0.4 mg). Sublingual NTG acts within 30–60 sec of administration, with peak effects at 4–5 min. Duration of action is 20–30 min. The tablets are administered at 5-min intervals.

    Long-term therapy with nitrates will usually include oral and/or topical routes of administration. These longer-acting agents help to decrease the frequency of pain episodes. The effects of isosorbide dinitrate (Isordil) PO begin within 15–30 min, peak within 45–120 min, and last 3–6 hr. A typical dose is 10–60 mg PO q 3–6 hr. Tolerance may develop with sustained administration of nitrates (IV or topical, but is less common with intermittent oral nitrates). Side effects are those associated with systemic vasodilatation (i.e., headache, flushing, dizziness, weakness, postural hypotension, perspiration, palpitations, tachycardia, etc.). The headache caused by nitrate administration is usually relieved by administration of acetaminophen, 325–650 mg PO q 4–6 hr as needed.

Topical NTG ointment acts within 15–30 minutes. Duration of action is variable, as it is slowly absorbed, but is usually 3 or more hr. It is applied on special measuring paper, spread into a uniform, thin layer (not using one's finger), and then secured to the body, avoiding areas used for defibrillator paddles in emergency situations. It is important to remove old Nitropaste before reapplication to avoid overdosage. Common side effects associated with use of NTG ointment include all those associated with administration of Isordil, and occasionally skin rash. A typical dose would be 1–2 inches applied every 4–6 hr.

Another form of nitrate therapy commonly administered to the USA patient is a continuous intravenous infusion. The NTG is diluted to the desired concentration in D_5W or NS, in a glass bottle. It is administered with an infusion pump using non-polyvinyl chloride tubing only. Onset of action with IV administration of NTG is 1–2 min. Peak effects will also be noted at 1–2 min, and duration of action is usually 3–5 min.

The dosage is measured in micrograms/minute, i.e.:

$$\frac{X \ \mu g \ NTG}{Y \ volume \ (ml) \ of \ diluent} \times \frac{Z \ infusion \ rate \ (ml/hr)}{60 \ (min/hr)} = \frac{W \ \mu g}{min}$$

The NTG infusion is usually started at 5 μg/min and increased by 5–10 μg/min every 5 min, with close monitoring of blood pressure for hypotension, until chest discomfort is relieved or the BP reaches a level predetermined by the physician, based on the patient's baseline BP. There is no fixed typical or optimum dose, as patient response to IV NTG is highly variable. Side effects include hypotension, headache, and those of vasodilatation as previously listed. Tolerance will invariably develop with sustained use of IV NTG.

8. **How do calcium channel blockers work?**
    (See Chapter 17, "Vasospastic (Prinzmetal's) Angina.")

9. **Why are β-blockers prescribed in the medical management of USA?**
    β-Blockers work by competing with β-receptor agonists at the adrenergic receptor sites to prevent the release of catecholamines. The resultant inhibition of cardiac response to the sympathetic nervous system causes a decrease in heart rate, force of myocardial contraction, arterial blood pressure, and cardiac output. These ef-

fects are beneficial to the USA patient, as they decrease myocardial oxygen demand, hopefully preventing myocardial ischemia. One potential disadvantage of β-blocker administration is coronary artery vasoconstriction. This is countered by the vasodilating effects of nitrates and calcium channel blockers given in conjunction with β-blockers.

Propranolol hydrochloride (Inderal) is a common β-blocker administered in USA. Given PO, onset of action is within 30 min, peak action is within $1-1\frac{1}{2}$ hr, and duration of action is 6 hr. A typical dose would be 10–20 mg PO TID or QID, increasing gradually to a total of 80–480 mg PO q day. Side effects include bradycardia, AV block, asystole, hypotension, bronchospasm, laryngospasm, fluid retention, and congestive heart failure. Propranolol may mask the signs and symptoms of hypoglycemia. β-blockers may also increase serum cholesterol and LDL levels. Administration in patients with heart failure, cardiogenic shock, bronchial asthma, bradycardia, AV block greater than first degree, or insulin-dependent diabetes mellitus should be avoided.

On the first evening of admission, Mr. Harris complained of a 15-min episode of "heartburn." The discomfort radiated from the center of his chest to his left neck. He also complained at this time of left jaw numbness, shortness of breath, and nausea. Nursing interventions included checking vital signs (BP, 150/90), obtaining a 12-lead ECG while the pain was present, administering two sublingual nitroglycerin tablets at 5-min intervals, and remaining with Mr. Harris in a calm, reassuring manner. Cardiac auscultation revealed the presence of an S_4. A repeat 12-lead ECG was obtained after the pain was relieved.

10. **Mr. Harris' 12-lead ECG during this anginal attack showed NSR with a normal axis, T wave inversion in leads I, AVL, V_2–V_6, and ST segment depression in leads V_4–V_6. His ECG at rest, without chest pain, showed all ST segments returned to baseline with continued T wave inversion in V_{2-6}. What are the typical ECG changes associated with USA? What is the underlying pathophysiologic basis for these ECG changes?**

Evidence of subendocardial myocardial ischemia, namely ST segment depression or, on rare occasion elevation, and T wave flattening or inversion, are the most common ECG changes associated with USA. Mr. Harris had evidence of ischemia in the anterior and lateral leads. These ECG changes would lead one to suspect an inadequate blood supply was being provided to the areas of the myocardium perfused by the left coronary artery. With rest and vasodilatation from nitrates, the myocardial oxygen supply was once again great enough to meet the demand. Spontaneous lysis of the platelet plug probably played a role in increasing the myocardial oxygen supply as well. The ischemia resolved, and the ECG tracing returned to the patient's baseline configuration.

In ischemic tissues, anaerobic metabolism ensues, producing inadequate amounts of energy (ATP) to properly regulate the movement of sodium and potassium ions in and out of myocardial cells. As sodium builds up in the cells and potassium continues to leak out of the cells, the normal sequence of depolarization and repolarization is disrupted, leading to the ST segment and T wave alterations characteristic of USA.

Mr. Harris' serum cardiac enzyme levels remained within normal limits for the first 24 hr of his admission, and myocardial infarction was therefore ruled out.

11. Why are serum cardiac enzyme levels within normal limits in USA?

Myocardial cells are rich in the cardiac enzymes creatine phosphokinase (CK), aspartate aminotransferase (AST) (formerly called serum glutamic oxyloacetic transaminase (SGOT)) and lactic dehydrogenase (LDH). With myocardial infarction, enzymes leak out of the cells and plasma levels of these enzymes are elevated. In USA, although ischemia occurs, cellular necrosis does not occur, so no enzymes leak out into the serum.

On the second day of hospitalization, Mr. Harris' nitrate therapy was changed to include Isordil, 20 mg PO TID, and NTG was decreased to only 1 inch topically QHS, to be removed each morning.

Mr. Harris had two episodes of angina the next morning, both of which were relieved by sublingual NTG. He was started on diltiazem and a continuous intravenous infusion of heparin at 1000 units/hr per infusion pump. He consented to a cardiac catheterization for coronary angiography for the next morning at 7:00 AM.

In preparation for cardiac catheterization, Mr. Harris was made NPO after midnight. All medications were administered as previously ordered, with the exception of the intravenous heparin infusion, which was discontinued at midnight. Blood was sent for group, screen, and hold so packed red blood cells (PRBCs) would be readily available for transfusion in the unlikely event Mr. Harris experienced massive blood loss during or after the procedure. On the following morning, Mr. Harris was premedicated with Benadryl, 50 mg PO to prevent potential allergic reactions to the contrast dye and Valium, 10 mg PO to allay anxiety prior to and during the procedure. He was then transported to the cardiac catheterization laboratory where the procedure was performed in a controlled environment, using fluoroscopy.

12. What is the purpose of coronary angiography in evaluation of USA?

The purpose of coronary angiography in this setting is to assess coronary artery anatomy. The location of atherosclerotic lesions and extent of coronary artery occlusion can be determined, as can the location and patency of collateral circulation.

13. What are the potential complications of cardiac catheterization and angiography?

Potential complications include dysrhythmias, vasospasm, myocardial infarction, pericardial tamponade, perforation of a heart vessel, systemic embolization, allergic reaction to the contrast medium, bleeding, infection at the puncture site, or loss of a pulse in the affected extremity distal to the puncture site. For postcatheterization care, see Chapter 17, "Vasospastic (Prinzmetal's) Angina.")

Mr. Harris' coronary angiography results were significant for:

Right coronary artery
  proximal ⅓   50% stenosis
  mid ⅓   25% stenosis
  distal ⅓   within normal limits
Left anterior descending artery
  mid ⅓   75% stenosis

The cardiologists recommended a percutaneous transluminal coronary angioplasty (PTCA) of the left anterior descending artery. Mr. Harris consented and the procedure was scheduled for the following morning at 7:00 AM.

14. What does the PTCA procedure involve?

PTCA is a method of revascularization for some patients with coronary artery disease. Access to the occluded coronary artery is obtained by passing a balloon-tipped dilatation catheter up through a sheath in the femoral artery. (Occasionally the brachial vessels will be used.) Intracoronary NTG may be given to prevent or reduce coronary artery spasm, as the balloon portion of the catheter is centered over the atheroma (plaque) using fluoroscopy. The balloon is inflated with a mixture of contrast medium and NS for 30–45 sec. This cracks the plaque and enlarges the vessel lumen. The balloon is deflated to visually assess the arterial dilatation, but may be reinflated several times within a matter of minutes to attempt plaque compression again. Heparin, 10,000 units by IV push, is given during the procedure to prevent thrombus formation. A heparin infusion should be continued for 24–48 hr afterward to prevent acute reocclusion.

15. How are PTCA candidates chosen?
In the past, the ideal PTCA candidate was age 60 years or less, had single vessel coronary artery disease (CAD) with a proximal, noncalcified lesion, and good collateral flow to the area normally supplied by the artery involved. Ideally the PTCA candidate would also be a candidate for coronary artery bypass grafting (CABG), have a history of stable angina for <1 year, and would have good left ventricular function. As technology improves, angioplasty is being successfully performed on candidates with multiple vessel CAD, single vessel CAD with multiple lesions, USA, acute myocardial infarction, and cardiogenic shock.

16. Are there any potential complications of PTCA?
Yes. Potential complications of PTCA include:

Emboli
Dissection or rupture of the coronary artery, resulting in need for emergency CABG
Angina (due to arterial occlusion while the balloon is inflated)
Myocardial infarction
Restenosis (2–6% within the first 24 hr after angioplasty)
Dysrhythmias
Bleeding
Infection
Death (overall mortality, less than 1%)

17. How is the success of a PTCA procedure determined?
There is not one widely accepted method of evaluating the success of PTCA. Angiography under fluoroscopy is commonly used to estimate the amount of residual stenosis. Successful PTCA would be considered an increase by 20% or greater in the diameter of the stenosed vessel or a residual stenosis of <50%. There are also computer-based methods that are capable of measuring the stenosed vessel diameter and lumen cross-sectional area. Success is also considered by some if the pressure proximal and distal to the lesion is within 10 mm Hg. Perhaps most importantly, the PTCA can be deemed successful if the patient resumes a life-style normal for him or her, relieved of the signs and symptoms of angina. An increased exercise capacity and improved myocardial perfusion per thallium-201 imaging should also be noted at this time.

Angioplasty of the left anterior descending coronary artery in Mr. Harris resulted in a decrease from 75 to 30% (estimated) stenosis. He suffered no complications, including chest pain, throughout the procedure.

Postangioplasty care of Mr. Harris was identical to that given postcardiac catheterization with one exception. Both the venous and arterial sheaths were left in place for 4 hr per post-PTCA routine, for easy access should restenosis occur. After the sheaths were removed, pressure was held at the site for at least 30 min, a pressure dressing was applied, and a sandbag was kept on the site for 6 hr. The affected extremity and site were then assessed per postcatheterization routine. Mr. Harris remained in CCU for cardiac monitoring for the next 24 hr. Patient teaching was done during this time to assist Mr. Harris in modifying his risk factors for CAD. He was discharged home the following day on a medication regimen including aspirin, diltiazem, Isordil, and Nitropaste.

18. What nursing diagnoses apply in this case?

Potential for altered cardiac tissue perfusion related to catheter placement during cardiac catheterization

Potential for cardiac dysrhythmias related to inadequate myocardial oxygen supply during USA attack

Pain related to ischemia resulting from USA attack

Anxiety related to strange environment

Knowledge deficit regarding diagnosis and treatments

Potential infection related to invasive procedures and invasive lines

Potential alteration in tissue perfusion related to thromboembolism post-PTCA.

SUGGESTED READINGS

Alspach JG, Williams SM. Core curriculum for critical care nursing. 3rd ed. Philadelphia: WB Saunders, 1985:160–161, 164–168.

Braunwald E, Isselbacher KJ, Petersdorf RG, Wilson JD, Martin JB, Fauci AS, eds. Harrison's principles of internal medicine. 11th ed. New York: McGraw-Hill, 1987:981–982.

Conti RC. Unstable angina before and after infarction: Thoughts on pathogenesis and therapeutic strategies. Heart Lung 1986;15(4):361–368.

Doenges ME, Jeffries MF, Moorhouse MF. Nursing care plans: Nursing diagnoses in planning patient care. Philadelphia: FA Davis, 1984:39–42.

Gahart BL. Intravenous medications—A handbook for nurses and other allied health personnel. 4th ed. St. Louis: CV Mosby, 1985:230–232, 360–362.

Galan KM, Hollman JL. Recurrence of stenosis after coronary angioplasty. Heart Lung 1986;15(6):585–587.

Heger JW, Niemann JT, Criley JM. Cardiology for the house officer. 2nd ed. Baltimore: Williams & Wilkins, 1987:123–127.

Hillis LD, Firth BG, Winniford MD, Willerson JT. Manual of clinical problems in cardiology. 3rd ed. Boston: Little, Brown & Co, 1988:72–76, 130–134, 333–359.

Kenner CV, Guzetta CE, Dossey BM. Critical care nursing: Body, mind, spirit. 2nd ed. Boston: Little, Brown & Co, 1982: 584–586.

Klein DM. Angina: Pathophysiology and the resulting signs and symptoms. Nursing 1988;18(7):44–46.

Popma JJ, Dehmer GJ. Care of the patient after coronary angioplasty. Ann Intern Med 1989;110(7):547–559.

Rippe JM, Csete ME, eds. Manual of intensive care medicine. 1st ed. Boston: Little, Brown & Co, 1983:62–63.

CHAPTER 17

Vasospastic (Prinzmetal's) Angina

Margaret A. Wegner, RN, BSN, CCRN

Albert Green, a 48-year-old construction worker, was admitted to the Coronary Care Unit with a diagnosis of vasospastic angina. He complained of substernal chest pressure immediately upon awakening, but before rising from bed, for the past 4 months. Initially the pain averaged only two occurrences per week, with frequency increasing over the past month to three to four episodes per week. The pain always occurred between 4:45 AM and 5:15 AM and lasted 10–15 min.

Significant medical history included smoking 1½ packs of cigarettes/day for the past 30 years and hypertension diagnosed 6 years ago. The patient stated that he had not taken his prescribed antihypertensive medications for the past 9 months. Mr. Green had been evaluated for these same complaints at a local hospital 2 months prior to arrival. He refused cardiac catheterization for coronary angiography at that time and was discharged home after 2 days. During that admission, he had no documented episodes of chest discomfort. Upon his wife's insistence, Mr. Green was seen in the outpatient clinic 3 days prior to this admission, where he presented with complaints of increasingly frequent episodes of early morning chest discomfort. He denied chest discomfort with physical exertion, after heavy meals, or at any other time of day or night. He also denied associated signs and symptoms such as nausea, diaphoresis, dyspnea, or radiation of the pain. As he was pain-free at the time of the clinic visit 3 days ago, he had been sent home with a 48-hr Holter monitor in place to assist with evaluation of his pain episodes.

QUESTIONS AND ANSWERS

1. **What is a Holter monitor?**

   A Holter monitor is an ambulatory electrocardiographic recording device worn on a shoulder strap or attached to the patient's belt. It provides a continuous ECG recording via chest leads, while the patient performs his or her activities of daily living. During Holter monitoring, the patient keeps a log of activities performed, symptoms noted (i.e., chest pain, dizziness, etc.), and times of each. The physician then compares the timed ECG recording with the patient's log of activities and/or symptoms to detect any associated ECG changes or dysrhythmias.

   Mr. Green's Holter monitor tracings revealed sinus bradycardia at 52–58 beats/min with first degree AV block (PR = 0.24). Two epi-

165

sodes of ST segment elevation were noted to correlate with times Mr. Green had documented early morning chest "aching" or "pressure." ST segment normalization was noted after each episode of pain subsided. During the second episode of pain, the Holter monitor showed second degree AV block-Mobitz I (Wenckebach) at 54 beats/min, which resolved with the cessation of chest discomfort.

Mr. Green was immediately contacted at his place of employment to arrange for CCU admission to rule out coronary artery vasospasm. Mr. Green's initial examination revealed a slightly overweight man in no apparent distress.

Admission vital signs were:

BP	184/104
HR	58
Resp	16, even and unlabored
Temp	36.9°C

Normal S_1 and S_2 were auscultated with no murmur, gallop, or rub.

Laboratory results were significant for normal electrolytes, CBC, ABG, cardiac enzymes, and thyroid function tests. Cholesterol and triglyceride levels were slightly elevated. Admission 12-lead ECG showed sinus bradycardia with first degree AV block, no ectopy, normal axis, and normal ST segments. Mr. Green denied any chest discomfort.

Admission orders included 12-lead ECG and cardiac enzyme levels every 6 hr for the first 24 hr, strict bedrest, and continuous cardiac monitoring. An intravenous line was placed with D_5W infusing at a TKO rate. Antihypertensive medications were resumed at previously prescribed doses.

At 4:50 AM the morning after admission, Mr. Green complained of severe substernal chest discomfort—"aching pressure, not sharp." He denied any associated symptoms. Twelve-lead ECG at this time revealed sinus bradycardia with first degree AV block at 54 bpm, no ectopy, and ST segment elevation in leads II, III, and AVF. BP was 150/90. Chest discomfort was relieved immediately with two sublingual nitroglycerin tablets (0.4 mg) administered at 5-min intervals. A repeat 12-lead ECG after resolution of chest pain revealed normalization of ST segments. The remainder of hospital day 2 was unremarkable. Cardiac enzyme levels remained within normal limits. Serial ECGs when the patient was without pain showed no changes from the baseline ECG.

2. **During rounds on the morning after Mr. Green's admission, the attending cardiologist mentioned Prinzmetal's angina as a possible diagnosis. What is Prinzmetal's angina?**

   In 1959, Prinzmetal and coworkers described a syndrome in which anginal pain occurred at rest rather than during physical exertion or emotional excitement. During the episodes of chest pain, the ECG demonstrated ST segment elevation. This completely resolved when the pain subsided, and the pain was easily relieved by sublingual nitroglycerin.

   Prinzmetal's angina has also been termed variant angina. The important differentiation between variant and classical angina is that it occurs at rest, rather than in response to an increase in myocardial oxygen demand, and is associated with ST segment elevation, not depression. Variant angina is due to coronary artery spasm and may occur in either normal or diseased coronary arteries.

3. **Prinzmetal's angina, which occurs at times of minimal or no exertion, has been demonstrated to be due to coronary artery spasm. Does coronary artery spasm ever occur during periods of increased myocardial oxygen demand?**

   Yes. Coronary artery spasm has been shown to play a role not only in Prinzmetal's angina, but also in the development of angina of effort, unstable angina, acute myocardial infarction, and sudden cardiac death. Coronary artery spasm can occur in both normal coronary arteries and in those with varying degrees of obstructive lesions. The term vasospastic angina implies that at least part of the oxygen supply/demand imbalance occurs secondary to transient, abrupt, marked reduction in the diameter of a coronary artery.

4. **What is the significance of cardiac enzyme levels remaining within normal limits after an episode of chest pain?**

   Myocardial cells release certain enzymes into the blood stream when heart muscle damage occurs. These enzymes are creatine phosphokinase (CK), lactic dehydrogenase (LDH), and aspartate aminotransferase (AST) (formerly termed serum glutamic oxaloacetic transaminase (SGOT)). Myocardial injury generally can be ruled out if these blood enzyme levels remain within normal limits.

Mr. Green again complained of moderate chest discomfort upon awakening at 5:05 AM the next morning. Twelve-lead ECG at this time again showed ST segment elevation in leads II, III, and AVF. BP was 156/98. ECG changes resolved and discomfort was relieved after administration of one sublingual nitroglycerin tablet (0.4 mg).

5. **What are the typical ECG changes associated with Prinzmetal's angina?**

ST segment elevation due to transmural myocardial ischemia is the most common ECG change associated with Prinzmetal's angina. The ECG may also show peaked T waves on rare occasion. The ECG typically returns to normal upon resolution of the pain.

Dysrhythmias, including bradycardia, varying degrees of AV block, bundle branch block, and ventricular tachycardia or fibrillation, are sometimes associated with Prinzmetal's angina and occur secondary to ischemia.

Mr. Green's baseline ECG showed sinus bradycardia with first degree AV block. His Holter ECG showed Mobitz I during an episode of chest pain. While hospitalized, 12-lead ECGs done during episodes of chest pain revealed ST segment elevation in leads II, III, and AVF, the inferior leads. These ECG changes would lead one to suspect coronary artery disease and/or spasm of the right coronary artery, which supplies blood to the AV node and inferior surface of the left ventricle.

On hospital day 3, Mr. Green agreed to have coronary angiography performed, with administration of intravenous ergonovine maleate to induce coronary artery vasospasm, if necessary. Prior to cardiac catheterization, Mr. Green was given nothing by mouth, except medications, for 8 hr. Calcium channel blockers and nitrates were withheld. (Note: Had Mr. Green been receiving an intravenous infusion of heparin, this would have been stopped 6–8 hr before the procedure began.) Blood was sent for group, screen, and hold so packed red blood cells (PRBCs) would be readily available for transfusion in the unlikely event Mr. Green experienced massive blood loss during or after the procedure. Informed consent was obtained by the cardiologist. Mr. Green was premedicated with Benadryl, 50 mg PO, to prevent potential allergic responses to the contrast medium used, and Valium, 10 mg PO, to allay anxiety prior to and during the procedure. He was then transported to the cardiac catheterization laboratory where the procedure was performed in a controlled environment.

6. **What is the role of coronary angiography in evaluation of Prinzmetal's angina?**

The purpose of coronary artery angiography in this setting is trifold:

a. *To assess the condition of the coronary arteries at baseline (i.e., while the patient is pain-free).* Coronary artery spasm causing

Prinzmetal's angina may occur at the site of an atherosclerotic lesion or in an anatomically normal ("clean") coronary artery.

b. *To assess the condition of the coronary arteries with spontaneous or induced vasospasm.* In the patient with Prinzmetal's angina, coronary arteriography performed during an episode of spontaneous or ergonovine-induced chest pain demonstrates total or near total occlusion of large epicardial coronary arteries. A 12-lead ECG performed during this episode of spasm would demonstrate the characteristic ST elevation associated with the syndrome.

c. *To assess the response of the coronary artery spasm to intracoronary, intravenous, or sublingual nitroglycerin administration.* Angiographic resolution of the coronary artery occlusion occurs quickly after nitroglycerin administration. Relief of symptoms and normalization of the electrocardiographic changes also occurs.

7. How is coronary artery vasospasm induced during coronary angiography?

Ergonovine maleate is the drug most commonly administered during coronary angiography to induce vasospasm. It is given intravenously as gradually increasing boluses of 0.02–0.20 mg every 3–5 min, until spasm is elicited or a maximum dose of 0.40 mg is given. Ergonovine maleate is an α-adrenergic agonist and, therefore, directly stimulates smooth muscle contraction causing coronary artery spasm. Induced vasospasm is usually severe and localized in one or more coronary arteries.

Coronary artery vasospasm can also be induced with administration of methacholine (a parasympathomimetic agent) or histamine, by exposure to cold, or by administration of an intravenous buffer solution while the patient hyperventilates. However, best results have been obtained using ergonovine.

8. Are there risks involved in artificially inducing coronary artery vasospasm?

Yes. Complications of this test include myocardial infarction secondary to severe ischemia and, upon rare occasion, death. Coronary angiography in Mr. Green revealed a 40% occlusion of the proximal portion of the right coronary artery (RCA). Ergonovine-induced spasm produced an 80–90% occlusion of the RCA at this site. The patient complained of severe substernal pressure at this time. Twelve-lead ECG showed ST segment elevation in leads II, III, and AVF as anticipated. The vasospasm was relieved after intracoronary administration of 200 μg of nitroglycerin. ST segment changes resolved and the patient denied any chest discomfort within 30 sec of nitroglycerin administration. Prinzmetal's angina secondary to coronary artery vasospasm was thus verified as the cause of Mr. Green's chest discomfort.

9. **What are the nursing care priorities following cardiac catheterization?**

Postcatheterization care of Mr. Green included monitoring his vital signs every 15 min for 2 hr, every 30 min for 1 hr, every hour for 3 hr, and then every 2 hr per CCU routine. The femoral access site was evaluated for hematoma formation and active bleeding every 30 min for 3 hr and then every hour for 3 hr. In the event of hematoma formation or bleeding, the physician would have been notified immediately. A sandbag was applied to the entry site for 6 hr and a pressure dressing was maintained at the site until the next morning to prevent hematoma formation. The affected leg, distal to the femoral puncture site, was also evaluated at these times for alterations in temperature, color, or peripheral pulses. The patient was instructed to keep his leg still and notify his nurse of any numbness, tingling, or pain in the affected extremity, or any chest pain. Mr. Green received 1 liter each of NS, ½ NS, and D_5W, consecutively, at a rate of 250 ml/hr, and oral fluids were encouraged to aid in complete clearance of the contrast medium. Diet and medications were resumed as previously ordered. Mr. Green was maintained on strict bedrest for 24 hr and instructed to keep the affected leg immobile during this time. Cardiac enzyme levels were ordered for 24 and 48 hr after catheterization to assess any myocardial tissue damage done during the procedure. A hematocrit level was checked 2 hr postcatheterization to assess for significant blood loss during cardiac catheterization.

Mr. Green was started on nifedipine, 20 mg PO TID.

10. **What is the treatment of choice for vasospastic angina?**

The goal in treatment of vasospastic angina is to prevent coronary artery constriction due to vasospasm. The treatment of choice involves administration of oral calcium channel blockers. The addition of nitrates may be useful in preventing spasm in those patients who continue to have symptoms despite treatment with calcium channel blockers. β-blocking agents are usually avoided, as they may interfere with intrinsic β-adrenergic mediated vasodilatation and exacerbate or prolong coronary vasospasm.

11. How do calcium channel blockers work?

Vascular smooth muscle contraction (i.e., coronary artery constriction) depends on the movement of calcium ions from extracellular to intracellular sites. Calcium channel blockers prevent this influx of calcium ions and produce vasodilatation. These agents help prevent coronary artery vasospasm and maintain maximal oxygen supply to the myocardium. They also antagonize the effects of calcium ions on the cardiac conduction system, causing a decrease in heart rate.

The most commonly prescribed calcium channel blockers and the recommended total daily oral dosage of each are:

verapamil	320–480 mg/day
nifedipine	60–120 mg/day
diltiazem	120–360 mg/day

Calcium channel blockers may cause bradycardia and hypotension. Therefore, close monitoring of vital signs is necessary during initiation of therapy. With continued administration of calcium channel blockers, the ECG should also be closely monitored for prolongation of the PR interval indicating development of first degree AV block, and the development of higher degree block (second or third degree AV block). Other common side effects include constipation, dizziness, flushing, nervousness, edema, and headache. Administration of these agents should be either avoided or implemented only with extreme caution in patients with severe heart failure, high grade conduction disease (second or third degree AV block), hypotension (systolic BP <90 mm Hg), bradycardia (HR <60 beats/min), or concomitant use of digoxin or β-blockers.

12. What are the pharmacological effects of nitrates?

(See Chapter 16, "Unstable Angina and Percutaneous Transluminal Coronary Angioplasty.")

13. What nursing diagnoses apply in this case?

Altered cardiac tissue perfusion related to inadequate myocardial oxygen supply during coronary artery vasospasm

Potential for cardiac dysrhythmias related to inadequate myocardial oxygen supply during coronary artery vasospasm

Pain related to ischemia resulting from coronary artery vasospasm

Anxiety related to strange environment

Knowledge deficit regarding diagnosis and treatment

Potential for injury related to noncompliance with antihypertensive medication regimen

SUGGESTED READINGS

Alspach JG, Williams SM. Core curriculum for critical care nursing. 3rd ed. Philadelphia: WB Saunders, 1985:165.

Conti RC. Unstable angina before and after infarction: Thoughts on pathogenesis and therapeutic strategies. Heart Lung 1986;15(4):361–368.

Heger JW, Niemann JT, Criley JM. Cardiology for the house officer. 2nd ed. Baltimore: Williams & Wilkins, 1987:123–137.

Hillis LD, Firth BG, Winniford MD, Willerson JT. Manual of clinical problems in cardiology. 3rd ed. Boston: Little, Brown & Co, 1988:63–67, 333–339.

Klein DM. Angina: Pathophysiology and the resulting signs and symptoms. Nursing 1988;18(7):44–46.

Perchalski DL, Pepine CJ. Patient with coronary artery spasm and role of the critical care nurse. Heart Lung 1987;16(4):392–402.

Rippe JM, Csete ME, eds. Manual of intensive care medicine. 1st ed. Boston: Little, Brown & Co, 1983:64–66.

Part II

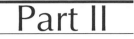

Pulmonary System

CHAPTER 18

Adult Respiratory Distress Syndrome

Barbara Clark Mims, RN, MSN, CCRN

Brian Davis is a 17-year-old boy who was brought to the Emergency Department following a near-drowning. He was driving his car to his high school graduation party when he missed a curve and plunged off the highway into a creek. His car was completely submerged, and he was not breathing when he was pulled from the wreckage by a passing motorist. CPR was administered by the motorist and Brian was awake when the paramedics arrived.

Upon arrival in the Emergency Department, Brian was oriented ×3 but extremely anxious. His BP was 124/82, heart rate 118, respirations 26/min. His breath sounds were diminished bilaterally with crackles and expiratory wheezes audible throughout all lung fields. He was receiving 40% O_2 via face mask, and his ABGs were as follows:

pH	7.48
$PaCO_2$	30
PaO_2	60
SaO_2	90%
HCO_3	24

All other laboratory values were normal, and except for some minor bruises and abrasions, no traumatic injuries were apparent. Brian was admitted to the Respiratory ICU with a diagnosis of near-drowning. He was stable for 24 hr, at which time he manifested dyspnea, tachypnea, tachycardia, and progressive hypoxemia. Despite increasing the FIO_2 via face mask, Brian's ABGs continued to deteriorate. Thirty hours after admission, his ABGs on 100% nonrebreathing mask were:

pH	7.50
$PaCO_2$	28
PaO_2	48
SaO_2	77%
HCO_3	24

He was intubated and placed on a volume ventilator at the following settings:

Mode	Assist control
Rate	12
FIO_2	0.60
Tidal volume	800
PEEP	5

His initial static effective compliance was 35 ml/cm H_2O, and his postintubation chest x-ray revealed appropriate endotracheal tube placement and bilateral, diffuse, patchy infiltrates. A fiberoptic pulmonary artery catheter was inserted, and the following data obtained:

Hemodynamic Parameters		ABGs	
PAP	25/10	pH	7.48
PAWP	8	$PaCO_2$	30
CVP	6	PaO_2	58
CO	7.5	SaO_2	89%
$S_{\bar{v}}O_2$	74%	HCO_3	24
		Hgb	15

Brian was diagnosed with the adult respiratory distress syndrome (ARDS).

QUESTIONS AND ANSWERS

1. What is ARDS? What are the diagnostic criteria for ARDS?

ARDS is a rapidly progressive respiratory insufficiency that is due to pulmonary edema of a noncardiac etiology. Precise criteria for diagnosis of ARDS vary, but it is generally agreed that the patient must have moderate to severe hypoxemia, bilateral diffuse infiltrates on chest x-ray, a clinical history compatible with ARDS, no evidence of left atrial pressure elevation, and a decreased static effective compliance.

2. What clinical conditions are commonly associated with ARDS?

Pulmonary Causes

> Aspiration of gastric contents
> Direct chest trauma
> Exposure to irritant gases
> Fat embolism
> Near-drowning
> Oxygen toxicity
> Pneumonia
> Smoke inhalation

Systemic (Endothelial) Causes

    Cardiopulmonary bypass
    Disseminated intravascular coagulopathy
    Heroin overdose
    Multiple transfusions
    Pancreatitis
    Sepsis
    Shock
    Snakebite
    Toxemia of pregnancy
    Trauma
    Uremia

There is usually a lag time of from several hours to 72 hr between the pulmonary insult and full-blown ARDS.

3. What are the major pathophysiologic alterations in ARDS?

The initial defect in ARDS involves damage to the pulmonary capillary endothelium, resulting in increased microvascular permeability. This may result from direct lung injury, as in the case of aspiration of gastric contents, inhalation of toxins, oxygen toxicity, or pulmonary contusion. A second mechanism of injury to the pulmonary capillary endothelium involves neutrophils. In ARDS, neutrophils are attracted to the interstitium of the lung, where they damage the pulmonary endothelium through the release of oxygen-free radicals, proteases, platelet-activating factor, and arachidonic acid metabolites (thromboxane A_2, prostaglandins E_2, F_2, and H_2, and leukotrienes). (See Appendix F.) As the endothelium is damaged, fluid and proteins leak into the interstitium and then into the alveoli. Various other cells and cellular debris leak into the interstitium. Enzymes such as collagenase and elastase disrupt the elastic and collagen fibers in the interstitium. The plasma proteins and protein by-products of interstitial fiber breakdown increase oncotic pressure, drawing more water into the interstitium. Both type I epithelial cells (gas-exchange pneumocytes) and type II pneumocytes (surfactant-producing cells) are damaged. Fluid pours into the alveoli from the interstitium, causing alveolar collapse. Loss of surfactant production leads to an increase in surface tension, which worsens the alveolar collapse and decreases the functional residual capacity. An intrapulmonary shunt develops, leading to refractory hypoxemia.

Various pulmonary perfusion defects also occur, leading to increased pulmonary vascular resistance and dead space.

4. **What are the clinical indicators of ARDS?**

> History of one or more risk factors
> Dyspnea
> Tachypnea
> Tachycardia
> Decreased lung volumes
> Bilateral, diffuse, patchy infiltrates on chest x-ray (occur 12–24 hr after other clinical indicators)
> Diffuse, fine rales
> PaO_2 < 60 mm Hg on FIO_2 0.40
> Shunt > 20%
> Static effective compliance < 50 ml/cm H_2O
> PAWP < 18 mm Hg (to rule out cardiogenic pulmonary edema)

5. **What is the usual cause of hypoxemia in ARDS?**

The usual cause of hypoxemia in ARDS is intrapulmonary shunting. A shunt exists when blood perfuses a capillary that interfaces with a completely unventilated alveolus. Because there is no contact between air and blood, no matter how much oxygen the patient is breathing, there will be no gas exchange in the shunt unit.

6. **What is the treatment for an intrapulmonary shunt?**

The patient who has an intrapulmonary shunt of >30% will usually require mechanical ventilation with positive end-expiratory pressure (PEEP). PEEP maintains the intraluminal airway pressure above atmospheric throughout exhalation, thereby increasing the functional residual capacity. This maneuver helps stabilize partially collapsed alveoli and may open up completely collapsed alveoli. This reestablishes contact between oxygen in the alveolus and blood in the pulmonary capillary, enabling gas exchange to take place.

PEEP is used to maintain adequate tissue oxygenation without having to use a toxic FIO_2. Although little definitive data exists to indicate the maximal safe FIO_2, a frequent practice is to use PEEP to keep the PaO_2 ≥60 mm Hg and SaO_2 ≥90% with an FIO_2 ≤0.60. However, the effects of PEEP on oxygen transport must also be considered and optimal assessment of PEEP therapy involves the calculation of oxygen transport each time the PEEP level is changed.

7. **How can PEEP affect oxygen transport?**

Oxygen transport is the amount of oxygen delivered to the tissues each minute. It is determined by the amount of oxygen in the blood, and the amount of blood pumped by the heart each minute, i.e., cardiac output.

PEEP can increase oxygen transport by decreasing the shunt and increasing the amount of oxygen in the blood.

PEEP can also decrease oxygen transport by decreasing cardiac output. The mechanisms by which PEEP is thought to decrease cardiac output include:

Decreased Venous Return. The positive pressure in the thorax is transmitted to the great vessels, impeding venous return.

Ventricular Dysfunction. The increased resistance in the pulmonary vasculature increases right ventricular afterload. The right ventricle must contract more vigorously, and the increased force of contraction causes a mechanical displacement of the interventricular septum. As the septum bulges into the left ventricle, left ventricular stroke volume decreases.

Humoral Myocardial Depressant Factor. The existence of a humoral myocardial depressant factor is theorized. It is thought that a chemical is released from the lungs of the patient on PEEP; the chemical circulates in the blood and causes a depression of myocardial contractility when it reaches the heart.

When Brian's first postintubation ABG came back with a PaO_2 of 58 mm Hg and an SaO_2 of 89%, the physician ordered the PEEP increased to 10 cm. Thirty minutes later, the following data were obtained:

Ventilator Settings		Hemodynamic Parameters		ABGs	
Mode	Assist Control	CVP	5	pH	7.46
Rate	12	PAP	25/10	$PaCO_2$	32
FIO_2	0.60	PAWP	8	PaO_2	65
Tidal volume	800	CO	7	SaO_2	90%
PEEP	10	$S_{\bar{v}}O_2$	75%	HCO_3	24
				Hgb	15

In the hopes that the FIO_2 could be decreased, the PEEP was increased to 15 cm and all other ventilator settings left the same. Relevant clinical data obtained 30 min later included:

Hemodynamic Parameters		ABGs	
CO	3.8	pH	7.46
$S_{\bar{v}}O_2$	70%	$PaCO_2$	33
		PaO_2	88
		SaO_2	95%
		HCO_3	24
		Hgb	15

8. **Was Brian's oxygen transport better with a PEEP of 10 or 15?**

His oxygen transport was better with a PEEP of 10, even though his PaO_2 and SaO_2 were higher on a PEEP of 15.

Oxygen Transport on PEEP 10

$$CaO_2 = (15 \times 1.39 \times 0.90) + (0.003 \times 65)$$

$$= 18.77 + 0.20$$

$$= 18.97 \text{ ml/dl}$$

$$O_2 \text{ transport} = 7 \times 18.97 \times 10$$

$$= 1328 \text{ ml/min}$$

Oxygen Transport on PEEP 15

$$CaO_2 = (15 \times 1.39 \times 0.95) + (0.003 \times 88)$$

$$= 19.81 + 0.26$$

$$= 20.07 \text{ ml/dl}$$

$$O_2 \text{ transport} = 3.8 \times 20.07 \times 10$$

$$= 763 \text{ ml/min}$$

The peep was decreased to 10 cm.

9. **Why are patients with ARDS prone to develop oxygen toxicity?**

The cellular metabolism of oxygen involves the stepwise reduction of oxygen to water. Along the way, substances referred to as oxygen-free radicals are produced. These free radicals are highly reactive and capable of damaging cell membranes. There are protective intracellular mechanisms, such as the enzyme superoxide dismutase, that protect the cell from accumulation of oxygen-free radicals at ambient conditions.

Exposure to high levels of FIO_2 causes rapid production of oxygen-free radicals, and the protective mechanisms are overcome. The pulmonary endothelium is damaged, and oxygen toxicity occurs.

In ARDS, neutrophils, mononuclear cells, and macrophages accumulate in the pulmonary interstitium. When activated, these cells release leukotrienes, which produce oxygen-free radicals and increase vascular permeability.

Leukotrienes attract polymorphonuclear leukocytes (PMNs), which adhere to the pulmonary endothelium. When activated, PMNs release proteases, which produce oxygen-free radicals and inactivate protective enzyme systems. Therefore, the patient with ARDS is at high risk for developing oxygen toxicity. PEEP is used to treat the hypoxemia with the least possible FIO_2.

10. **Following intubation and institution of mechanical ventilation, Brian was in a respiratory alkalosis. Is this typical?**

Yes. The initial response to hypoxemia is hyperventilation, resulting in a respiratory alkalosis. In addition, the interstitial edema in ARDS stimulates the J receptors, which results in a rapid, shallow breathing pattern and contributes to the respiratory alkalosis. Once the $PaCO_2$ starts to rise, it usually signifies an increase in V_D/V_T, and is often a preterminal event. However, correctable causes of hypercapnia, such as pneumothorax, right mainstream intubation, or inadequate minute ventilation must be ruled out.

11. **Brian's static effective compliance was 35 ml/cm of H_2O. What is the clinical significance of this value?**

Compliance has been defined as the change in volume divided by the change in pressure. The concept of compliance relates to the lungs' ability to stretch; the more compliant, the less pressure needed to distend the lungs and deliver the tidal volume.

In ARDS, as previously described, the alveoli fill with fluid and collapse. They become very boggy, stiff, and difficult to expand. The compliance is decreased. The normal textbook static effective compliance is 100 ml/cm H_2O. In clinical practice, 50 ml/cm H_2O is considered normal. In ARDS, the compliance will be <50 ml/cm of H_2O.

Brian's compliance was 35 ml/cm of H_2O, which was significantly below normal. Because his lungs were stiff, the work of breathing was significantly increased. In addition, higher than normal pressures would be required to deliver his ventilator breaths.

The term "elasticity" is sometimes mistakenly used to mean compliance. Elasticity refers to the tendency of the lung to return to its resting state after it has been inflated, not the ability of the lung to stretch. Elasticity and compliance are opposites, or reciprocals. The more elastic, the less compliant the lung, and vice versa.

12. **Before the diagnosis of ARDS was made, a pulmonary artery catheter was inserted. Why?**

In order to rule out cardiogenic causes of pulmonary edema, a pulmonary artery wedge pressure of <18 mm Hg should be evidenced. The pulmonary artery catheter is invaluable in monitoring hemodynamics in ARDS, and the $S\overline{v}O_2$ obtained via the fiberoptic lumen gives an indication of the balance between oxygen supply and demand.

13. Brian appears restless, and the nurse notes that he is "bucking" the ventilator. Why is this a concern in the patient with ARDS?

Bucking refers to a pattern of breathing that is out of phase with the ventilator; the patient breathes out during the ventilator's inspiratory phase. This is a significant concern in the patient with ARDS for two reasons. First, the increased respiratory muscle activity results in increased work of breathing and increased oxygen consumption. This may be disastrous in the hypoxemic patient with limited cardiovascular reserve. Second, bucking may result in high peak airway pressures, thereby increasing the likelihood of barotrauma.

Brian undergoes a complete clinical assessment, including ABGs, which are essentially unchanged. The chest x-ray taken that morning was reviewed for proper endotracheal tube (ETT) placement, which was verified at 3 cm above the carina. If the tube had been in any further, it would have been withdrawn slightly by the physician. Because the chest x-ray is usually taken with the patient at end-inspiration, the ETT may appear to be above the carina on the film, only to fall down and rest slightly on the carina upon expiration. The carina is exquisitely sensitive to touch, and stimulation of the carina may precipitate violent paroxysms of coughing and ventilator bucking. ETT placement should be checked before neuromuscular blockade is considered for ventilator control.

Brian receives Valium, 10 mg by IV push with careful checks of his BP after each 2 mg is given. Although he relaxes for a short while, he begins breathing out of phase again. The decision is made to begin pharmacologic paralysis with the neuromuscular blocker Pavulon.

14. What does neuromuscular blockade accomplish?

Administration of neuromuscular blockers results in complete skeletal muscle paralysis. The patient is completely flaccid and does not perform any of the work of breathing. This reduces oxygen consumption, which may be beneficial in the critically ill, hypoxemic patient.

The patient's complete state of relaxation enables the ventilator to deliver the tidal volume at lower mean airway pressures, thereby decreasing the chance of barotrauma.

The decision to begin neuromuscular blockade should only be made after all other methods to achieve patient relaxation and synchronous breathing with the ventilator have been exhausted. The attendant risks of this regimen are significant.

15. **What are the two most essential nursing responsibilities when caring for mechanically ventilated patients on neuromuscular blockers?**

Once neuromuscular blockade is started, the health care team assumes full responsibility for maintaining the patient's ventilation. If the patient comes off the ventilator, or if the ventilator fails, apnea will occur. Both ventilator and cardiac alarms must be set correctly and checked for proper functioning at least q 4 hr. The patient should be under direct observation of a qualified, professional nurse at all times. A complete Ambu bag must be set up and ready for immediate use in case of ventilator failure or accidental extubation.

Neuromuscular blockers paralyze all skeletal muscle but do not affect smooth muscle or the level of consciousness. It is essential that adequate sedation be given to dull the patient's awareness and help him or her relax under these stressful, anxiety-producing circumstances. If the patient has been injured or had surgery, analgesics should also be administered. Maintaining safety and sedation are paramount in caring for patients who are on neuromuscular blockers.

After the initial dose of Pavulon, Brain's BP is 150/90 and heart rate is 132. Even after Valium, 10 mg, his BP remains 140/86, heart rate 126. The physician orders Pavulon discontinued and Norcuron substituted.

16. **What is Norcuron? What are its advantages and disadvantages?**

Norcuron is a nondepolarizing muscle relaxant that is similar to Pavulon. It is 1–1.5 times as potent, but has ⅓ as long the duration of action of Pavulon.

Advantages of Norcuron

> Minimal cardiovascular effects
> Does not produce hyperkalemia as does succinylcholine in patients with burns
> Can be used in severe renal disease
> Has shorter duration of action than Pavulon or Curare
> Has little histamine-releasing activity
> Produces less cumulative properties than other nondepolarizing muscle relaxants

Disadvantages of Norcuron

> Norcuron is largely eliminated in the bile, and dose reduction is required in patients with hepatic disease.
> Norcuron has a longer onset of action than succinylcholine, and is not the agent of choice when emergency intubation is required.

The dosage of Norcuron must be carefully adjusted according to individual requirements and response.

17. **Morphine sulfate was not used in Brian's case because of a reported allergy to the drug. However, morphine is an excellent drug for respiratory control in mechanically ventilated patients with ARDS. Why?**

    Morphine sulfate has three features that make it useful in achieving respiratory control in patients with ARDS. These include:

    > It depresses the patient's mental perception of dyspnea and increases patient comfort while decreasing the respiratory drive.
    > It causes venous vasodilatation, thereby decreasing preload. This reduces the transudation of fluid into the alveoli and decreases the pulmonary edema.
    > It is rapidly reversible with Narcan. If there is a question about an acute neurological event having occurred, the drug effects can be rapidly eliminated and a neurological assessment performed.

18. **After Brian is stabilized on Norcuron and Valium, he does relatively well for several hours. Subsequently, the nurse at the bedside notes that his peak inspiratory pressure has increased from 30 to 50 cm H_2O. His breath sounds are diminished on the right side, and there is hyperresonance to percussion. Faint subcutaneous emphysema is palpable over the lower third of the right side of Brian's chest. What is the most likely problem? What should be done?**

    The most likely problem is a pneumothorax, as barotrauma is a frequent complication of PEEP. The physician should be notified immediately, and the equipment for a chest tube insertion assembled. In cases of tension pneumothorax, where cardiac or respiratory compromise is obvious, the physician may insert a large bore over-the-needle-catheter into the anterior chest to relieve the pressure.

19. **Brian's BP drops to 90/58, CVP to 2 mm Hg, PAWP to 4 mm Hg, and urine output to <30 ml/hr. What therapy is appropriate?**

    Cautious infusion of a crystalloid solution such as normal saline is appropriate, with checks of Brian's BP, HR, and PAWP every 30 min. Maintenance of intravascular volume is important, as preload is a determinant of cardiac output. Cardiac output is a determinant of oxygen transport.

    Crystalloids are generally chosen over colloids in ARDS because of the leaky alveolocapillary membrane. If colloid moved out of the vessel into the pulmonary interstitium, water would follow and worsen the pulmonary edema. However, the issue of colloids versus crystalloids remains controversial, and colloids are currently being used in some centers.

    Careful monitoring of the PAWP is essential to avoid vascular overload in patients with ARDS. An important note regarding fluid administration in the patient with ARDS is the linear relationship between PAWP and the amount of lung water in this patient population. At any given PAWP, if the PAWP increases, the amount of lung water increases. For this reason, the patient with ARDS should be kept "optimally dry," with as low a PAWP as is sufficient to maintain hemodynamic stability.

20. Brian was started on enteral feedings on the second day in the unit. Why is nutrition important in the patient with ARDS?

The patient with ARDS is typically on the ventilator for several days to weeks. His or her energy expenditure during this time may be high due to increased work of breathing, anxiety, pain, fever, infection, wound healing, etc. Continuous and unabated catabolism significantly increases the incidence and severity of the metabolic and infectious complications occurring in ARDS. The patient may actually catabolize his or her own respiratory muscles. The return to spontaneous and unassisted ventilation may be possible only following a substantial period of anabolism. Patients with ARDS generally require 35–45 kcal/kg/day. Protein is especially important, as is elemental phosphorus. Dietary fat should also be supplied. It should be noted that overfeeding may lead to volume overload, hepatic dysfunction, and CO_2 retention.

21. What is the leading cause of death in patients with ARDS?

Sepsis is the leading cause of death in ARDS patients. Fever should be reported to the physician promptly so appropriate cultures can be obtained. Some practitioners advocate the use of antibiotic paste in the mouth and nose to reduce oropharyngeal bacteria, which is one source of nosocomial pneumonia.

22. What nursing diagnoses apply in this case?

Impaired gas exchange related to alveolar collapse
Potential for inadequate cardiac output related to decreased venous return
Potential for multisystem organ failure related to inadequate tissue oxygenation
Ineffective breathing pattern related to decreased lung compliance
Ineffective airway clearance related to retained secretions
Potential for infection related to presence of invasive lines
Sleep pattern disturbance related to environmental stimuli
Impaired verbal communication related to presence of endotracheal tube
Impaired physical mobility related to pharmacologic paralysis
Impaired social interaction related to ICU environment

184 / *Pulmonary System*

SUGGESTED READINGS

Bernard GR, Bradley RB. Adult respiratory distress syndrome diagnosis and management. Heart Lung 1986;15(3):250–255.

Bradley RB. Adult respiratory distress syndrome. Focus Crit Care 1987;14(5):48–59.

Brandstetter RD. The adult respiratory distress syndrome—1986. Heart Lung 1986; 15(2):155–164.

Hechtman HB, Valeri CR, Shepro D. Role of humoral mediators in adult respiratory distress syndrome. Chest 1984;86(4):623–627.

Martin C, Saux P, Albanese J, Bonneru J, Govin F. Right ventricular function during positive end-expiratory pressure thermodilution evaluation and clinical application. Chest 1987;92(6):999–1003.

Mims BC. Fat embolism: A variant of ARDS. Orthop Nurs, 1989;8(3):22–27.

Raffin T. ARDS: Mechanisms and management. Hosp Pract 1987;22(11):65–80.

Snyder JV, Pinsky MR. Oxygen transport in the critically ill. Chicago: Year Book, 1987:3–15, 396–404.

Tennenberg SD, Jacobs MP, Solomkin JS, Ehlers NA, Hurst JM. Increased pulmonary alveolar-capillary permeability in patients at risk for adult respiratory distress syndrome. Crit Care Med 1987;15(4):289–293.

Weiland JE, Davis WB, Holter JF, Mohammed JR, Dorinsky PM, Gadek JE. Lung neutrophils in the adult respiratory distress syndrome clinical and pathophysiologic significance. Am Rev Respir Dis 1986;133:218–225.

CHAPTER 19

Chronic Obstructive Pulmonary Disease

Barbara Clark Mims, RN, MSN, CCRN

Todd Cox is a 69-year-old retired geologist who was diagnosed with chronic obstructive pulmonary disease 5 years ago. He is widowed, lives alone, and manages the activities of daily living with minimal difficulty. He smoked cigarettes heavily for 40 years, but has not smoked for the past 10 years. Although he is mildly short of breath with almost any exertion, he has never been in frank respiratory failure. He is maintained on oral theophylline and an inhaled bronchodilator.

Shortly after a visit from his daughter and three grandchildren, Mr. Cox began to experience a low grade fever, productive cough, and feelings of malaise. His shortness of breath worsened, and he developed palpitations. He was taken by a neighbor to the Emergency Department of his community hospital.

Mr. Cox's physical examination showed a thin, asthenic, white man who was sitting up on the side of the stretcher, leaning forward, bracing his arms on the overbed table. He was using his accessory muscles and breathing through pursed lips. His cardiac monitor showed multifocal atrial tachycardia (MAT) at a rate of 126 beats/min. His breath sounds were diminished, with prolonged expiration and faint, high-pitched rhonchi. His heart sounds were distant. A 12-lead ECG showed right axis deviation, P-pulmonale, and right ventricular hypertrophy. He was diaphoretic, anxious, and short of breath.

Blood was drawn for ABGs, electrolytes, CBC, and theophylline level. His vital signs and relevant laboratory values were as follows:

Vital Signs		ABGs (room air)	
BP	164/94	pH	7.30
HR	126	$PaCO_2$	62
Resp	30	PaO_2	48
Temp	99.8°F	SaO_2	80%
		HCO_3	30
Hct	51	Theophylline level 2.5 $\mu g/ml$	
Hgb	16.5		

Oxygen was started at 24% via Venti-mask. An IV line of D_5W was started at 75 ml/hr, and a loading dose of aminophylline, 3 mg/kg, was given over 30 min, followed by a constant infusion of 0.3 mg/kg hr. Alupent was given by updraft nebulizer and was to be repeated every 4 hr. Solu-Medrol,

185

35 mg, was given by IV push. Following collection of a sputum specimen, ampicillin, 500 mg PO every 6 hr was started. Percussion and postural drainage every 2 hr was ordered, and Mr. Cox was transferred to the Respiratory ICU (RICU).

Upon admission to the RICU, Mr. Cox's nurse greeted him with a calm, reassuring approach. She encouraged him to maintain his sitting position and to slow his breathing down. She supported his coughing efforts and explained to him the importance of clearing the secretions from his airways.

Four hours after admission to the RICU, Mr. Cox stated that he was breathing easier. His cardiac monitor still showed MAT at a rate of 120, and he was still using his accessory muscles to breathe. His ABG drawn on 0.24% Venti-mask showed:

pH	7.35
$PaCO_2$	55
PaO_2	50
SaO_2	83%
HCO_3	30

The FIO_2 was increased to 0.28 Venti-mask. Mr. Cox was coughing up moderate amounts of thick, yellow sputum. Small amounts of oral fluids were offered at frequent intervals. After 6 more hr of intensive pulmonary hygiene, monitoring, and psychological reassurance, Mr. Cox was resting comfortably. His monitor showed sinus tachycardia at a rate of 108 with frequent PACs. On 0.28 Venti-mask, his ABGs showed:

pH	7.35
$PaCO_2$	55
PaO_2	56
SaO_2	87%
HCO_3	30

Mr. Cox was able to sleep when left alone but was easily arousable and oriented ×3. After a relatively restful night, he was examined by his attending physician and transferred to the pulmonary rehabilitation floor 16 hr after admission.

QUESTIONS AND ANSWERS

1. What is COPD?

Chronic obstructive pulmonary disease is a condition in which there is a chronic obstruction to airflow due to chronic bronchitis and/or emphysema. The degree of obstruction may be less when the patient is free from respiratory infection and may improve with bronchodilators; however, some obstruction is always present.

COPD includes chronic bronchitis and emphysema. Chronic bronchitis is a condition associated with excessive tracheobronchial mucous production sufficient to cause cough with expectoration for at least 3 months of the year for more than 2 consecutive years.

Emphysema is distention of the air spaces distal to the terminal bronchiole with destruction of alveolar septa. Lung recoil is decreased. Most patients exhibit a combination of bronchitis and emphysema.

2. **Mr. Cox is receiving oxygen via Venti-mask. Why is this the preferred O_2 administration device in the patient with COPD?**

Patients with COPD may have chronically elevated $PaCO_2$ levels. As a result, the responsiveness of the medullary respiratory centers to CO_2 stimulation may become dulled, causing the patient to breathe off his hypoxic drive. If too much oxygen is administered, the hypoxic drive may be suppressed, and the patient may hypoventilate or become apneic.

Using a Venti-mask allows a precise FIO_2 to be delivered. In most other oxygen administration devices, such as a nasal cannula or simple face mask, the FIO_2 is quite variable. It is prudent to start out with a 0.24 Venti-mask, and gradually increase the FIO_2 if the PaO_2 remains unacceptably low and the $PaCO_2$ does not rise.

3. **Why does the patient with COPD breathe best sitting upright, leaning forward?**

The chronic air trapping and loss of elasticity in COPD cause the functional residual capacity to increase. Over the course of years, the chest wall becomes deformed, as the increased anterior posterior diameter results in a "barrel chest." As the chest gets bigger, the diaphragm flattens out. Now when it contracts, the diaphragm doesn't move very much, so the accessory muscles in the neck and upper chest are used to maintain ventilation. When the patient leans forward and rests on a table, it makes his or her shoulder girdle more efficient in moving the chest cage up and down.

The viscous resistance caused by the abdominal contents pressing up against the diaphragm is greater in the supine position. When the patient sits up, gravity displaces the abdominal contents away from the diaphragm, and the viscous resistance is less. Keeping the patient pulled up in bed with the head elevated, or better yet, sitting up in a chair, can significantly improve ventilation.

When a patient with COPD lies down at night to sleep, secretions may move into the central airways from the peripheral airways and obstruct airflow. Coughing helps clear the airways and improve ventilation; patients frequently awaken themselves with vigorous coughing several hours after retiring.

4. **What are the accessory muscles of ventilation? What is the significance of accessory muscle use?**

   Many clinicians mistakenly categorize the intercostal muscles as accessory muscles. In actuality, the intercostal muscles are primary ventilatory muscles, as they elevate the anterior ends of the ribs and increase the anterior-posterior diameter of the thorax.

   The accessory muscles for inspiration include the scalene, sternocleidomastoid, trapezius, and pectoralis muscles.

   The accessory muscles for expiration are the abdominal muscles, including the external oblique, rectus abdominis, internal oblique, and transverse abdominis.

   Since COPD is an obstructive defect, the major problem occurs on expiration, and the abdominal muscles may be seen to vigorously contract in an attempt to force air out through the obstructed airways. However, this extra muscular effort causes high intrathoracic pressures, causing airway collapse and worsening expiratory obstruction. Therefore, use of the abdominal muscles may not improve expiratory air flow over that which occurs with quiet expiration.

   Normally, only about 2–5% of the available oxygen is used to support the work of the ventilatory muscles. With accessory muscle use, the increase in ventilatory muscle work may consume as much as 20% of the available oxygen. This deprives other vital organs, such as the heart, brain, kidneys, etc., of needed oxygen. If the patient is hypoxemic, this increased work of breathing and oxygen deprivation to vital organs may have significant consequences.

5. **Mr. Cox's hematocrit was 51%. Why does polycythemia occur in COPD?**

   The amount of oxygen present in the arterial blood depends on the partial pressure of oxygen, the oxygen saturation, and the hemoglobin. The exact number of milliliters of oxygen in 100 ml of arterial blood is termed the oxygen content and can be determined as follows:

   $$\text{Oxygen content} = (\text{Hgb} \times 1.39 \times \text{SaO}_2) + (0.003 \times \text{PaO}_2)$$

   If the PaO_2 and SaO_2 are low, the body increases the hemoglobin level by increasing red blood cell production. This increases the oxygen content. In Mr. Cox's case, the elevated Hgb resulted in an almost normal arterial O_2 content even though the PaO_2 and SaO_2 were quite low.

   $$
   \begin{aligned}
   \text{CaO}_2 &= (16.5 \times 1.39 \times 0.80) + (0.003 \times 48) \\
   &= 18.35 + 0.14 \\
   &= 18.5 \text{ ml/dl}
   \end{aligned}
   $$

This is a compensatory mechanism, but if taken to extreme, can cause problems. If the hematocrit gets too high, the hyperviscosity of the blood can impede blood flow to the tissues. If the hematocrit reaches >55–60%, phlebotomy is indicated.

6. What is the relationship between hypoxemia and myocardial workload?

The pulmonary vasculature constricts in response to hypoxemia. When the vessels constrict, the pulmonary vascular resistance rises. The right ventricle must pump harder to eject blood out the pulmonic valve into the pulmonary artery, and myocardial work goes up. This may lead to cor pulmonale.

7. Mr. Cox's monitor showed multifocal atrial tachycardia. What are the ECG criteria for this dysrhythmia?

Multifocal atrial tachycardia occurs when impulses originate from three or more atrial ectopic foci at a rate over 100 beats/min (Fig. 19.1). The most common cause is severe, systemic hypoxia, especially in patients with severe chronic lung disease. MAT is resistant to drug therapy, and the most effective treatment is correction of hypoxia.

The ECG criteria include:

Three or more different P wave morphologies
Irregular R to R and P to P intervals
Variable PR interval
Normal QRS
Rate > 100 beats/min

8. What are the typical ECG changes associated with COPD?

ECG changes in emphysema include (*a*) right axis deviation; (*b*) right ventricular hypertrophy, or rS complexes across the precordium; (*c*) P-pulmonale (small P in lead I with tall, pointed P in 2, 3, and AVF, and (*d*) low voltage QRS in precordial leads (Fig. 19.2).

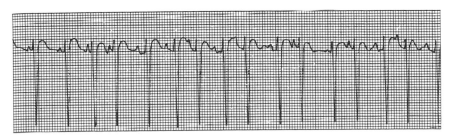

Figure 19.1. Multifocal atrial tachycardia.

9. **Why was provision of adequate hydration a priority of care in Mr. Cox's case?**

    The mucus in patients with COPD, especially with a superimposed respiratory infection, is extremely viscous, sticky, and difficult to clear. When secretions become inspissated in small airways, alveoli distal to those airways become underventilated and may eventually collapse. This results in a low $\dot{V}/\dot{Q}$ ratio and hypoxemia.

    Providing adequate systemic hydration and humidification of mucus with nebulization or aerosol therapy decreases sputum viscosity and facilitates mucociliary clearance. Percussion and postural drainage may help mobilize secretions. Inability to clear pulmonary secretions may necessitate intubation.

10. **Mr. Cox was started on ampicillin before any culture results were available. Is this a common practice?**

    Yes. Empirical administration of broad-spectrum antibiotics without culture and sensitivity results is common clinical practice in patients with COPD and superimposed respiratory infections. Common pathogens include *Haemophilus influenzae* and *Streptococcus pneumoniae*.

11. **What are the pharmacologic effects of aminophylline?**

    Aminophylline is a bronchodilator and also has a mild respiratory stimulant effect.

    As mentioned earlier, patients with COPD typically have a mixture of bronchitis and emphysema. Bronchitis may respond to bronchodi-

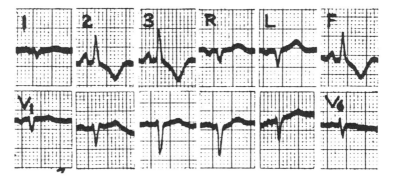

Figure 19.2. From a patient with emphysema. Note: right axis deviation (+95°) with rS complexes all across the precordium. The ST-T pattern of right ventricular "strain" is fully developed in leads 2, 3, and AVF. The P wave pattern suggests P-pulmonale with an axis of +80° and pointed, though not very tall, P waves in 2, 3, and AVF. (From Marriott HJL. Practical electrocardiography. 8th ed. Baltimore: Williams & Wilkins, 1977:57.)

latation, whereas pure emphysema does not. It may be helpful to evaluate the patient's FEV_1 with spirometry before and after bronchodilator administration. (See Chapter 24, "Status Asthmaticus.") Also of benefit is an empirical trial with various bronchodilators, using the patient's subjective response to evaluate efficacy.

12. What is the normal dose of aminophylline?

A loading dose of 6 mg/kg should be given over 20–30 min, followed by a constant infusion of 0.3–0.5 mg/kg hr. If the patient has been taking theophylline preparations at home, resulting in near therapeutic levels, the loading dose should be lowered or skipped. If the patient is on cimetidine, erythromycin, or propranolol, drug interactions with aminophylline may elevate the serum level. If the patient has proven or potential liver disease, as is the case with this patient due to his cor pulmonale, the maintenance dose should be reduced to ⅓ to ½ the usual infusion rate.

13. What is a therapeutic serum concentration of theophylline?

A therapeutic serum concentration of theophylline is 10–20 $\mu g/ml$.

14. What are the signs and symptoms of theophylline toxicity?

Theophylline toxicity may be manifested by nausea and vomiting, seizures, and dysrhythmias.

15. How do β_2-agonists such as Alupent work?

β_2-Agonists increase cyclic AMP by increasing levels of the enzyme adenyl cyclase. Cyclic AMP causes bronchodilatation. β_2-Agonists are relatively selective for the lungs, so cardiac side effects are minimized; however, they can cause tremors, palpitations, and dysrhythmias. β_2-Agonists include Ventolin, Bronkosol, Alupent, and Metaprel.

16. Why are steroids given in COPD?

Although the mechanism of action is not clear, intravenous administration of Solu-Medrol, 0.5 mg/kg every 6 hr for 72 hr, has been shown to decrease airway resistance in acute exacerbations of COPD. Patients who are most likely to benefit include those with a prominent bronchospastic component, sputum eosinophilia, or history of allergy. Administration of sucralfate for prevention of peptic ulcer is advisable in the patient receiving steroids.

17. What are the indications for mechanical ventilation in a patient with COPD?

Because it is frequently difficult to wean patients with COPD from the ventilator, intubation is avoided. However, in the case of a PaO_2

below 45 mm Hg or pH below 7.30, despite rigorous therapy, or a depressed mental status, intubation and mechanical ventilation should be considered.

18. Describe the paradoxical abdominal respiratory movements that are sometimes seen in patients with emphysema. What is the clinical significance?

The following pattern of abdominal movement is sometimes seen in the patient with COPD:

> Outward movement of the chest wall and inward movement of the epigastrium during inspiration, indicating diaphragmatic paresis or paralysis
>
> Inward movement of the chest wall with outward movement of the epigastrium during expiration

This pattern of paradoxical respirations is associated with an increased mortality rate.

19. What nursing diagnoses apply in this case?

> Ineffective airway clearance related to ineffective cough and mucociliary mechanisms
>
> Impaired gas exchange related to shallow breathing and tenacious mucus
>
> Ineffective breathing pattern related to decreased diaphragmatic function and increased lung volumes
>
> Potential for cardiac dysrhythmias related to hypoxia
>
> Anxiety related to difficulty breathing and the unknown
>
> Hopelessness related to irreversible nature of the disease

SUGGESTED READINGS

Bates DV. Respiratory function in disease. 3rd ed. Philadelphia: WB Saunders, 1989: 172–213.

COPD: Grasping for breath. Emerg Med 1987, Feb 15;19(3):86–92, 101–103, 106–107.

Holloway NM. Nursing the critically ill adult. 3rd ed. Menlo Park, CA: Addison-Wesley, 1988:177–179.

Hudson LD. Management of COPD: State of the art. Chest 1984, June;85(suppl):765–815.

Kersten LD. Comprehensive respiratory nursing—A decision making approach. Philadelphia: WB Saunders, 1989:107–112.

Laureau S, Larson JL. Ineffective breathing pattern related to airflow limitation. Nurse Clin North Am 1987, Mar;22(1):179–191.

Matus VW, Glennon SA. Respiratory disorders. In: Kinney MR, Packa DR, Dunbar SB. AACN's clinical reference for critical care nursing, 2nd ed. New York: McGraw-Hill, 1988:806–810.

Welch MH. Obstructive diseases. In: Guenter CA, Welch MH, eds. Pulmonary diseases. 2nd ed. Philadelphia: JB Lippincott, 1982:664–709.

CHAPTER 20

Pneumonia

Terry L. Jones, RN, BSN, CCRN

Raymond Johnson is a 72-year-old man who presented to the Emergency Department with a 4-day history of shortness of breath. He reported having experienced flu-like symptoms for the past 7 days with a sudden onset of fever, a shaking chill, and a cough productive of thick, rust-colored sputum for 2 days prior to admission. He further complained of a sharp, nonradiating pain in his left lateral chest that seemed worse with inspiration and was at least partially relieved by lying on his left side. His past medical history included an inferior MI 10 years ago and adult-onset diabetes controlled by oral hypoglycemics. He stated that he uses alcohol only socially and has smoked approximately 2 packs of cigarettes/day for the last 50 years.

Physical examination revealed coarse crackles and rhonchi over the left lung fields with increased tactile fremitus and a pleural friction rub. Vital signs and laboratory work revealed the following clinical data:

Vital Signs		ABGs (room air)	
BP	150/84	pH	7.49
HR	118	PaCO$_2$	32
Resp	24	PaO$_2$	68
Temp	38.8°C	SaO$_2$	92%
		HCO$_3$	27

CBC				Glucose	
WBC	14.4	Monos	7	164	
Polys	82	Eosinophils	1		
Bands	4	Hgb	15		
Lymphs	6	Hct	45		

Mr. Johnson was given O$_2$ per nasal cannula at 4 liters/min, and an IV line of D$_5$½NS was started and infused at a rate of 200 ml/hr. His sputum was Gram-stained and sent for culture. The Gram stain revealed short chains of Gram-positive cocci. After two sets of blood cultures were obtained, he was started on penicillin G 2 million units IV piggyback every 4 hr. Mr. Johnson was admitted to the hospital with a tentative diagnosis of community-acquired pneumococcal pneumonia. His condition deteriorated over the next 24 hr, as evidenced by the following serial ABGs.

Time	FIO_2	pH	$PaCO_2$	PaO_2	SaO_2	HCO_3
10:00 AM	4 liters of nasal O_2	7.45	38	54	90%	26
11:30 AM	40% face mask	7.45	37	53	89%	26
12:30 PM	50% face mask	7.49	33	66	94%	26
6:30 PM	50% face mask	7.49	32	50	87%	26
7:30 PM	100% nonrebreathing mask	7.46	35	86	95%	25

A chest x-ray taken at 6:00 AM the second hospital day revealed left upper lobe and left lower lobe infiltrates. His breath sounds were coarse with crackles and rhonchi present throughout the left lung fields. His fever rose to 39.8°C and his heart rate to 141 beats/min with a BP of 180/100. His respiratory rate at times reached 60 and his respirations were labored. An ABG on 100% nonrebreathing mask at 7:00 AM on day 2 revealed worsening hypoxemia:

pH	7.44
$PaCO_2$	31
PaO_2	58
HCO_3	22
SaO_2	89%

Mr. Johnson became disoriented and combative and was consequently transferred to the Respiratory ICU where he was orally intubated with an 8-mm endotracheal tube and placed on a volume ventilator. Acceptable ABGs were initially obtained with the ventilator settings of assist control rate 12, tidal volume 1000 ml, and FIO_2 0.50. Pulmonary hygiene was enhanced with frequent suctioning, percussion, and postural drainage.

QUESTIONS AND ANSWERS

1. **Define pneumonia.**

    Pneumonia is an acute inflammation of the lung parenchyma (alveolar spaces and interstitial tissue), which is caused by an infectious agent and leads to alveolar consolidation.

2. **What are the differences between community-acquired and hospital-acquired pneumonia?**

    Community-acquired pneumonia is typically much less virulent than hospital-acquired pneumonia. Patients who require hospitalization as a result of community-acquired pneumonia are usually elderly and suffer from underlying diseases such as COPD, diabetes mellitus, or cardiac disease.

    Hospital-acquired (nosocomial) pneumonia is usually much more serious than community-acquired pneumonia, as many of the causative organisms are resistant to antibiotic therapy.

3. What are the major causes of pneumonia?

> Bacteria
> Virus
> Mycoplasma
> Legionnaires' disease in some geographic areas

In addition to the above causes of pneumonia, aspiration of gastric contents can evoke a similar response, particularly when the pH of the aspirate is <2.5. This type of aspiration can cause diffuse damage to the lung parenchyma, including degeneration of bronchial epithelium as well as type I and II pneumocytes. Pulmonary edema, atelectasis, and consolidation are the result.

4. What are the normal pulmonary defense mechanisms against pulmonary infections?

> Ciliary action
> Mucus secretion
> Coughing
> Alveolar macrophages
> Neutrophils
> Immunoglobulins IgA and IgG
> Lymphatic system

5. What are the mechanisms through which pulmonary infections can occur?

> Aspiration
> Colonization of the tracheobronchial tree
> Direct spread from adjacent sites
> Hematogenous spread

Aspiration of pathogenic organisms from the oropharynx is the mechanism most often responsible for pneumonia and in the normal host the most likely flora responsible include *Streptococcus pneumoniae, Haemophilus influenzae,* and *Staphylococcus aureus.* Circumstances that seem to predispose one to aspiration include a diminished cough or gag reflex, esophageal disorders, endotracheal intubation, nasogastric intubation, and tracheostomy. Most of the time the mucociliary clearance is quite efficient in the removal of aspirated microorganisms. However, a pneumonia may result if the aspiration is massive, the organism is especially virulent, or the normal defense mechanisms are compromised.

6. **What conditions can compromise pulmonary defense mechanisms?**

   Viral infections
   Cigarette smoking
   Aspiration of acidic gastric contents
   Endotracheal intubation
   Acidosis (depressing antibacterial activity of alveolar macrophages)
   Hypoxia
   Edema
   COPD
   Malnutrition
   Diabetes
   CHF
   Alcoholism

7. **Which of the above conditions were present in Mr. Johnson prior to the appearance of symptoms?**

   Viral infection
   Cigarette smoking
   Diabetes mellitus

8. **Mr. Johnson presented with fever, chills, pulmonary infiltrate, productive cough, pleural chest pain, and elevated WBC. Is this a typical presentation for someone with bacterial pneumonia?**
   Yes. These are the classic clinical findings in bacterial pneumonia.

9. **A differential blood count was done on Mr. Johnson. What kind of information does this simple diagnostic test yield?**
   While the WBC measures the total number of leukocytes, a differential identifies the presence of specific types of leukocytes and determines what percentage each contributes to the WBC. Because each type of leukocyte has a unique function and consequently is released in response to specific disease categories, elevation of the differential components can offer valuable information with regard to potential etiology. Mr. Johnson's differential blood count revealed an elevation of polymorphonuclear leukocytes, suggestive of a severe infection. The presence of bands, the immature form of polymorphonuclear leukocytes released when the mature reserve is depleted, further suggests that the infection is acute rather than chronic. This pattern in a differential blood count is sometimes referred to as a "shift to the left."

10. What procedures are most frequently used to make a diagnosis of pneumonia?

Sputum for culture and microscopic analysis (Gram stain)
Chest x-ray

11. What are the major pathophysiological changes associated with pneumonia?

Alveolar inflammation
Increased capillary permeability
Increased interstitial and alveolar fluid
Alveolar consolidation with exudate consisting of fluid, fibrin, bacteria, polymorphonuclear leukocytes, and red blood cells
Intrapulmonary shunting

12. Upon arrival in the Emergency Department, Mr. Johnson's room air ABG revealed hypoxemia (PaO_2 68). Is this typical for pneumonia? What is the mechanism responsible for hypoxemia in pneumonia?

Hypoxemia is very typical in a patient with pneumonia. The decrease in PaO_2 is a result of a decreased $\dot{V}/\dot{Q}$ ratio and subsequent venous admixture effect. Pneumonia is an infectious process involving the alveoli. As in any other infectious condition, the body responds with the inflammatory response. Consequently, serum, RBCs, polymorphonuclear leukocytes, and macrophages flood the site of infection, in this case the alveoli, to aid in the defense. In situations where the infection is severe, the alveoli become completely filled with fluid and debris, and a condition of consolidation is said to occur. As a result of this consolidation, the affected alveoli are perfused but not adequately ventilated, thus creating a $\dot{V}/\dot{Q}$ mismatch and, if severe, an intrapulmonary shunt. In a shunt, blood perfuses a capillary bed adjacent to a completely nonventilated alveolus (e.g., consolidated alveolus) and no gas exchange occurs. Upon return to the left heart, this blood, which is essentially venous in nature, combines with the oxygenated blood having perfused ventilated alveoli. The result is a venous admixture causing a decrease in PaO_2.

13. What was the most likely etiology of Mr. Johnson's chest pain?

The lungs are covered by two membranes known as the visceral and parietal pleurae. The visceral pleura adheres to the lung itself, whereas the parietal pleura, containing pain receptors, lines the thoracic cavity. Normally, the pleurae are separated by a thin layer of fluid that allows the surfaces to glide over one another during the act of breathing without stimulation of the pain receptors. Should an inflammatory process, such as that in a pneumonia, involve the parietal pleura, the pain receptors will be stimulated, especially during inspiration. This condition is commonly called pleurisy and at times can be heard as a pleural friction rub as the inflammed pleura rub against each other. When Mr. Johnson was positioned on his left side, a splint effect was created which decreased his pain.

After a couple of days, Mr. Johnson's pleurisy disappeared and his breath sounds were slightly diminished in the left base. A chest x-ray revealed a left pleural effusion. A thoracentesis was done and approximately 800 ml of cloudy serous fluid was removed.

15. Describe the mechanism responsible for a pleural effusion in Mr. Johnson.

As part of the vascular response to inflammation, capillary permeability is increased and fluid from the pulmonary capillaries diffuses into the pleural cavity separating the pleural layers.

16. Even after intubation and mechanical ventilation, Mr. Johnson's PaO$_2$ would vary throughout the day. The nurse noticed that his best ABG values seemed to occur when he was positioned on his right side. What is a possible explanation for this apparent correlation between body position and oxygenation?

Recent studies suggest that in unilateral lung disease, oxygenation is best when the patient is positioned with the "good" or unaffected lung down. This is because gravity increases perfusion in the dependent areas. With the good lung down, more blood goes to the healthy lung tissue, and gas exchange is optimized.

17. One mechanism thought to contribute to the rapid, shallow breathing pattern exhibited by patients with pneumonia is stimulation of the J receptors. What are the J receptors?

Juxtapulmonary-capillary receptors or J receptors are believed to be present in the interstitial tissue between the pulmonary capillaries and the alveoli. It is thought that stimulation of such receptors triggers a CNS reflex causing rapid, shallow breathing. Conditions believed to activate this reflex are pulmonary capillary congestion or hypertension, alveolar wall edema, humoral agents, lung deflation, and emboli. Both alveolar wall edema and lung deflation from atelectasis may be present in pneumonia and result in stimulation of the J receptors. Other mechanisms that probably contribute to the rapid, shallow breathing pattern in patients with pneumonia include stimulation of peripheral chemoreceptors sensitive to decreased PaO$_2$ levels, decreased lung compliance, and the chest pain and anxiety that are often present.

18. **Despite prompt initiation of antibiotic therapy with penicillin, Mr. Johnson's fever persisted and his condition deteriorated. Blood cultures, sputum cultures, and Gram-stain were repeated. Why?**

Because there is a plethora of pathogens that can cause pneumonia, definite etiologic identification can be difficult and time-consuming. With the help of sputum stains, empiric antibiotic therapy is recommended while cultures are pending. The goals of such empiric therapy are to treat the most likely etiologic pathogen while avoiding toxicity, superinfection, and unnecessary cost. Failure to respond to such therapy may indicate that the chosen antibiotic regimen does not appropriately cover all of the etiologic pathogens or that a new source of infection has developed.

19. **Appropriate antibiotic therapy is crucial in the treatment of acute pneumonia. Such medications, however, are not without potential adverse effects. What are some examples of the more common adverse effects associated with the various classifications of antimicrobial agents?**

The major adverse effect of the penicillin family is hypersensitivity, which can be minimized with documentation of reported allergies, skin testing, and test doses. One other potential adverse effect is hemolytic anemia, resulting in a positive direct Coombs' test. Ticarcillin, an extended range penicillin, is especially noted for its high salt content, as well as its association with platelet dysfunction. Nafcillin, a semisynthetic drug, is commonly associated with neutropenia. Consequently, close attention to CBC results becomes important when administering these agents in high doses or for a prolonged period of time. The aminoglycosides are associated with dose-related nephrotoxicity, which is usually mild and reversible. Fortunately, this adverse effect can be minimized with frequent peak and trough levels and appropriate dosage adjustments. Unfortunately, however, the ototoxicity resulting from damage to the inner ear is thought to be both irreversible and unavoidable.

20. **What are some complications associated with pneumonia?**

Empyema
Pleural effusions
Bacteremia
ARDS
Sepsis

21. **Mr. Johnson's clinical course was complicated by bacteremia. Which of the above complications does this make him especially susceptible to?**

    Sepsis
    ARDS

22. **What nursing diagnoses might apply to Mr. Johnson?**

    Ineffective airway clearance related to airway infection
    Ineffective breathing pattern related to decreased lung expansion
    Ineffective airway clearance related to artificial airway
    Social isolation related to impaired verbal communication
    Impaired gas exchange related to body position
    Anxiety related to perceived powerlessness
    Sleep pattern disturbance related to environmental stimuli

SUGGESTED READINGS

Alspach J, Williams S. Core curriculum for critical care nursing. Philadelphia: WB Saunders, 1985.

Cosenza J, Cilentano N. Secretion clearance: State of the art from a nursing perspective. Crit Care Nurse 1986;6(4): 23–37.

Des Jordins, T. Clinical manifestations of respiratory disease. Chicago: Year Book, 1984.

Hanley MV, Tyler ML. Ineffective airway clearance related to airway infection. Nurs Clin North Am 1987;22(1):135–151.

Hopp LJ, Williams M. Ineffective breathing pattern related to decreased lung expansion. Nurs Clin North Am 1987;22(1): 193–205.

McFarland G, Nasehinski C. Impaired communication. Nurs Clin North Am 1985; 20(4):775–785.

Norton L, Conforti C. The effects of body position on oxygenation. Heart Lung 1985;14(1):45–52.

Sahn S. Pulmonary emergencies. New York: Churchill Livingstone, 1982.

Shekleton M, Nield M. Ineffective airway clearance related to artificial airway. Nurs Clin North Am 1987;22(1):167–179.

Shoemaker W, Ayers S, Ohe G, Holbrook P, Thompson W, eds. Textbook of critical care. 2nd ed. Philadelphia: WB Saunders, 1989.

Stratton C. Bacterial pneumonias: An overview with emphasis on pathogenesis, diagnosis and treatment. Heart Lung 1986; 15(3):226–240.

Traver G. Ineffective airway clearance: Physiology and clinical application. Dimens Crit Care Nurs 1985;4(4):198–208.

CHAPTER 21

Pulmonary Contusion

Wendy L. Baker, RN, MS, CCRN

Joshua Martin is a 78-year-old driver of a car that became airborne and crashed into another car. Mr. Martin was found ambulating at the scene of the accident and claims to have been wearing a seat belt. He was transported by ambulance from the scene of the accident, hemodynamically stable and denying any loss of consciousness. He arrived at the Emergency Department complaining of shortness of breath and bilateral chest pain.

Physical examination revealed an elderly white man with an obvious left flail chest. Pulse was 108, respirations were 28, and blood pressure was 136/70 mm Hg. There was a 3-cm laceration over the left eyebrow. Pupils were equal and reactive to light in spite of recent cataract surgery to the left eye.

Examination of the chest revealed breath sounds that were clear but decreased bilaterally. The rest of the physical examination was unremarkable.

The past medical history was positive for hypertension (medications unknown), cholecystectomy, and smoking.

Relevant clinical data were as follows:

ABGs	**(40% face mask)**	**HCT**	46
pH	7.44	**Chest x-ray**	
$PaCO_2$	35	Bilateral pneumotho-	
PaO_2	72	races and multiple	
SaO_2	94%	fractured ribs (5th–8th	
HCO_3	24	right, 5th–7th left)	

Treatment

Bilateral chest tubes were inserted with a return of 150 ml of bloody fluid on the left side and 450 ml on the right side.

A thoracic epidural catheter was placed for pain control in the 6th thoracic epidural space. Thirty micrograms of fentanyl were injected, producing good pain relief and allowing the patient to use an incentive spirometer to about 1 liter. The patient confirmed pain control, stating he hurt "only when he coughed."

Mr. Martin was admitted to the Surgical Intensive Care Unit for observation on 40% face mask and with the epidural catheter in place.

Hospital Course

Three days after admission, Mr. Martin demonstrated progressive respiratory distress. He appeared "tired," and on a 100% nonrebreathing mask his arterial blood gases were: pH 7.46, $PaCO_2$ 32, PaO_2 56. His pulse increased from 110 to 130 beats/min, blood pressure was 102/52 mm Hg, temperature was 99.4°C, respiratory rate was 28, and arterial oxygen saturation fell from 94 to 88%. A large, persistant air leak was noted through the right chest tube. Wheezing was noted bilaterally on auscultation of the lungs. A size 8.0 oral endotracheal tube was placed and Mr. Martin was put on a volume ventilator at FIO_2 0.40, tidal volume 1000 ml, SIMV 4, and pressure support 10. A pulmonary artery catheter was inserted: PAP 38/17 mm Hg, PAWP 12 mm Hg, CO 12 liters/min, SVR 1296.

ABGs drawn 1 hr after mechanical ventilation was started were:

pH	7.40
$PaCO_2$	40
PaO_2	58
SaO_2	88%
HCO_3	24

PEEP 10 cm was added. ABGs 2 hr later were:

pH	7.42
$PaCO_2$	38
PaO_2	58
SaO_2	88%
HCO_3	24

Oxygenation did not improve until PEEP levels reached 16 cm H_2O.

QUESTIONS AND ANSWERS

1. **Is Mr. Martin's injury pattern typical of people who receive chest injury from blunt trauma?**

   No. Isolated chest injury is uncommon. Although chest wall injuries range from relatively trivial to fatal, significant chest wall injury is present in about one-third of the patients admitted with severe trauma. Associated injuries are present approximately 80% of the time. These injuries commonly include (in order of frequency of occurrence): cerebral concussion, cerebral contusion, extremity trauma, spine injury, abdominal injury, and pelvic injury. Many blunt chest injuries are of moderate severity and, like Mr. Martin's, rarely require surgical intervention. Chest trauma ranks third behind head and extremity trauma as the cause of death in major accidents in the United States.

2. What kind of chest wall injuries commonly accompany pulmonary contusion and how severe are they?

These injuries can range from fatal to relatively trivial. In blunt trauma, there is a direct correlation between the number of fractured ribs and both intrathoracic injury and death rates. Pulmonary contusion rarely occurs in isolation and is often accompanied by pain, pneumothorax, or a flail chest (two or more ribs broken in two or more places). This proved true in Mr. Martin's case; his chest trauma, which involved seven ribs, injured the lung to the point of a bronchopleural fistula (ongoing large air leak on the right side). Scapular fracture is a reliable clinical clue to ipsilateral lung contusion.

Chest compliance varies greatly, and patients who have a very compliant chest wall may have a tremendous amount of force transmitted to the lungs. This results in severe, bilateral contusions with little in the way of bony injury to the chest wall itself. Chest walls of older patients, like Mr. Martin, are less compliant and may break more easily, although the underlying lung injury is less severe.

3. How does pulmonary contusion actually damage the lung tissue and what is the range of injury to the lung?

Pulmonary contusion may be minor to severe, ranging from localized bruising, to parenchymal laceration, to pulmonary hematoma. In its simplest form, pulmonary contusion represents suffusion of air and blood from disrupted vessels into the surrounding parenchyma. In addition to being a hemorrhagic process, contusion causes interstitial and alveolar edema. Hemorrhage and edema occur within the area of contusion and gradually involve surrounding tissue in the inflammatory process. When there is no disruption of the pulmonary parenchyma, resorption is prompt.

With tearing of the pulmonary parenchyma, blood vessels and air passages may be disrupted. Subsequent developments partially depend on whether the laceration connects with the pleura. If a communication exists, a hemothorax, pneumothorax, or pneumohemothorax occurs. In blunt trauma, parenchymal disruptions are often localized near the intermediary bronchus, so that extravasated blood and air accumulate in the space created by the parenchymal laceration, causing pulmonary hematoma or cystic cavities.

Pulmonary hematoma occurs when blood extravasates into the space created by the parenchymal contusion at the time of the contusion, in contrast to after contusion, as is true with parenchymal laceration.

When associated injuries or shock are present, secondary lung injury may occur. (See Chapter 18, "Adult Respiratory Distress Syndrome.")

4. **What are the main physiological abnormalities associated with pulmonary contusion? Did Mr. Martin's course reflect these?**

   Relative hypoxemia, increased pulmonary vascular resistance, decreased pulmonary vascular flow, pulmonary vascular "shunting" through consolidated areas, decreased compliance, and hyperventilation with hypocarbia may be associated with pulmonary contusion. Also, in the dog model, decreased lung bacterial clearance occurs, suggesting that contused lungs are more susceptible to bacterial infections. Three days after injury Mr. Martin exhibited a falling PaO_2 (to 56), a decreasing $PaCO_2$ (to 32), an arterial oxygen saturation of 88%, and an increasing respiratory rate (to 28). Perhaps most importantly, Mr. Martin indicated he was tired. Although during the first few days after injury he had achieved 1 liter on the incentive spirometer, this volume dropped to 400 ml on the third postinjury day.

5. **What are the risk factors for developing traumatic wet lung (adult respiratory distress syndrome (ARDS)) after pulmonary contusion?**

   Although no data clearly indicates who will develop ARDS, it is probably related to the severity of the initial injury and the patient's age. Researchers generally agree that higher morbidity and mortality result in the presence of: high injury severity scores (multiple body systems involved), initial Glasgow Coma Scores of <7, transfusion of more than 3 units of blood, frank shock, falls from heights, or the combination of pulmonary contusion and flail chest. The presence of a closed glottis at the moment of impact has also been implicated.

6. **Was Mr. Martin's clinical decline typical?**

   Yes. Often, although blunt chest trauma creates pain and hypoventilation, true respiratory failure does not occur until 48–72 hr after the injury. After a variable period of delay, patients usually develop an ineffective cough, progressive hyperpnea, and dyspnea. Sputum is usually thick, bloody, and difficult to remove. Scattered, fine rales are often auscultated, which usually do not completely clear on coughing. Local areas of wheezing are common. The overall picture resembles pulmonary edema associated with a degree of bronchospasm.

7. **How is pulmonary contusion diagnosed?**

   The radiologic diagnosis of pulmonary contusion has been based on the classic findings of a pulmonary infiltrate seen within hours of trauma. In the past, it has been repeatedly written that the clinical and radiographic alterations of pulmonary contusion are often absent on the initial evaluation because these reports were based on chest x-rays. However, this is not true in CT, where the pulmonary laceration and the surrounding hemorrhage are seen immediately.

8. Which nursing interventions facilitate oxygenation of the injured lung and may prevent intubation and mechanical ventilation?

Treatment is based on the severity of injury and symptoms. Supplemental oxygen and vigorous pulmonary toilet are the cornerstones of treatment for pulmonary contusion. The level of oxygen provided will depend on the amount of shunt present. Mr. Martin required increasing support, from 40% face mask to 100% nonrebreathing mask before he was intubated. An important part of pulmonary toilet, besides incentive spirometry to limit atelectasis, is mobilizing the patient, as other system injuries allow. Early fixation of orthopaedic injuries is an essential component of trauma pulmonary care. Unfortunately, when even a few fractured ribs are present, tremendous pain prevents even the most well-intentioned patients from adequate coughing. Thus, if an intercostal nerve block or epidural pain control is ineffective or contraindicated, intubation with mechanical ventilation may be necessary.

9. Why was Mr. Martin's ventilatory management difficult?

Several factors made Mr. Martin's ventilatory management difficult: (*a*) he had an unstable chest wall (bilateral fractured ribs); (*b*) he had a large air leak (bronchopleural fistula) on the right side, which was exacerbated by the PEEP required to overcome his shunt; and (*c*) in spite of attempts to control peak airway pressures (and theoretically limit barotrauma) by using pressure support ventilation with a low SIMV rate, peak inspiratory pressures remained high.

10. What is the rationale underlying fluid management of patients with pulmonary contusions like Mr. Martin's?

Blood and crystalloid infusions are titrated to maintain peripheral perfusion and urine output. Mr. Martin's central venous pressure, blood pressure, pulmonary artery pressure, and urine output were monitored to prevent fluid overload.

It is generally accepted that excessive fluid administration must be avoided so the pulmonary edema present with pulmonary contusion is not exacerbated. However, serial CT scans demonstrate that the pulmonary infiltration and consolidation seen on chest roentgenograms, which is known as "pulmonary contusion," is a pulmonary laceration surrounded by intraalveolar hemorrhage, without significant interstitial injury. Thus, contusion can be treated without steroids, diuretics, and severe fluid restriction.

11. Why is airway clearance a nursing priority?

With pulmonary contusion, secretions are often thick and bloody. Thick, bloody secretions can encrust and partially block an endotracheal tube, increasing the work of breathing. Atelectasis is the frequent result of pulmonary contusion when secretion clearance is inadequate. Infection often follows atelectasis, so monitoring patient temperature, sputum appearance, and white blood cell count is important.

12. What makes chest wall injuries so painful?

Trauma to the parietal pleura, bony structures, and especially the intercostal nerves is very painful.

13. How can pain contribute to respiratory failure?

When breathing is painful, respiratory effort becomes shallow, and tachypnea and hypoventilation occur. This results in a relative increase in dead space, decreased cough effectiveness, and retained secretions. If uncorrected, these conditions may progress to hypercarbia, hypoxia, and later, infection.

14. Is epidural pain control a good way of managing pain in chest wall trauma? What are the nursing implications?

Intravenous morphine, either administered by the nurse or via patient controlled analgesia pump, can be effective in the pain control of blunt chest trauma. However, it is often difficult to maintain a balance between pain control and ventilation, at least in the early stages of pulmonary trauma, when pain is severe. Patients early after injury may not remember to push the button for pain control with patient controlled analgesia. The epidural catheter may be more effective. When rib fractures are high (i.e., first and second ribs), epidural pain control is dangerous because of the proximity to the phrenic nerve. In these cases, local intercostal rib blocks are a safer procedure.

Patients receiving epidural morphine should be carefully observed for respiratory depression and an ampule of Narcan should be kept at the bedside.

15. What other factors contributed to Mr. Martin's respiratory failure?

Factors contributing to Mr. Martin's respiratory failure included his age, bilateral pneumothoraces, ineffective cough and retained secretions, and intraalveolar edema secondary to pulmonary contusion.

16. **What abdominal injury should be suspected with fracture of the sixth and seventh ribs?**

    Liver laceration and ruptured spleen should be suspected when these ribs are fractured. These injuries did not occur in Mr. Martin, who was hemodynamically stable throughout transport and the early stages of his hospitalization. If the liver or spleen are injured, there is usually bleeding severe enough to cause hemodynamic instability requiring operative intervention. Monitoring the hematocrit over the first several days postinjury is therefore important.

17. **What does fracture of the first and/or second rib imply?**

    Because a greater force is required to fracture the first or second ribs than other ribs, a more severe lung injury may be present.

18. **When is a nasogastric tube inserted in blunt chest trauma and why?**

    When multiple ribs (especially the seventh through the tenth) are injured, a nasogastric tube is mandatory. If gastric distention occurs, further restriction of breathing, vomiting, and aspiration may occur.

19. **Which nursing diagnoses are commonly used in pulmonary contusion?**

    Ineffective airway clearance related to pain and inability to cough
    Impaired gas exchange related to consolidation and alveolar collapse
    Pain related to chest wall injury
    Anxiety related to air hunger
    Potential for infection related to proteinaceous intraalveolar edema

SUGGESTED READINGS

Clark GC, Schecter WP, Trunkey DD. Variables affecting outcome in blunt chest trauma: Flail chest vs pulmonary contusion. J Trauma 1988;28(3):298–304.

Hurn PD. Thoracic injuries. In: Cardona VD, Hurn PD, Mason PJB, Scanlon-Schilpp AM, Veise-Berry SW, eds. Trauma nursing: From resuscitation through rehabilitation. Philadelphia: WB Saunders, 1988:449–490.

Johnson JA, Cogbill TH, Winga ER. Determinants of outcome after pulmonary contusion. J Trauma 1986;26(8):695–697.

LoCicero J, Mattox KL. Epidemiology of chest trauma. Surg Clin North Am 1989;69(1):15–19.

Olsson GL, Leddo CC, Wild L. Nursing management of patients receiving epidural narcotics. Heart Lung 1989;18(2):130–138.

Pate JW. Chest wall injuries. Surg Clin North Am 1989;69(1):59–69.

CHAPTER 22

Pulmonary Embolism

Kimmith M. Jones, RN, BS, CCRN

Jeff Moore is a 32-year-old man who fell asleep while driving and was involved in a motor vehicle accident. Although there was extensive damage to the front of his car, Mr. Moore was wearing a seat belt, and he was awake when the ambulance arrived. A Philadelphia collar was applied, and he was placed on a backboard and transported to the hospital.

Mr. Moore's injuries included a fractured pelvis, a fractured right tibia and ankle, and a fractured left knee with ligamentous injury. A below the knee cast was placed on the right leg along with a full length knee immbolizer on the left.

Mr. Moore's course in the Surgical ICU was uneventful until the 5th day when his nurse noticed swelling of his left thigh while giving him a bath. The primary physician was notified and a Doppler flow study was performed. The results revealed a left femoral-popliteal deep venous thrombosis. Mr. Moore was placed on bed rest and anticoagulation therapy via a continuous heparin infusion. He did well on the heparin for 2 days, after which time he began complaining of shortness of breath, left anterior chest pain that worsened with deep inspiration, and a feeling of impending doom. Physical assessment revealed the following:

BP	160/88
HR	120
Resp	34 and labored
Temp	99°F

A stat chest x-ray showed left lower lobe atelectasis.

Mr. Moore was started on O_2 via nasal cannula at 4 liters/min and an arterial blood gas was drawn. The following results were obtained:

pH	7.52
$PaCO_2$	28
PaO_2	131
SaO_2	99%

A ventilation perfusion scan performed that afternoon revealed perfusion defects of the anterior and posterior segments of the left upper lobe. Ventilation was normal, and a pulmonary embolus (PE) was suspected. Mr. Moore was scheduled for a pulmonary angiogram the next morning.

208

On the morning of the scheduled angiogram, Mr. Moore's PT and PTT were as follows:

PT	16.7 sec	PTT	46.9 sec
Control	1.7 sec	Control	25.3 sec

The angiogram was postponed pending reversal of the anticoagulation. Six units of fresh frozen plasma were administered.

Several hours later, Mr. Moore exhibited tachycardia, diaphoresis, and cyanosis. His SaO_2, which was being monitored by pulse oximeter, dropped to 81%. He was placed on a 100% nonrebreathing mask. An ABG was drawn after 30 min, and the results were as follows:

pH	7.48
$PaCO_2$	30
PaO_2	45
SaO_2	81%

Mr. Moore was intubated and placed on a volume ventilator. A moderate amount of blood-tinged secretions were suctioned from his endotracheal tube. A pulmonary angiogram done that day revealed emboli in the left upper lobe lingular and right main pulmonary arteries. Bilateral iliac vein Greenfield filters were placed under fluoroscopy and anticoagulation therapy was resumed. Once the prothrombin times were in the therapeutic range, Coumadin was started. Mr. Moore was extubated 24 hr after the filters were placed and the heparin was discontinued after 72 hr. He made steady progress and was discharged on Coumadin therapy several days later.

QUESTIONS AND ANSWERS

1. **What alterations in gas exchange occur following a pulmonary embolus? How does a pulmonary embolus cause hypoxemia?**

   The pathophysiologic alterations in gas exchange that occur following a PE are complex and multifaceted. The following is a brief description:

   a. Obstruction of blood flow through the lung region distal to the embolus creates dead space, or areas of wasted ventilation. No contact between blood and air occurs in the dead space, so no gas exchange can take place. Dead space increases the work of breathing, as the patient must increase his or her minute ventilation in order to maintain adequate gas exchange. However, desaturated blood does not flow from the dead space into the left heart.

    b. Because blood cannot flow past the obstruction created by the embolus, flow is diverted to the nonembolized lung regions. These regions receive more blood than normal, resulting in a low $\dot{V}/\dot{Q}$ ratio. Blood flowing through areas of low $\dot{V}/\dot{Q}$ does not become fully saturated, so some desaturated blood flows into the left heart. Hypoxemia is the result.

    c. Vasoactive amines and other humoral substances are released from the platelets in the embolus itself or from the pulmonary vascular endothelium distal to the embolus. These chemicals cause stiffening and constriction of the alveolar ducts and small bronchioles. Airway resistance increases, and the vital capacity and functional residual capacity decrease. As ventilation decreases, areas of low $\dot{V}/\dot{Q}$ are created. This results in a widened alveolar-arterial oxygen gradient and progressive hypoxemia.

    d. The mechanical obstruction of blood flow through the pulmonary circuit creates an increase in pulmonary vascular resistance. This is exacerbated by vasoconstrictive substances released from the platelets within the thrombus. In addition, the pulmonary vasculature constricts in response to hypoxemia, increasing pulmonary vascular resistance even further. The workload of the right ventricle is significantly increased by the increased pulmonary vascular resistance. The hemodynamic effects of the increased right ventricular workload depend on the patient's cardiopulmonary status prior to the embolus. Right ventricular failure with inadequate cardiac output is a possibility. When cardiac output is reduced, the venous oxygen reserve is used; that is, because less blood is delivered to the tissues each minute, the tissues extract more oxygen than normal to maintain adequate tissue oxygen utilization. This causes a reduced venous oxygen content, as less oxygen remains in the venous blood entering the right heart and pulmonary artery. The reduction in $\dot{V}/\dot{Q}$ ratio in combination with a decreased venous oxygen content results in a widened alveolar-arterial oxygen gradient and hypoxemia.

    e. Early in pulmonary embolism (PE), the $PaCO_2$ is low, as the patient hyperventilates secondary to hypoxemia. Later in the course, the $PaCO_2$ may rise due to increased CO_2 production from increased work of breathing.

    A common misconception regarding the pathophysiology of PE is that the hypoxemia is a direct result of the increased physiologic dead space. Although the dead space created by a PE contributes to the work of breathing, it is not the primary cause of hypoxemia.

2. **What are the four major types of pulmonary emboli? What are the risk factors for each type?**

   Venous Thromboembolism
   Risk factors:
   Blood stasis
   Immobility
   Obesity
   Congestive heart failure
   Atrial fibrillation
   Venous wall abnormalities
   Venous punctures
   Trauma
   Atherosclerosis
   Bone fractures with vessel injury
   Surgery
   Obstetric manipulations
   Clotting abnormalities
   Oral contraceptives
   Dehydration
   Polycythemia
   Malignancies
   Pregnancy

   Air Embolism
   Risk factors:
   Air in IV lines (especially disconnection of subclavian catheters)
   Ruptured pulmonary artery catheter balloon
   Surgery on peritoneal cavity
   Neurosurgical procedures
   Open chest wounds

   Fat Emboli
   Risk factors:
   Long bone or pelvic fractures
   Sternal splitting incisions

   Catheter Emboli
   Risk factors:
   Broken IV catheters
   Reinsertion of stylets through catheters

   Other less common types of pulmonary emboli include amniotic fluid, tumor, septic, and parasitic emboli.

3. **What are the signs and symptoms of a pulmonary embolism?**

   Dyspnea
   Pleuritic chest pain
   Syncope/collapse (indicates massive PE)

Fever (with pulmonary infarction)
Tachycardia (almost always present)
Pleural friction rub
Tachypnea
Rales and rhonchi
Accentuated P_2, caused from the increased pressure in the pulmonary
  artery
S_3, S_4
Hemoptysis
Sudden development of pulmonary hypertension in the hemodynami-
  cally monitored patient
Decreased ventilation of affected side

The classic triad of symptoms for a pulmonary embolus includes dyspnea, pleuritic chest pain, and hemoptysis. However, these symptoms are present in only 20% of patients who have sustained a major PE. The presentation is often nonspecific, and the clinical indicators may be quite subtle.

Many patients in the ICU are intubated and on mechanical ventilators. Progressive hypoxemia, hypercarbia, and respiratory acidosis in the sedated patient receiving controlled mechanical ventilation may indicate the occurrence of a PE.

4. **What causes a thrombus to dislodge from a peripheral vein and travel to the lung?**

  Although there is little data to support this, clinical evidence indicates that movement of the leg, the Valsalva maneuver, quickly changing from a sitting to standing position, or hyperventilation may facilitate embolization of a thrombus.

5. **Is pulmonary infarction a common complication of pulmonary embolism?**

  No. The lung has a dual blood supply, consisting of arterial blood from the bronchial artery and venous blood from the pulmonary artery. A PE obstructs a portion of pulmonary arterial flow, but bronchial artery perfusion continues and supplies oxygenated blood to the lung tissue. Pulmonary infarction occurs in approximately 10–15% of patients sustaining PE.

6. **Are PEs usually single or multiple? What areas of the lung are most likely to be affected?**

  Pulmonary emboli are almost always multiple. When a thrombus travels from the peripheral veins to the right heart, the churning action of the blood breaks it into fragments that then travel to branches of the pulmonary artery. These fragments may create a partial or complete obstruction to blood flow. Most commonly, some blood is forced around the embolus when pulmonary artery pressure increases during systole.

The lower lobes are the most likely to be affected, as blood flow is greatest in these areas.

8. Is phlebitis a common finding in patients who develop pulmonary emboli?

It is true that thrombophlebitis predisposes the patient to a pulmonary embolus. The risk is lowest when only the calf veins are involved, and highest when the thrombus is located in the proximal thigh veins and the iliac veins. Interestingly, only about 50% of patients with pulmonary emboli have clinical evidence of phlebitis prior to the embolus.

9. What diagnostic tests can be used to determine the presence of a PE?

Chest X-ray.   Chest x-rays are not definitive for the diagnosis of a pulmonary embolus. An elevated diaphragmatic dome may be seen secondary to decreased lung volumes, which may be caused by peripheral bronchoconstriction, infiltrates, atelectasis, and pleural effusions. Although both pleural effusions and/or atelectasis may occur, they are nonspecific diagnostically.

Electrocardiogram.   Changes include inverted T waves, depressed ST segments, right axis deviation, and a right bundle branch block pattern. The classic S_1Q_3 ECG pattern is rarely seen and usually occurs with massive PE.

Pulmonary Scintigraphy ($\dot{V}/\dot{Q}$ Scan).   This test measures pulmonary blood flow. The absence of perfusion with normal ventilation suggests the presence of a PE. As discussed earlier, pulmonary vascular occlusion does produce bronchoconstriction and atelectasis, but the decrease in ventilation will not be as significant as the decrease in perfusion portion of the scan. $\dot{V}/\dot{Q}$ scans are most commonly indeterminate and are frequently of limited value in the presence of preexisting lung disease (especially COPD).

Pulmonary Angiography.   This test is the "gold" standard diagnostic tool for PE. It is indicated whenever embolectomy, thrombolytic therapy, or vena cava interruption is being considered, or $\dot{V}/\dot{Q}$ scan is inconclusive. Contrast media is injected into the pulmonary artery, and even small emboli are visualized.

10. **Mr. Moore's pulmonary embolus was caused from a venous thrombo-embolism. What four therapeutic modalities are used in the management of a pulmonary embolus caused from venous thromboembolism?**

Anticoagulation. This is the cornerstone of therapy. Anticoagulants do not dissolve the thrombus but do prevent further thrombus formation and further propagation of the existing thrombus. Heparin is the drug of choice for achieving anticoagulation. Heparin works by combining with antithrombin III (AT-III) to prevent the conversion of fibrinogen to fibrin and prothrombin to thrombin. This allows the body to remove the emboli by its own fibrinolytic mechanisms. AT-III is a glycoprotein that is made in the liver. It neutralizes coagulation factors II, IX, X, and XI that have been activated. Heparin requires the presence of AT-III for its anticoagulant action. Therefore, patients who are deficient in AT-III who have thromboembolic disease should not be treated with heparin but should be treated with Coumadin instead.

Heparin should be started as soon as the diagnosis of deep vein thrombosis (DVT) is made and should be continued for 7–10 days. The goal of therapy is to prolong the PTT to 1½–2 times the control value.

A loading IV bolus of 5000 units is given initially, followed by a continuous infusion of 1000 units hr. Continuous infusion adjusted by measuring serial PTT values is the method of administration that carries the least risk of bleeding complications. The two main complications of heparin therapy include hemorrhage and thrombocytopenia. Therefore, invasive procedures should be avoided and strict monitoring of the patient's platelet count is mandatory.

The PTT should initially be checked every 4 hr to make sure acceptable anticoagulation is being achieved. If the PTT is not 1½–2 times the control value, the infusion rate should be increased.

Contraindications to heparin therapy include active internal bleeding, intracranial bleeding, recent major surgery, preexisting bleeding disorders, and uncontrolled, severe hypertension.

Coumadin therapy is usually started on or around day 3 or 4 of heparin therapy. Coumadin also interferes with blood clotting, inhibits further formation of existing clots, and prevents new clots from forming. It is given by mouth, has a longer duration of action, and is monitored by the PT instead of the PTT. The PT is maintained at 1½–2 times the control value. Combined Coumadin and heparin therapy is given for several days, and the heparin is then stopped. The duration of Coumadin therapy is individualized and depends upon the risk factors for further emboli. Treatment can range from 3 weeks to lifelong.

Thrombolytic Enzymes. Unlike anticoagulants, thrombolytic enzymes actually dissolve recent emboli as well as inhibit the formation of new ones. While thrombolytic enzymes are in use, it is recommended that the patient remain in bed, have no invasive procedures performed, receive no IM injections, and have no other anticoagulants or antiplatelet agents administered. When these precautions are followed, the incidence of bleeding is no higher than for a patient on heparin or Coumadin.

The indications for thrombolytic therapy include: obstruction of more than 50% of the pulmonary artery bed, hemodynamically unstable patients that are not responding to other therapies, or patients with PE who have severe cardiopulmonary disease.

Contraindications to this therapy include recent CVA, TIAs, tumors, AV malformations, bleeding ulcers, recent invasive procedures where local control of potential bleeding cannot be obtained (e.g., subclavian puncture), and uncontrolled hypertension.

The two substances currently being used are streptokinase (SK) and urokinase (UK). SK is a protein from the group C β-hemolytic streptococci. It has the ability to cause allergic reactions, being a foreign protein derived from bacteria. Its half-life is about 80 min. UK comes from purified human urine or human fetal kidney cell cultures and is unlikely to cause allergic reactions. It has a half-life of about 16 min. Both substances are usually given by continuous infusion. The goal of therapy is to decrease the fibrinogen level to ½ of the pretherapy value and to double the thrombin time. Thrombolytics are administered for about 24 hr for PEs and for about 48–72 hr for DVTs. Two to four hours after SK or UK has been discontinued, heparin therapy is usually started to avoid rethrombosis. A loading dose may or may not be given, depending upon the PTT value.

Inferior Vena Cava Interruption (IVC). Indications for IVC interruption include contraindications to anticoagulants or complications with anticoagulants, recurrent PEs despite anticoagulation, chronic embolization, as an adjunctive procedure with an embolectomy, or the presence of a propagating iliofemoral vein thrombus with a mobile clot.

The device most commonly used is the Greenfield filter. It is a cone-shaped device that was designed to catch emboli larger than 3 mm. It is placed transvenously, most often via the internal jugular vein. The filter is positioned infrarenally unless the source is located above the renal veins.

Embolectomy. This is usually reserved for massive emboli. With the transvenous technique, a cap device is inserted into the femoral vein and placed just distally to the embolus using fluoroscopy. Suction is then applied to the cap device, which attracts the clot. The cap and clot are then withdrawn.

11. What nursing measures can decrease the chance of a PE?

Identify patients at risk
Identify signs and symptoms of DVT and PE
Apply pneumatic compression devices as ordered
Administer prophylactic anticoagulants as prescribed (usually heparin 5000 units SC every 12 hr)
Elevate lower extremities when patients are out of bed to facilitate venous return
Perform active and/or passive ROM exercises
Promote early mobilization of patients
Change the patient's position frequently—avoid constant Fowler's position
Avoid venipunctures in leg veins
Maintain adequate hydration

12. List the nursing diagnoses pertaining to this case.

Impaired gas exchange related to ventilation/perfusion mismatch
Potential impaired skin integrity related to right leg cast and left knee immobilizer
Impaired verbal communication related to endotracheal intubation
Impaired social interaction related to hospitalization
Impaired physical mobility related to lower extremity injuries and anticoagulant therapy
Potential for sleep pattern disturbance related to ICU environment
Anxiety related to knowledge deficit of disease process

SUGGESTED READINGS

Belenkie I. Pulmonary vascular diseases. In: Guenter CA, Welch MH, eds. Pulmonary medicine. 2nd ed. Philadelphia: JB Lippincott, 1982:476–498.
Fahey VA. Life threatening pulmonary embolism. Crit Care Q 1985;8(2):81–88.
Kersten LD. Comprehensive respiratory nursing: A decision making approach. Philadelphia: WB Saunders, 1989:155–157.
Long BC, Phipps WJ, eds. Medical-surgical nursing: The nursing process approach. St Louis: CV Mosby, 1989.
Tsapegas MJ. Pulmonary embolism. Part I.

Incidence, pathophysiology, and diagnosis. Ala J Med Sci 1987;24(4):405–411.
Tsapegas MJ. Pulmonary embolism. part II. Management. Ala J Med Sci 1988;25(1):59–66.
Tsapegas MJ. Venous thrombosis. Part I. Etiology, diagnosis, and prevention. Ala J Med Sci 1987;24(2):176–182.
Tsapegas MJ. Venous thrombosis. Part II. Management. Ala J Med Sci 1987;24(3):301–305.
Valenzuela TD. Pulmonary embolism. Ann Emerg Med March, 1988;17(3):209–213.

CHAPTER 23

Stab Wound to the Chest

Kimmith M. Jones, RN, BS, CCRN

Brad Fox is a 27-year-old man who was stabbed with a 4-inch knife during a fight at a local bar. He sustained three wounds on the right side of his chest. The wounds were located in the third intercostal space (ICS) midclavicular line, the fifth ICS anterior axillary line, and the sixth ICS anterior axillary line.

Upon arrival in the Emergency Department, Mr. Fox was awake, anxious, and confused, but able to follow commands. His skin was cool and clammy. His BP was 92/68, heart rate 128, and respirations 38 and labored. Breath sounds were absent on the right side, which was also dull to percussion. The patient had subcutaneous emphysema from the third to the seventh right intercostal space. A 36F chest tube was placed in the fifth intercostal space midaxillary line on the right side. Immediately after insertion, 1750 ml of bloody fluid drained into the collection chamber and an air leak was noted in the water seal chamber. The chest tube was sutured in place and an occlusive dressing was applied. Occlusive dressings were also applied to the stab wound sites.

Two large bore IV lines were placed and 2 liters of Ringer's lactate was rapidly infused. Mr. Fox's blood pressure made no significant change following this infusion. Two units of O negative blood were rapidly infused.

Mr. Fox went to the Operating Room for exploration of his wounds and ligation of bleeding blood vessels. During surgery, the third and fourth intercostal arteries were ligated. The wound in the sixth ICS revealed a tract downward, which nicked the diaphragm and produced a 1.5-cm tear, which was also repaired. A peritoneal lavage was performed with negative results.

Upon admission to the Surgical ICU, Mr. Fox's vital signs and ventilator settings were:

BP	120/88	Mode	Assist control
HR	115	Rate	16
Resp	18	FIO$_2$	0.40
Temp	98°F	Tidal volume	1000
		PEEP	5

Mr. Fox's right chest tube was draining 50 ml/hr of serosanguinous fluid, and intermittent bubbling in the water seal chamber was noted. Two hours following admission, his chest tube drainage stopped and his peak inspiratory pressure (PIP) rose from 30 to 55 cm H_2O, causing the ventilator's high pressure alarm to sound. The patient's blood pressure dropped to 90/66. Breath sounds were absent on the right side and unequal chest excursion was noted.

QUESTIONS AND ANSWERS

1. **What was the most probable cause of this problem?**

   Tension pneumothorax

2. **What are the causes of a tension pneumothorax?**

   Fractured ribs
   Rupture of bronchus, bronchiole, or alveolus
   Occluded open pneumothorax
   Mechanical ventilation

3. **What are the signs and symptoms of a tension pneumothorax?**

   Respiratory distress
   Tracheal deviation away from the affected side
   Unilateral absence of breath sounds
   Distended neck veins (unless the patient is severely hypovolemic)
   Hyperresonance to percussion on ipsilateral side
   Shift of mediastinum away from affected side

   Tension pneumothorax is a clinical diagnosis and not a radiographic diagnosis. Therefore, treatment should begin when signs and symptoms are initially observed and not delayed until a chest x-ray is obtained.

4. **What is the initial and the definitive treatment for a tension pneumothorax?**

   Initially, a 14- or 16-gauge over-the-needle catheter is placed into the second intercostal space in the midclavicular line. The inner needle stylet is then removed to allow reexpansion of the lung without further trauma to the lung tissue. This procedure releases the trapped air and converts the tension pneumothorax to an open pneumothorax. The catheter is placed in the midclavicular line in order to avoid cannulation of the mammary artery. The intercostal arteries and veins can be avoided by inserting the catheter directly in the middle of the intercostal space.

   Definitive treatment involves the placement of a chest tube.

5. **How does a tension pneumothorax occur?**

   Air enters the pleural space via a tear in either the visceral or parietal pleura. The pleura acts as a one-way valve, allowing air to enter the pleural space but not exit. The intrapleural pressure exceeds atmospheric pressure, causing collapse of the affected lung. If left untreated, this pressure continues to accumulate. Compression of the heart and great vessels occurs, leading to a mediastinal shift away from the affected side. The result is an inability to ventilate and a decrease in venous return and cardiac output.

6. What are the 12 conditions, also called the "dirty dozen," most commonly associated with chest trauma?

Airway obstruction	Cardiac contusion
Flail chest	Aortic rupture
Open pneumothorax	Diaphragmatic rupture
Tension pneuomothorax	Esophageal rupture
Massive hemothorax	Tracheobronchial tree rupture
Cardiac tamponade	Pulmonary contusion

75% of penetrating chest trauma results from stabbings. When the chest wall and pleural cavity have been entered, damage to deep, underlying structures must be ruled out.

Injuries are not always obvious on the initial clinical examination or chest x-ray. Delayed pneumothoraces and hemothoraces may develop. If the initial clinical and radiographic findings are negative, inspiratory and expiratory chest films should be obtained at that time and 6 hr later. If these films are normal, the patient may be sent home; however, he or she should be reevaluated in 24 hr.

7. What defines a massive hemothorax?

1500 ml or more of blood in the chest cavity. This is usually discovered when shock is associated with the absence of breath sounds and/or dullness to percussion is heard over one side of the chest. This volume of blood is approximately 15–30% of the total blood volume in an average size adult.

8. What injuries may precipitate the development of a massive hemothorax?

Injuries to the heart, great vessels, major systemic arteries, or intercostal arteries may precipitate a massive hemothorax.

9. What is the treatment for a massive hemothorax?

The patient who sustains a massive hemothorax will require operative management to locate the source of bleeding and to repair the injury. Prior to surgery, emergency treatment procedures include chest tube insertion and administration of fluids and blood. Generally, 2 liters of Ringer's lactate will be given, followed by O negative blood until type-specific blood can be obtained.

10. **What are the two most common complications of chest trauma?**

Empyema. Empyema occurs when pus or necrotic tissue accumulates between the pleural layers. Signs and symptoms of empyema include fever, dyspnea, decreased breath sounds, an increased WBC count, and thick, cloudy, purulent drainage. The patient may also complain of pleuritic chest pain. This type of pain is characteristically sharp and nonradiating and intensifies during a deep inspiration.

Treatment for empyema may include a thoracentesis, if the purulent drainage is not too thick, or insertion of a chest tube for continual drainage of the pleural space. The goal of therapy is to remove the debris and approximate the visceral and parietal pleurae. Antibiotics specific to the offending organism will also be started. Other treatments include converting the closed system drainage to an open empyema tube that then drains into a dressing, open tube drainage and rib resection, and thoracotomy and decortication.

Atelectasis. Atelectasis can be caused from pressure being applied directly to the lung. (i.e., pleural effusion), from an internal obstruction of the airways, or from poor excursion due to pain or splinting. Signs and symptoms include moist rales, decreased breath sounds, fever, increased heart rate, dyspnea, and abnormal arterial blood gases.

Treatment includes removing the outside pressure by insertion of a chest tube or removal of the airway obstruction. Maneuvers to remove an airway obstruction include chest physiotherapy and postural drainage, frequent suctioning, bronchoscopy, and mobilization of the patient.

11. **What should be included in assessing the proper function of a chest tube?**

Start at the patient and move toward the collection device.

Palpate around the dressing and insertion site for subcutaneous emphysema.

Assess the dressing for occlusiveness and dryness.

Assess the drainage coming from the chest tube noting its color, consistency, and amount.

Make sure that all connections are tight and secured with tape.

Note the presence or absence of fluid fluctuation in the water seal chamber. Suction will decrease the amount of fluctuation that will be seen. Therefore, suction should be removed when assessing fluctuation.

Note the presence or absence of an air leak in the water seal chamber. The physician should be notified if a new leak develops.

Assess the suction control chamber to make sure the desired amount of suction is being applied. The suction being applied is regulated by the amount of water in the suction control chamber and not by the wall suction unit. The amount of bubbling in the suction control chamber has no effect on the amount of suction being applied. Therefore, only a mild continuous bubbling is needed to achieve the desired suction.

12. What is the difference between milking and stripping a chest tube?

The primary goal of milking or stripping a chest tube is to prevent occlusion of the tube. The frequency of milking and stripping varies according to the primary physician's preference.

Milking a chest tube involves progressively squeezing and releasing the chest tube tubing using a hand-over-hand technique. Milking results in a smaller amount of negative pressure being generated in the pleural space.

Stripping involves occluding the chest tube tubing with one hand. The other hand is then used to occlude the tube below that point. The lower hand is then moved along the tube maintaining occlusion of the tube. After a portion of the tube has been stripped, the upper hand is removed. This results in negative pressure being generated in the pleural space. Stripping the whole length of the chest tube tubing can generate a negative intrapleural pressure in excess of 400 cm of water pressure. Stripping only a few centimeters of tubing can produce a negative pressure of 100 cm H_2O. The amount of negative pressure that is generated appears to be directly related to the amount of tube that is stripped at one time.

There is no objective data, to date, that supports the stripping of chest tubes. Side effects of stripping chest tubes include an increase in negative pressure in the pleural space, tissue damage from lung tissue being entrapped in the chest tube eyelets, and persistent pneumothoraces from air leaks that have not sealed off due to the increase in negative pressure.

Each chest tube should be evaluated for the amount and frequency of milking or stripping that is needed. If the chest tube was placed for the purpose of relieving a pneumothorax, milking or stripping most likely would not be needed. If, however, the thoracostomy tube was placed because of a hemothorax, the tube should be evaluated for clots and milking should be done. In order to prevent the occlusion of thoracostomy tubes, they should be positioned so that there are no dependent loops or kinks.

13. During which phase of the respiratory cycle will an air leak be noted if the patient is connected to a mechanical ventilator?

Inspiration. If the patient is connected to a mechanical ventilator, an air leak will be noted on inspiration. When a ventilator delivers a

222 / Pulmonary System

breath, positive pressure is exerted to the thoracic cavity. The air will travel through the defect in the lung and out the chest tube.

This is just the opposite for a patient who is breathing on his or her own. During inspiration, an increased negativity in the thoracic cavity develops. Therefore, during inspiration the column of water in the water seal chamber will rise. During expiration this increased negativity diminishes. Air will follow the path of least resistance and travel through the defect in the lung and an air leak will be noted.

14. What does bubbling in the water seal chamber indicate?

Bubbling in the water seal chamber indicates the presence of an air leak. Initially upon insertion, continuous bubbling in the water seal chamber may be present due to the release of trapped air from the thoracic cavity. This continuous bubbling should subside within a few minutes. Intermittent bubbling will be present in the water seal chamber until the defect in the lung seals.

15. What are the indications for clamping a chest tube?

One indication for clamping a chest tube is during the investigation of an air leak in the system. This clamping is intermittent and done for a few seconds only, beginning at the chest tube dressing. The clamp is progressively removed and applied to the tube until the continuous bubbling in the water seal stops. The air leak is located distal to the point where the clamp is applied and the bubbling stops. If the bubbling stops when pressure is applied over the chest tube dressing, the air leak is at the insertion site or in the patient's chest. Pressure can be maintained around the dressing in an attempt to stop the leak. If the bubbling stops, the leak was at the insertion site and a more occlusive dressing is needed.

Another indication for clamping a chest tube is during the change of the collection device. The new system should be prepared, the clamp applied, and the system changed. The clamp should not have to remain in place for longer than 30 sec.

The final indication for clamping is if the chest tube becomes disconnected from the collection device. However, if the patient has an air leak the tube should not be clamped, because the build-up of pressure in the pleural space can lead to a tension pneumothorax.

Chest tubes should not be clamped during patient transport to other areas of the hospital. If an air leak in the lung is present, clamping the chest tube allows a build-up of positive pressure in the thoracic cavity and can lead to a tension pneumothorax.

When transporting a patient with a chest tube, the drainage system must remain lower than the thorax. This prevents fluid from flowing backward into the pleural space.

16. **What are the indications for discontinuing a chest tube?**

Less than 100 ml of drainage in a 24-hr period
Chest x-ray reveals a totally inflated lung
No air leak is present in the water seal chamber
Fluctuations stop. When no air remains in the pleural space, the lung wall closes off the eyelets in the chest tube and fluctuations stop.

17. **What nursing diagnoses pertain to Mr. Fox's case?**

Potential for infection related to stab wounds
Fluid volume deficit related to hemothorax
Impaired gas exchange related to tension pneumothorax
Impaired verbal communication related to intubation
Impaired social interaction related to hospitalization
Sleep pattern disturbance related to ICU environment
Knowledge deficit related to diagnosis and invasive tubes
Pain related to stab wounds and chest tube

SUGGESTED READINGS

Alspach JG, Williams SM. Core curriculum for critical care nurses. 3rd ed. Philadelphia: WB Saunders, 1985.

Cardona VD. Trauma nursing. New Jersey: Medical Economics Co., Inc., 1985.

Hurn PD. Thoracic injury. In: Cardona VD, Hurn PD, Mason PJ, Scanlon-Schilpp AM, Veise-Berry SW, eds. Trauma nursing from resuscitation through rehabilitation. Philadelphia: WB Saunders, 1988: 449–490.

Civetta JM, Taylor RW, Kirby RR. Critical care. Philadelphia: JB Lippincott, 1988.

Duncan C, Erickson R. Pressures associated with chest tube stripping. Heart Lung, 1982;11(2):166–171.

Lim-Levy F, Babler SA, De Groot-Kosolcharoen J, Kosolcharoen P,

Dronche GM. Is milking and stripping chest tubes really necessary? Ann Thorac Surg July, 1986;42(1):77–80.

Long BC, Phipps WJ. Medical-surgical nursing, a nursing process approach. 2nd ed. St. Louis: CV Mosby, 1989.

Palau D, Jones S. Test your skill at troubleshooting chest tubes. *RN* 1986;49(10): 43–45.

King TC, Smith CR. Chest wall, pleura, lung, and mediastinum. In: Schwartz SI, Shires GT, Spencer FC, eds. Principles of surgery. 5th ed. New York: McGraw-Hill, 1989:627–770.

Weigelt JA, Aurbakken CM, Meier DE, Thal ER. Management of asymptomatic patients following stab wounds to the chest. J Trauma April, 1982;22(4):291–294.

CHAPTER 24

Status Asthmaticus

Terry L. Jones, RN, BSN, CCRN

Tom Smith is a 15-year-old boy with a history of asthma dating from early childhood, who presented to the Emergency Department with a chief complaint of shortness of breath. His mother reports that he had been in his usual state of health until today when he awoke with mild wheezing. Tom had assisted his brother in cleaning the garage the day previously. Ms. Smith further reported that Tom has always been compliant with his medications, which included Theo-Dur, 300 mg PO TID, terbutaline, 2.5 mg PO TID, and Alupent inhaler, two puffs q 4 hr PRN, and that in addition he had taken a total of five Bronkosol treatments within the past 10 hr at home without significant improvement. Physical examination upon arrival in the Emergency Department revealed bilateral breath sounds with pronounced inspiratory and expiratory wheezing throughout all lung fields. Tom was extremely anxious, exhibited use of accessory muscles of ventilation, and could speak only a few words at a time. Vital signs, ABGs, and initial pulmonary function tests (PFTs) were as follows:

Vital Signs		ABG (room air)		PFTs	
BP	112/80 expiration	pH	7.50	FEV_1	1.1 liters (31% predicted)
BP	102/80 inspiration	$PaCO_2$	28		
		PaO_2	70		
HR	116	SaO_2	91%		
Resp	28	HCO_3	24		
Temp	36°C				

Oxygen was administered by nasal cannula at 4 liters/min, and Tom was immediately treated with 0.3 ml of 1 : 1000 dilution subcutaneous epinephrine and 0.5 ml of Bronkosol in 3 ml of NS by nebulizer. Blood was drawn and sent for electrolytes, CBC, and theophylline level, and a peripheral IV was started for infusion of aminophylline, 270 mg in 1 liter of NS at 100 ml/hr. Tom was also given Solu-Medrol, 125 mg IV push at this time. The subcutaneous epinephrine was repeated in 20 min along with 0.5 ml of subcutaneous terbutaline. Bronkosol treatments followed by PFTs were also repeated every hour, with the following results:

Time	4:00	5:00	6:00	7:00
Liters	1.1	1.2	1.0	0.8
% Predicted FVC	31%	34%	28%	23%

When Tom failed to respond to treatment and his initial theophylline level came back 10 μg/ml, a bolus of aminophylline, 200 mg, was given IV piggyback over 20 min. However, his condition continued to deteriorate. He became diaphoretic and disoriented and exhibited the following clinical data:

Vital Signs		ABGs		Physical Examination
BP	150/100	pH	7.38	Faint wheezing
	expiration	PaCO$_2$	43	15 mm Hg paradox
BP	135/100	PaO$_2$	56	Hyperresonant chest
	inspiration	HCO$_3$	24	to percussion
HR	130	O$_2$ saturation	88%	
Resp	35			

Tom was orally intubated with a size 8 endotracheal tube, placed on mechanical ventilation, and transferred to the Respiratory ICU. His initial ventilator settings included: assist control 12, tidal volume 800 ml, FIO$_2$ 0.60. Although the aminophylline drip and Bronkosol nebulizer treatments were continued after initiation of mechanical ventilation, the peak inspiratory pressures (PIP) remained consistently between 80 and 90 cm H$_2$O. Tom developed subcutaneous emphysema that began with his neck and spread to his face and trunk. A chest x-ray revealed a left pneumothorax, for which a chest tube was inserted and placed to 20 cm H$_2$O suction. Following the chest tube insertion, there was minimal change in the PIP. Tom was kept paralyzed and sedated with a combination of Pavulon and Valium.

QUESTIONS AND ANSWERS

1. **What are the major pathophysiological changes during an acute asthmatic episode?**

    The major problem in asthma is a reduction in the airway diameter resulting from constriction of bronchial smooth muscle, mucosal edema, and excessive production of thick, tenacious mucus. As the cross-sectional diameter of the airways drops, airway resistance increases, which causes a reduction in forced expiratory volumes and flow rates, hyperinflation of the lungs and thorax, increased work of breathing, and abnormal distribution of both ventilation and perfusion.

2. **How is status asthmaticus different from an acute asthmatic attack?**

    Status asthmaticus is a severe, unrelenting asthma attack that fails to respond to conventional therapy with hydration and bronchodilators.

3. **Tom's admission ABG (room air) included pH 7.50, PaCO$_2$ 28, PaO$_2$ 70, HCO$_3$ 24, and SaO$_2$ 91%. Is this typical of a patient experiencing an acute asthmatic attack?**

   Yes. It is common to see a respiratory alkalosis with mild hypoxemia during an acute asthmatic attack. The bronchoconstriction and mucus plugging result in underventilation of some alveoli, with diversion of blood flow to more normally ventilated alveoli. Even so, a $\dot{V}/\dot{Q}$ mismatch develops, resulting in hypoxemia. Unlike the patient with other types of obstructive lung defects, the asthmatic does not usually present with hypercapnia. In fact, once the PaCO$_2$ exceeds 40, the patient is likely to be tiring and approaching respiratory failure. Intubation should be strongly considered at this point. Failure of the clinician to recognize the serious implications of a PaCO$_2$ >40 can result in disastrous consequences for the asthmatic.

4. **Tom's PFTs demonstrated a progressive decline in FEV$_1$. What did this indicate?**

   Failure of PFTs to improve or deterioration of PFTs despite aggressive bronchodilator therapy is diagnostic of status asthmaticus and indicates the potential need for endotracheal intubation. FEV$_1$ (forced expiratory volume in 1 sec) is the maximum volume of gas that the patient can exhale in 1 sec. Normally this equals approximately 75 to 83% of the forced vital capacity (maximum volume of gas exhaled following a maximal inhalation). PEFR (peak expiratory flow rate), also known as PFR (peak flow rate) is the maximum flow rate that the patient can generate. The average PEFR for healthy adults is approximately 600 liters/min. An FEV$_1$ of <30% of the predicted value and/or a PEFR of <100–200 liters/min are risk factors for respiratory failure and indicate that intubation with mechanical ventilation may be imminent.

5. **Tom's initial assessment revealed pronounced inspiratory and expiratory wheezing throughout all lung fields, but after three Bronkosol treatments, the wheezing became faint. Was this a good prognostic sign?**

   No. If a patient experiencing a severe asthmatic attack exhibits a disappearance of wheezing with accompanying diminished breath sounds, it may indicate that the bronchospasm has worsened and the patient is not even moving enough air to generate wheezing. Therefore, the disappearance of wheezing with overall diminished breath sounds in an acute asthmatic episode may indicate worsening of the ventilatory defect.

6. **As Tom's condition deteriorated, he developed pulsus paradoxus of 15 mm Hg. What is the mechanism believed to be responsible for this?**
   Pulsus paradoxus occurs when one's systolic BP on inspiration is ≥10 mm Hg lower than on expiration. The greater negative intrapleural pressure created during inspiration when accessory muscles are used causes pulmonary vasodilatation, leading to pooling of blood and decreased left ventricular return. As a result, there is a transient decrease in CO and BP. During expiration, on the other hand, use of accessory muscles creates a very high intrapleural pressure, which results in a squeezing effect on the pulmonary vasculature. Consequently, left ventricular filling is facilitated and BP and CO are increased.

7. **List the therapeutic modalities generally employed to treat status asthmaticus.**
   Oxygen
   Sympathomimetics
   Methylxanthines
   Corticosteroids
   Antimicrobials
   Hydration
   Intubation with mechanical ventilation
   Sedation with paralytic therapy (postintubation only)

8. **In an effort to reverse his increased airways resistance, Tom was given sympathomimetics to enhance bronchodilatation. What are the recommended routes and dosages of the commonly used sympathomimetics?**
   Epinephrine, 1 : 1000 0.3 ml SC q 20–30 min for a maximum of three doses. Epinephrine should be used cautiously, if at all, in patients over 40 years of age.
   Terbutaline sulfate, 0.25–0.5 ml SC q 30 min for a maximum of three doses.
   Bronkosol, 0.5 ml in 3 ml of NS via nebulizer q 30 min times 2–3 then q 1–2 hr.
   Alupent, 0.3 ml in 3 ml of NS via nebulizer q 1–2 hr.

   Effectiveness of these drugs should be monitored with serial PFTs to assess for improvement in FEV_1.

9. **Aminophylline, a methylxanthine, is also an integral part of the treatment for status asthmaticus. What is the recommended dosage of aminophylline for the patient in status asthmaticus?**
   If the patient has been taking theophylline at home, he or she should not be given a loading dose of aminophylline until serum lev-

els have been checked. The therapeutic theophylline level is 10–20 μg/ml. While the level is pending, a continuous IV infusion of 0.6–0.9 mg/kg/hr in young patients or 0.5 mg/kg/hr in older patients should be initiated. Once the level is obtained, a half loading/bolus dose of 3.0 mg/kg can be infused over 20–30 min if indicated. A full loading dose of 6.0 mg/kg over 20 min should be given prior to the continuous infusion if the patient has not been receiving theophylline.

10. **What is the rationale for administration of steroids in status asthmaticus?**

Although the exact mechanism of action is not completely clear, the two known effects of corticosteroids believed to be of benefit in status asthmaticus include their anti-inflammatory effects and potentiation of β-adrenergic medications. Approximately 10–20% of asthmatics receive steroids chronically and therefore must have prompt administration of steroids during an acute attack.

11. **Why is adequate hydration an important consideration in the management of status asthmaticus?**

The increased work of breathing in status asthmaticus results in tachypnea and diaphoresis, both of which increase insensible water loss. In addition, patients in status asthmaticus often have decreased oral intake, and all of these factors contribute to dehydration. This may be reflected in an increased hematocrit and increased urine specific gravity.

The patient experiencing an acute asthma attack produces a large volume of viscous mucus. If the patient is dehydrated, the secretions will be even more tenacious. There is frequently a defect in the mucociliary apparatus, which results in inadequate clearing of bronchial secretions. All of these factors contribute to the formation of mucus plugs. These thick, tenacious mucus plugs can completely occlude the airways and have been implicated as an important cause of mortality in status asthmaticus. Maintenance of adequate hydration helps liquefy the secretions so that they can be mobilized and cleared. Using a humidifier on the oxygen administration device is important for similar reasons.

12. **What indicated the need for mechanical ventilation in Tom's case?**

Decreased pH
Increased $PaCO_2$
Disorientation
FEV_1 <1 liter/<30% of predicted value

Failure to respond to bronchodilators
Markedly diminished breath sounds associated with cessation of
wheezing

Tom was intubated via the oral route with a large ETT (size 8) and
placed on a volume ventilator. Because his initial peak inspiratory
pressures were significantly elevated, reaching 80–90 cm H_2O, he
was kept sedated and paralyzed with a combination of Valium and
Pavulon.

13. **Why is a large endotracheal tube desired for intubation of an asthmatic? What other considerations are pertinent regarding intubation of an asthmatic?**

    The cross-sectional diameter of the airway is one of the factors that
    determines airway resistance. The smaller the tube, the greater the
    airway resistance. This constriction of the airway proximal to the
    patient compounds the problems in ventilator management. Further,
    it is difficult to suction the viscid secretions through a small endotracheal tube.

    Intubation may be difficult in the asthmatic, as the patient is frequently alert, fearful, and severely dyspneic. Struggling and increased fear during intubation may worsen the bronchospasm. Sedation is frequently required, and a manual resuscitator bag must be
    set up and ready. The assistance of an anesthesiologist may be
    needed.

14. **Although Tom had been highly anxious since his arrival in the Emergency Department, he was not sedated until he was intubated. Was this an oversight?**

    No. Opiates, sedatives, and tranquilizers can depress alveolar
    ventilation and are absolutely contraindicated in the nonintubated
    asthmatic patient (with the exception of immediately prior to intubation by a skilled physician). Sedative administration in status
    asthmaticus has been associated with respiratory arrest. In addition,
    the available sedatives have been shown to have one or more of the
    following adverse effects: cough suppression, histamine release, and
    mucosal drying.

15. **Despite aggressive treatment with bronchodilators and controlled ventilation, Tom's bronchospasm persisted for several hours, resulting in peak pressures of 80–90 cm H_2O. The anesthesia service was consulted and Tom was given halothane anesthesia in the unit. What was the rationale for this therapeutic modality?**

    For that small portion of patients who exhibit profound persistent
    bronchospasm accompanied by respiratory acidosis despite in-

tubation with mechanical ventilation and other conventional modalities, halothane has been used to relieve bronchospasm. Halothane anesthesia has a potent bronchodilator effect without stimulation of respiratory secretions. It is not, however, without side effects, as it is a known myocardial depressant, causes vasodilatation, and has the ability to increase ventricular irritability. Patients receiving such treatment must be closely monitored with frequent vital signs.

16. **Although the only ECG abnormality noted on Tom was sinus tachycardia, what other ECG changes might you expect in the older patient in status asthmaticus?**

The stress of hypoxia during status asthmaticus may cause ECG changes indicative of myocardial ischemia and/or infarction. The pulmonary artery responds to hypoxia by constricting, creating an increase in pulmonary vascular resistance and subsequent right heart strain. Consequently, right axis deviation, P-pulmonale, ST depression, right bundle branch block, and PVCs may occur.

17. **What is the rationale for initiation of pharmacologic paralysis?**

Due to the presence of alveolar hyperinflation, the patient in status asthmaticus is at increased risk for barotrauma. The risk is further exaggerated in the patient receiving mechanical ventilation with high peak inspiratory pressures. In addition, such patients require prolonged expiratory times to adequately exhale due to their extremely constricted airways. The inspiratory flow must be sufficiently fast to ensure sufficient time for exhalation. In order to achieve this, without further increasing peak inspiratory pressure with a rapid peak flow rate, it is necessary to ventilate the patient at a lower rate than his or her spontaneous rate. When the patient is pharmacologically paralyzed and sedated, controlled ventilation can be achieved, resulting in an increase in ventilator efficacy, decreased tissue oxygen demands, relief of muscle fatigue, and decreased risk of barotrauma (pneumothorax). One must remember that the bronchospasms causing status are not reversed simply by intubation, and even the intubated asthmatic will continue to be extremely anxious and tachypneic. The patient may breathe asynchronously with the ventilator, which heightens anxiety and worsens tachypnea. In addition, breathing out of phase with the ventilator elevates mean airway pressure, increasing the risk of barotrauma.

18. **What nursing diagnoses might have been applicable for Tom?**

Ineffective breathing pattern related to respiratory muscle fatigue
Ineffective airway clearance related to artificial airway

Impaired gas exchange related to airway constriction
Potential for injury in case of ventilator disconnection
Powerlessness related to pharmacologic paralysis
Fear related to perceived inability to control breathing pattern
Social isolation related to impaired verbal communication

SUGGESTED READINGS

Alspach J, Williams S. Core curriculum for critical care nursing. 3rd ed. Philadelphia: WB Saunders, 1985.

Cosenza J, Cilentano N. Secretion clearance: State of the art from a nursing perspective. Crit Care Nurse 1986;6(4):23–37.

Des Jordins T. Clinical manifestations of respiratory disease. Chicago: Year Book, 1984.

Larson J, Kim M. Ineffective breathing pattern related to respiratory muscle fatigue. Nurs Clin North Am 1987;22(1):207–223.

McFarland G, Naschinski C. Impaired communication. Nurs Clin North Am 1985;20(4):775–785.

Rochester D. Respiratory muscle function in health. Heart Lung 1984;13(4):349–353.

Sohn S. Pulmonary emergencies. New York: Churchill Livingston, 1982.

Schwartz S. Treatment of status asthmaticus with halothane. JAMA 1984;251(6):2688–2689.

Shekleton M, Nield M. Ineffective airway clearance related to artificial airway. Nurs Clin North Am 1987;22(1):167–179.

Shoemaker W, Ayres S, Ohe G, Holbrook P, Thompson W, eds. Textbook of critical care. 2nd ed. Philadelphia: WB Saunders, 1989.

Traver, G. Ineffective airway clearance: Physiology and clinical application. Dimensions Crit Care Nurs 1985;4(4):198–208.

Part III

Neurological System

CHAPTER 25

Arteriovenous Malformation

Susan Nevins, RN, MA, CNRN

Mark Johnson is a 27-year-old single, right-handed male musician who lives with his parents and two younger sisters in a cooperative apartment in a large metropolitan city. Mr. Johnson teaches music theory and string instrumentation in a private high school. While conducting a sonata practice for a spring concert, he experienced a twitching of the right side of his mouth that progressed down his right arm and leg and lasted about 45 sec. He was startled and embarrassed, but ignored the incident because he thought it was related to his increased work schedule and stress related to organizing the concert. Several evenings later, he was using a rowing machine at home when he experienced a sudden, severe headache, blurred vision, and sensitivity to light followed by a stiffening of his neck muscles. He vomited and felt some relief of his headache. However, the headache soon intensified and involved the entire left side of his head. He took two aspirin with little relief. His sister, a registered nurse, became concerned and urged him to go to the Emergency Department of the nearest hospital.

Upon arrival in the Emergency Department, Mr. Johnson was examined by a neurologist. Based on his history and neurological examination, an emergency contrast enhanced CT scan was ordered. The scan revealed a subarachnoid hemorrhage (SAH), a diffuse enlargement of the ventricles (communicating hydrocephalus), no evidence of an intracerebral hematoma, but a moderate sized, left frontoparietal mass suggestive of a cerebral arteriovenous malformation (AVM).

QUESTIONS AND ANSWERS

1. **What is an AVM?**

    An AVM is a congenital vascular abnormality that occurs as a result of fetal maldevelopment of the primitive capillary system and vascular plexus. Blood shunts directly from arteries into veins without an intervening capillary system. Vessels adjacent to the AVM provide collateral circulation. These vessels eventually become a tortuous conglomeration of dilated thickened or thinned, fragile vessels. The mass of abnormal vessels comprising the AVM has been commonly called a "bag of worms."

AVMs have been known to increase in size over the long history of the disorder; however, most stabilize over time. Additional arterial feeders are thought to be responsible for the change in AVM mass as well as enlargement of the venous channels, as they are required to manage an increased load of shunted blood (1).

The intravascular dynamics of an AVM involve a system of abnormally high flow, low resistance. This results in alterations in autoregulation and the possible consequence of intracerebral steal phenomenon.

2. **Describe the intracerebral steal phenomenon and the two schools of thought concerning it.**

The concept of intracerebral steal phenomenon has been researched and debated in the literature extensively. Its advocates consider intracerebral steal to be a physiological consequence of cerebral AVMs. Cerebral ischemia and/or necrosis is thought to develop in the healthy cerebral tissue from which blood is shunted to supply the AVM. Cerebral perfusion is not considered to be supported as well by the AVMs nidus, its feeding vessels or draining veins. According to Rosenblum (2), a promising new technique known as laser Doppler velocimetry can measure cerebral blood flow intraoperatively. These authors consider this technique a reliable measure to support cerebral steal phenomenon. On a microcirculatory level, it assesses cerebral perfusion to brain tissue adjacent to an AVM pre- and postexcision.

Some authors argue against the intracerebral steal phenomenon. They claim that if decreased perfusion (ischemia) were really a consequence of steal, then proximal ligation, carotid ligation, or embolization of AVM feeders should result in increased neurological dysfunction (3). In such cases, however, patients have been reported to have an unchanged or improved neurological state. They allege this creates speculation and weakens the case for the steal phenomenon.

Regardless of whether cerebral ischemia related to cerebral AVMs is caused by steal, thrombosis, or increased venous perfusion, it is a significant factor causing progressive neurological deficits. Additional causations of neurological dysfunction include increased ICP, hemorrhage, and compression of neural tissue.

3. **What are the most common sites of cerebral AVMs?**

An AVM can be located in any part of the cerebral hemispheres, brainstem, or cerebellum, and can range in size from a few millimeters to > 4–5 cm. It can be found on the surface of the brain, the cerebral cortex, the ventricular system, or deep within the cerebral hemispheres (4).

4. **How common are AVMs?**

The most comprehensive study on vascular malformations was reported by Sarwar and McCormick in 1978 (5). It cites the prevalence of cerebral AVMs as 0.6% in over 4000 autopsy cases. The incidence is reported as slightly higher in male than in female subjects.

Mr. Johnson was transferred directly from CT scan to the neurosurgical step-down unit for close observation and monitoring. Admission assessment data included:

Alert and oriented ×3
Normal mental status
Moderate left-sided headache
Slight nuchal rigidity
Photophobia
No diplopia, no nystagmus, no blurred vision
Pupils equal bilaterally, 5 mm, reacting briskly to direct and consensual
    light
Motor strength full 5+ in all extremities
Sensory examination normal
Cerebellar examination normal
Reflexes normal
Cranial nerves intact including no papilledema

5. **What distinctions should the critical care nurse recognize between an ischemic (occlusive) versus hemorrhagic cerebrovascular accident (CVA)?**

A hemorrhagic CVA is most commonly caused by bleeding from congenital vascular anomalies, such as a ruptured intracranial aneurysm or cerebral AVM. Bleeding occurs directly into the subarachnoid space and/or into brain tissue, causing a sudden onset of neurological dysfunction. There is usually an absence of warning signs.

An embolic CVA is caused by an embolus that develops outside the brain. The heart, neck, and thorax are common sites for embolic development. As in a hemorrhagic CVA, neurological deficits occur within seconds or minutes and there is an absence of warning signs. Collateral circulation may be achieved earlier than in a hemorrhagic CVA.

An ischemic or occlusive CVA is most commonly caused by acquired conditions such as cerebral thrombosis or embolism, but may occur secondary to intracerebral steal phenomenon in AVM. Thrombosis is usually the result of arteriosclerosis, and the following progression of symptoms is common: transient ischemic attack (TIA), reversible ischemic neurological episode, stroke in evolution, and a completed stroke. Headaches resulting from AVMs are more generalized, recurrent, severe, and disabling.

Mr. Johnson spent the first 4 days of his admission uneventfully. His neurological status remained stable and the meningeal signs progressively cleared. However, a global left-sided headache persisted despite a stronger analgesic. On day 5, a right cerebral angiogram was performed, which revealed a moderate sized left frontoparietal AVM. He tolerated the procedure well with no complications.

6. **Describe the type of headaches associated with cerebral AVMs, classic "migraine," and subarachnoid hemorrhage.**
   Headaches associated with cerebral AVMs have sometimes been called atypical migraines. As in migraines, vomiting and visual disturbances can accompany an AVM headache. This is particularly likely with an occipital lobe AVM. Headaches resulting from AVMs are more generalized, recurrent, severe, and disabling. The degree of discomfort probably results from the dural involvement of the AVM. Important distinctions include the fact that AVM headaches remain on the same side of the head, unlike migraines, which tend to switch sides. Other differences include the fact that migraine attacks may be precipitated by fatigue, stress, the menstrual cycle, and dietary intolerances (e.g., wine, chocolate, cheese). The headache associated with a SAH from an intracranial aneurysm rupture is usually described as more explosive or bursting in nature than an AVM bleed. The AVM headache also tends to become intractable. Both AVM and aneurysm bleeds cause vomiting, visual deficits, an impaired level of consciousness in some cases, and meningeal signs (photophobia, nuchal rigidity, low grade fever).

On the evening of day 6, Mr. Johnson experienced a focal seizure of similar pattern to the one prior to admission. Seizure progression followed, which resulted in a loss of consciousness, incontinence, and tonic-clonic convulsive movements without respiratory embarrassment. The patient received Valium, 10 mg IV push, and was taken for an emergency CT scan. Following the seizure he had some expressive aphasia and a mild right-sided hemiparesis. The CT scan showed a left frontal hematoma. Mr. Johnson was sent to surgery for emergency evacuation of the hematoma and a complete resection of his AVM.

7. **What are the major complications of a cerebral AVM?**

    Common sequelae of an AVM include increased ICP, cerebral ischemia, compression of brain tissue, bleeding, and hydrocephalus.

8. **What are the two most common clinical manifestations of a cerebral AVM?**

    Seizure activity and hemorrhage represent the most common presenting clinical manifestations (3). Focal (partial) or generalized seizures can occur, depending on the size and location of the AVM. Focal seizures may be simple or complex. (See Chapter 30, "Status Epilepticus," for a discussion of seizures.)

    Hemorrhage occurs in 50% of all patients with AVMs (6) and is the most common presenting sign in childhood. There is subarachnoid extension and subsequently SAH in at least half of these cases. Furthermore, AVM bleeds are more likely to be intraparenchymal, because of their degree of location within cerebral tissue.

9. **Identify other clinical manifestations of an AVM.**

    Other focal symptoms include aphasias, contralateral hemiparesis, and/or hemisensory deficits, and visual impairments; e.g., diplopia, field cuts (hemianopsias). Scalp hemangiomas are sometimes present. Carotid, mastoid or ocular systolic bruits are less frequently diagnosed now, owing to earlier AVM detection by advances in neurodiagnostics such as the CT scan and MRI. Vein of Galen malformations can cause an obstructive hydrocephalus.

10. **Discuss the neurodiagnostic studies used to identify Mr. Johnson's AVM.**

    The contrast enhanced CT scan can diagnose all but the most minute cerebral AVMs. The AVM's site and size are identified, as well as any evidence of SAH, intracerebral hematoma, and/or signs of hydrocephalus. Mr. Johnson's admission CT scan revealed a left frontoparietal AVM and blood in the cisterns suggestive of a SAH. The diffuse enlargement of the ventricular system demonstrated communicating hydrocephalus, which was related to the SAH. There was no evidence on admission of any intracerebral bleed. A repeat CT scan when the patient's neurological status changed, however, revealed a small left frontal intracerebral bleed. Four-vessel cerebral angiography was performed to evaluate Mr. Johnson's complete vertebral and carotid cerebrovascular system. This contrast study is done to identify the operative problem, inspect cerebral blood flow, and evaluate collateral and compensatory blood supply. In addition, the arterial feeders, the nidus, and the venous drainage of the AVM could be assessed.

MRI can add useful information in evaluating nervous system disorders. It can provide localization information about cerebral AVMs. However, Mr. Johnson could not undergo an MRI due to the presence of metal pins implanted in his right wrist following an orthopaedic injury years ago.

11. What are the objectives of surgical resection of cerebral AVMs?

The primary objectives of surgical resection are to prevent further AVM bleeds, to decrease ICP, to alleviate progression in neurological deficits, and to eliminate seizure foci. Surgical excision is also done to treat intractable headaches, which can be disabling in some cases. AVM excision is generally considered the treatment of choice and involves the removal of the arteriovenous shunt. AVMs of the brainstem or diencephalon present the greatest risk, because of their proximity to vital structures of the nervous system. Without operative intervention, however, these patients can suffer serious bleeds, severe disability and/or death.

The microneurosurgical resection of a cerebral AVM is usually an elective procedure. Patients like Mr. Johnson are usually permitted time to recover from a hemorrhagic incident and then careful evaluation is performed. If an intracerebral bleed occurs, however, earlier surgical intervention is required.

Consistent with this practice, Mr. Johnson underwent an emergency CT scan when his neurological status deteriorated. This was followed by immediate neurosurgical intervention, involving evacuation of the left frontal intracerebral hematoma and total resection of the AVM.

12. What is normal perfusion breakthrough phenomenon and how can it be prevented or managed?

The normal perfusion breakthrough is described as a phenomenon that occurs immediately following cerebral AVM excision. Autoregulation fails when normal cerebral blood flow and perfusion is suddenly restored to dilated cortical vessels adjacent to the AVM. These vessels cannot constrict in response to the sudden hyperemic state. This can cause massive cerebral edema and postoperative hematomas in excessively large AVMs (2).

Some neurosurgeons recommend embolizing very large AVMs prior to operative resection or performing AVM excision in stages. Others suggest avoiding this complication by using a protocol of induced hypotension in the immediate postoperative period. This permits critical time for the normal cerebrovasculature to respond to intravascular changes. A dehydration protocol would accompany this measure.

13. **What is the role of embolization in the treatment of cerebral AVMs?**

    Embolization for the treatment of cerebral AVMs was introduced by Luessenhop in the 1960s. Embolization today is used as an adjunctive therapy done prior to the resection of large AVMs or as the treatment of choice for surgically inaccessible lesions. As an adjunctive treatment, it is thought to prevent or decrease the perfusion breakthrough in resection of large AVMs. As an alternative choice of treatment to surgical resection of accessible AVMs, it is considered controversial. Before embolization can be advocated as a primary treatment for cerebral AVMs, certain issues must be resolved. Included are the need for more extensive patient follow-up postembolization, for further advancement in embolization techniques, and long-term evaluation of patients' neurological outcome from embolization versus resection.

    Cerebral embolization has used several different methods. Some involve the injection of particulate matter (Gelfoam pellets, Silastic spheres, etc.) into the vessels feeding the AVM. Gelfoam is less commonly used, because it is difficult to make radiopaque and is reabsorbed in several weeks. Silastic spheres are radiopaque, easy to direct, and generally well tolerated; however, they are not thrombogenic (7). The major problem with either substance is that collateral circulation can develop around feeders that have been embolized. A more promising technique involves the injection of various glues into the nidus of the AVM. Potential complications include: glue reflux into normal cerebral arteries leading to neurological deficits, glue advancement into the venous drainage of the AVM causing hypertension and bleeding, and glue creating technical difficulties during an AVM resection (8). The long-term effects on cerebral tissue need to be researched. In any event, the technique of cerebral embolization is rapidly advancing.

    Mr. Johnson arrived in the Neurosurgical ICU alert and oriented ×3, extubated, with a global aphasia, expressive greater than receptive, and a right-sided hemiparesis and Babinski. Otherwise, he was neurologically intact.

14. **Differentiate between an expressive versus receptive versus global aphasia and the implications for the critical care nurse and describe Mr. Johnson's aphasia from AVM rebleed and resection.**

    Expressive or motor aphasia involves a dysfunction of Broca's area for speech in the frontal lobe. It is characterized by a nonfluent, telegraphic pattern of speech. The patient's comprehension is intact as is his or her ability to read; however, there is an impairment in verbal and written communication. The patient recognizes the errors, which increases his or her concern and feelings of frustration. It is important to acknowledge the patient's communication problems and emphasize the fact that comprehension is intact. Speak to the patient in a slow, relaxed manner and permit sufficient time for him or her to respond. Listen carefully and teach the patient alternative communication methods. Mr. Johnson experienced expressive aphasia when he rebled from his AVM and developed a left frontal intracerebral hematoma.

Receptive or sensory aphasia involves a dysfunction of Wernicke's area of speech in the parietotemporal lobes. It is marked by a fluent, illogical speech pattern. The patient's comprehension and ability to read is impaired, even though he or she may write or speak fluently.

Global aphasia involves components of both expressive and receptive impairments. Patients may have varying degrees of both. Global aphasia is a more common presentation for patients with larger AVMs involving the dominant hemisphere for speech. Mr. Johnson experienced a global aphasia from AVM resection with expressive more marked than receptive. The location of his AVM was in his dominant hemisphere, i.e., a left frontoparietal lesion affecting expressive and receptive speech components.

Mr. Johnson had the usual dehydration protocol and antihypertensive management.

15. Describe the postoperative care of patients following AVM excision.

Many aspects of postoperative care following AVM excision closely parallel the care administered to any patient post craniotomy. Neurological signs and vital signs are closely monitored every hour or more frequently if indicated. Seizure precautions are instituted. Total systems assessment and support are strictly followed with emphasis on blood gases, serum electrolytes, hematocrit, and clotting times. During the first 24 hr the nurse ensures the patient's readiness for immediate and emergent transport to CT scan or the Operating Room.

The two major postoperative complications of AVM excision are swelling and hemorrhage.

Protocol of Care: Swelling

Parameter. Elevate head of bed 15–30°.

Rationale. Cortical veins have no valves, and are therefore responsive to gravity drainage.

Parameter. Maintain neck in alignment with body using small pillows.

Rationale. Poor head and neck alignment decreases venous outflow and increases swelling.

Parameter. Fluid management should be based on the hemodynamic (BP >90 systolic, HR <120) and renal status (urine output >30 ml/hr) of the patient. Deviations from this protocol are appropriate in patients with underlying disease processes or when an AVM is accompanied by the rupture of an aneurysm. (See Chapter 26, "Cerebral Aneurysm.")

Rationale. Rehydrating the fluids lost from the intraoperative administration of mannitol and Lasix based on central venous or pulmonary artery wedge pressure readings can cause intracerebral edema. If blood volume must be replaced, consider Lasix administration also.

Parameter. Maintain blood pressure in the range of 90–100 systolic with vasodilators such as Nipride.

Rationale. Increased blood pressure results in increased cerebral blood flow. Increased cerebral blood flow increases intracerebral edema.

Protocol of Care: Hemorrhage

Parameter. Maintain blood pressure in the range of 90–100 systolic with vasodilators such as Nipride. Sedatives and anesthetic agents may be added to control blood pressure in the patient who responds poorly to vasodilation or whose activity level is problematic.

Rationale. Postoperative bleeds of all etiology are seen in patients post-AVM excision. (See Chapter 28, "Epidural Hematoma"; Chapter 31, "Subdural Hematoma"; and Chapter 26, "Cerebral Aneurysm" for further management strategies.) AVM excision is further complicated with the normal perfusion breakthrough phenomenon and the loss of autoregulation. (See information previously mentioned in this chapter.)

Parameter. Observe the site and distal pulses of the angiography site.

Rationale. AVM excision is always followed by cerebral angiography to confirm complete removal. In the event the patient is unstable, the angiography may be delayed.

No systems complications occurred, and Mr. Johnson was transferred to the neurosurgical step-down unit on the fourth postoperative day. There he underwent intensive speech, physical, and occupational therapy. He made very steady, progressive neurological improvement and eventually continued his therapies on an outpatient basis. He was able to resume a career in music.

16. Identify pertinent nursing diagnoses in Mr. Johnson's case.

Alteration in cerebral tissue perfusion related to cerebral edema
Fluid volume deficit related to postoperative dehydration protocol
Potential for injury related to seizures
Impaired physical mobility related to right-sided hemiparesis
Impaired verbal/written communication related to global aphasia
Role disturbance related to neurological deficits
Social isolation related to global aphasia
Alteration in family dynamics due to patient's neurological deficits.

REFERENCES

1. Stein BM, Wolpert SM. Arteriovenous malformations of the brain. I. Current concepts and treatments. Arch Neurol 1980;37:1–5, and Part II 1980;37:69–75.
2. Rosenblum BR. Pathophysiology of cerebral arteriovenous malformations: Recent advances in analysis and therapy. In: Rosenblum BR, ed. Neurosurgery: State of the art reviews on cerebral and spinal arteriovenous malformations. Vols. 1 and 3, Philadelphia: Hanley & Belfus, 1988: 1–11.
3. Malis LI. Arteriovenous malformations of the brain. In: Yomans JR, ed. Neurological surgery, Vol. 3. Philadelphia: WB Saunders, 1982:1787–1806.
4. Adams RD, Victor M. Principles of neurology. 3rd ed. New York: McGraw-Hill, 1985.
5. Sarwar M, McCormick WF. Intracerebral venous angioma. Arch Neurol 1978; 35:323–328.
6. Rudy EB. Advanced neurological and neurosurgical nursing. St. Louis: CV Mosby, 1984:211.
7. Michelsen WJ, Hilal SK. Interventional neuroradiology. In: Yomans JR, ed. Neurological surgery, Vol. 3. Philadelphia: WB Saunders, 1982:1194–1203.
8. Ojemann RG, Heros RC, Cromwell RM. Surgical management of cerebrovascular disease. 2nd ed. Baltimore: Williams and Wilkins, 1988:347–411.

SUGGESTED READINGS

Dembo M. Arteriovenous malformations of the brain: A review of the literature since 1960. Arch Phys Med Rehab 1982;63:565–568.

Hickey J. The clinical practice of neurological and neurosurgical nursing, 2nd ed. Philadelphia: JB Lippincott, 1986.

Merritt HH. A textbook of neurology. 7th ed. Philadelphia: Lea & Febiger, 1984.

Nevins S. Specific disorders affecting the central nervous system. In: Kneisl CR, Ames SW, eds. Adult health nursing: A biopsychosocial approach. Menlo Park, Ca: Addison-Wesley, 1986:1158–1162, 1164, 1167–1168.

Pallett PJ, O'Brien MT. Textbook of neurological nursing. Boston: Little, Brown & Co., 1985:260–261, 291.

Parkinson D, Bachers G. Arteriovenous malformations summary of 100 consecutive supratentorial cases. J Neurosurg 1980;53:285–299.

Vinter HV, Lundi MJ, Kaufman CE. Long-term pathological follow-up of cerebral arteriovenous malformations treated by embolizations with bucrylate N Engl J Med 1986;314:477–483.

Walter W. Conservative treatment of cerebral arteriovenous angiomas. In: Pia HW, Cleave JRW, Grote E, Zierski J, eds. Cerebral angiomas. Advances in diagnosis and therapy. New York: Springer-Verlag, 1975:271–278.

CHAPTER 26

Cerebral Aneurysm

Venita Dasch, RN, BSN

Barbara Lee is a 42-year-old homemaker who experienced the sudden onset of severe headache while working in her garden. Ms. Lee summoned the help of her husband and was taken to the Emergency Department of her community hospital.

On admission to the Emergency Department she describes the headache as "explosive" and "without warning." She reports slight nausea, sensitivity of her eyes to light, and blurred vision. She describes the headache as "the worst headache of my life."

Her examination reveals the following:

Vital Signs

BP	168/94
HR	88
Resp	20
Temp	37.4°C

Neurological. Pupils equal and reactive. Awake, alert, and oriented to person, place, and time. Speech clarity and content intact. Facial symmetry intact. Follows complex commands. Moves all extremities with equal power and a negative drift. Her neck is stiff and painful with positive Kernig's and Brudzinski's sign.

Psychosocial. Patient is restless; concerned that her headache has not been relieved by Demerol, 75 mg IM; and frequently asks, "What is wrong with me?"

All other systems are intact.

Ms. Lee's physician orders a CT scan, which shows a small collection of subdural blood in the area of the juncture of the posterior communicating artery and the internal carotid artery. She has no shift or further abnormal findings. Her physician obtains consent and performs a lumbar puncture on Ms. Lee. The results of her spinal tap are as follows:

Pressure	High normal at 160 mm H_2O in the lateral recumbent position
Appearance	Bloody
Cells	Increased at >5 lymphocytes
Protein	Increased at 95 mg/100 ml
Glucose	68 mg/100 ml

QUESTIONS AND ANSWERS

1. **Given the information obtained from Ms. Lee and the physical examination results, which factors indicate that she has suffered a subarachnoid hemorrhage?**

   Ms. Lee, at age 42, is within the most prevalent age range for subarachnoid hemorrhage, i.e., 35–60 years. Her headache presented without warning and was described as "explosive." The description of the headache as being "the worst headache of my life" is a universal statement made by individuals who have suffered a subarachnoid hemorrhage.

   In a subarachnoid hemorrhage, blood comes into contact with the meninges, producing Ms. Lee's symptoms of photophobia, blurred vision, restlessness, irritability, and positive Kernig's and Brudzinski's signs. Kernig's sign is elicited by flexing the patient's leg at the hip and knee and then straightening the knee and noting any resistance or pain. Brudzinski's sign is confirmed by flexing the recumbent patient's neck forward and observing for flexion of the knees and hips in response to this maneuver.

   Her spinal fluid results also indicate the probability of a subarachnoid hemorrhage. A review of spinal fluid parameters is as follows:

   Normal Pressure. Lateral recumbent 60–180 mm H_2O.
   SAH. Within normal limits to extreme increase.

   Normal Appearance. Clear.
   SAH: Pink to grossly bloody. Spinal fluid discolored by red cells is labeled xanthochromic.

   Normal Cells. 0–5 lymphocytes.
   SAH: Red blood cells increased. White blood cells increased.

   Normal Protein. 15–45 mg/100 ml.
   SAH: Increased.

   Normal Glucose. 60–80% of true blood sugar; 40–80 mg/100 ml.
   SAH. Within normal limits to a marked decrease.

   Ms. Lee is admitted to the Neurosurgical ICU with a diagnosis of Grade II subarachnoid hemorrhage. She is ordered on subarachnoid hemorrhage precautions, and a neurosurgeon is notified for consultation. Her headache and photophobia remain severe and she is now complaining of double vision. Her vital signs are:

BP	144/88
HR	76
Resp	16
Temp	37.6°C

2. **What system is used to classify SAH?**

   Grade I (Minimal Bleed). Asymptomatic; alert with minimal headache, slight nuchal rigidity, and no neurological deficit.
   Grade II (Mild Bleed). Alert, mild to severe headache, nuchal rigidity, minimal neurological deficit such as cranial nerve dysfunction.
   Grade III (Moderate Bleed). Drowsy or confused, nuchal rigidity; may have mild focal deficits.
   Grade IV (Moderate to Severe Bleed). Stupor; mild to severe hemiparesis; nuchal rigidity; possible early decerebration.
   Grade V (Severe Bleed). Deep coma; decerebrate rigidity; moribund appearance.

3. **What are subarachnoid hemorrhage precautions?**
   Subarachnoid hemorrhage precautions are instituted to provide the patient with a nonstimulating environment, thereby preventing the elevation of blood and intracranial pressures. The degree of anxiety created by severe limitations on physical activity should be assessed on every patient and the plan altered accordingly. In general, SAH precautions include:

   Precaution. Private room or cubicle. Lights dim. Complete bed rest. Physical care such as feeding and bathing is performed by the nurse. No television, radio, or phone. Visitors are kept to a minimum.
   Rationale. To prevent increases in blood pressure.

   Precaution. The patient must be cautioned against coughing, sneezing, or straining of any kind. No enemas are given. Stool softeners and mild laxatives are administered.
   Rationale. Valsalva maneuvers greatly increase intracranial pressure. Enemas increase intraabdominal pressure and subsequently increase intracranial pressure.

   Precaution. Head of the bed is elevated 30–45°.
   Rationale. The head of the bed is elevated to promote venous drainage and thus lower the intracranial pressure. Cerebral veins do not contain valves. Therefore, drainage is significantly enhanced by gravity.

   Precaution. Mild sedation for control of headache. Phenobarbital or codeine compounds are commonly used.
   Rationale. Pain results in restlessness with elevations of blood and intracranial pressures. However, the amount of sedation should allow the patient to be easily awakened for neurological and vital sign evaluation.

   Precaution. Vital and neurological sign evaluation is done hourly or more frequently when indicated.

Cerebral Aneurysm / **245**

Rationale. Blood pressure control is imperative for a successful outcome. Neurological changes must be reported immediately to the physician.

Precaution. Skin care. Pressure mattress. Heel protectors. Elastic stockings.

Rationale. Pressure sores and emboli are always a threat to the patient on complete bed rest.

Precaution. Routine seizure precautions.

Rationale. Seizure activity is common after a subarachnoid hemorrhage.

Ms. Lee is evaluated by a neurosurgeon and permission is obtained for a cerebral angiogram, the results of which show a berry aneurysm of the posterior communicating artery.

4. **What is an aneurysm?**

A cerebral aneurysm is a dilatation of the arterial wall. It results from a weakness in the wall. Berry aneurysms are the most prevalent and are so called because they have a stem and a neck. Aneurysms can also be giant (fusiform), behaving like space-occupying lesions in the brain. Mycotic aneurysms are created by septic emboli and are rare. Charcot-Bouchard are microscopic aneurysms associated with hypertension and affect the brainstem and basal ganglia. Traumatic aneurysms can occur after head injury. Most aneurysms occur at the point of bifurcation of the arterial vessels.

Ms. Lee remains in the Neurosurgical ICU under subarachnoid hemorrhage precautions. Her blood pressure is controlled between 130 and 150 systolic with Apresoline. She is loaded on 1 gm of Dilantin and started on 100 mg every 8 hr. Her surgery is scheduled for 1 week; however, on day 5 postbleed she complains of increased headache and becomes drowsy and confused. She develops ptosis of the left eye and a pronator drift. Ms. Lee's neurosurgeon is notified immediately and a CT scan is ordered. While being scanned she becomes stuporous and develops a right hemiparesis. Her scan shows a moderate accumulation of intraventricular and intracerebral blood. She is transferred directly to the Operating Room for evacuation of the hematoma and aneurysm clipping.

5. **With the serious consequences of rebleed, why was Ms. Lee's surgery to be delayed for 1 week?**

Rebleeding occurs most frequently from days 3–11, with a peak occurrence around day 7 after the initial bleed. Therefore, early surgical intervention would seem indicated. However, it has been documented that patient outcome is poor when subjected to early surgery due to complications such as intracerebral edema and vaso-spasm. Many physicians recommend a waiting period of 5 days to 3 weeks postbleed for patients with subarachnoid hemorrhage of Grade II or higher. Others opt for early clipping to eliminate the complication of rebleed for all Grade I or II and stable Grades III and IV.

6. **What is a "drift," and what is the neurological significance?**
    Drift assessment should be performed on all neurosurgical patients who have no detectable hemiparesis and are capable of following commands. The development of a drift heralds the very early compromise of the motor strip. It detects an early evolving muscular weakness so that intervention can be initiated before permanent damage from infarction occurs. The development of a drift requires the immediate notification of the patient's neurosurgeon. To assess a patient for a drift the nurse should:

    > Place the patient on his or her back. The head of the bed can be elevated or flat.
    > Ask the patient to extend both arms with palms toward the ceiling.
    > Ask the patient to spread the fingers.
    > Ask the patient to close his or her eyes. The nurse can shield the eyes if necessary.
    > Ask the patient to count backwards from 10. The nurse can estimate 10 sec if necessary.

    A negative drift is noted when the arms remain parallel; the palms remain upward; and the fingers remain open. Drifts are further classified as follows:

    Pronator Drift. The fingers of one hand curl or close. The wrist pronates.
    Drift with a Capture. The hand closes; wrist pronates; the arm drifts toward the body. The patient recovers the drift, bringing it back to the parallel position.
    Drift. The hand closes; wrist pronates; arm drifts toward the body without return to the original position.
    Frank Drift. The arm falls to the bed.

7. **Describe the surgical intervention for cerebral aneurysms.**
    Intracranial aneurysmal surgery is usually accomplished by a combination of microsurgical technique, hyperventilation, dehydration, and controlled systemic hypotension. Dehydration, usually achieved by drugs such as mannitol, reduces the brain mass, allowing better visualization of the aneurysm. Hypotension induced with peripheral vasodilators such as nitroprusside causes the aneurysm to collapse

slightly and control bleeding. Self-closing spring clips are then placed to occlude the stem of the aneurysm. Those aneurysms that cannot be clipped are wrapped with a gauze material coated with an acrylic substance. Postoperative cerebral angiography is obtained to confirm the occlusion of the aneurysm while maintaining arterial blood flow.

Postoperatively Ms. Lee is readmitted to the Neurosurgical ICU. The results of her physical examination are:

Vital Signs

BP	138/72
HR	80
Resp	14
Temp	38.2°C

Neurological. Opens eyes to pain. Follows commands with the left extremities. Localizes with the right extremities. Nods to questions. Oriented to person.

CV. Warm; dry; no edema. Capillary refill brisk; monitor shows NSR. Normal heart sounds. CVP 6.

Ventilator Settings		**ABGs**	
Mode	Assist control	pH	7.49
Rate	14	$PaCO_2$	28
FIO_2	0.40	PaO_2	136
Tidal volume	1000	SaO_2	97%

GI. Abdomen soft, flat, nontender. Bowel sounds absent. NG to low suction.

GU. Foley catheter in place draining clear yellow urine. Notify physician if urine output falls below 30 ml/hr or exceeds 200 ml/hr.

Metabolic

Temp	99°F
Na	138
K	4.2
Gluc	132
Creat	0.4
Hct	33

Musculoskeletal. Turban dressing in place. Dry and intact. An epidural drain was placed in the surgical flap to remove postoperative accumulations of blood, spinal fluid, and galeal fluid.

Ms. Lee was hyperventilated for 72 hr. She was then weaned and extubated without incident. Her vital signs remained stable. Her CVP was maintained between 6 and 10 with fluid boluses and Plasmanate. She continued to run a low grade fever despite negative cultures and clear chest films. Neurologically, she was awake and following commands with equal strength. Her speech was clear. However, she remained disoriented.

8. **What is the rationale for the order to notify the physician for a urine output < 30 ml/hr or > 200 ml/hr?**

Diuretics are used during many craniotomies to reduce brain mass and allow the surgeon better visualization of the aneurysm. Therefore, the patient's volume status must be closely monitored postoperatively or dehydration may occur. Furthermore, due to the proximity of many aneurysms to the hypophysis, transient diabetes insipidus often occurs. (See Chapter 38, "Diabetes Insipidus.")

9. **Why is Ms. Lee's CVP maintained in the 6–10 range?**

Studies have shown that hypovolemia contributes to the development of vasospasm and cerebral ischemia.

10. **What is the probable source of Ms. Lee's fever?**

Contact between blood and meningeal tissue causes fever in many patients.

On day 8 post-initial bleed, Ms. Lee developed a drift of her right arm. She was lethargic and her speech was slightly slurred. She also began to complain once again of headache.

11. **Given these signs and symptoms, what is the most probable diagnosis?**

All of these neurological changes are indicative of vasospasm. Vasospasm is defined as a narrowing of an artery or branch of an artery to a diameter less than that of the corresponding vessel on the other side of the brain. Vasospasm is confirmed by angiography. The peak incidence for vasospasm is 7–10 days after the initial bleed. The clinical manifestations result from compromised cerebral blood flow.

12. **What causes vasospasm?**

Vasospasm is thought to be due to an influx of calcium ions into the vascular smooth muscle. This shift of calcium ions is precipitated by many naturally occurring substances, including the by-products of blood breakdown, prostaglandins, serotonin, and catecholamines.

Ms. Lee's neurosurgeon was notified immediately and a CT scan obtained. The CT scan results were negative for hematoma or swelling. A pulmonary artery catheter was inserted. Fluids were administered to raise the PAWP to the 18–20 mm Hg range. Ms. Lee initially responded to treatment by becoming less lethargic and demonstrating an improvement in her speech. She remained confused with a pronator drift of the right arm. However, 4 hr after the onset of symptoms, she became aphasic with an evolving right hemiparesis. Ms. Lee was started on a dopamine infusion to elevate her blood pressure. Consequently, her urine output began to exceed 200 ml/hr, causing a decrease in her PAWP and only a marginal increase in blood pressure. Vasopressin (aqueous Pitressin), 5 units IM, was given to decrease her urine output. Her blood pressure increased to 180 systolic, causing stimulation of pressure-sensitive receptors in the carotid sinus and aorta. The result was vagal stimulation of the vasomotor center in the brainstem. The resultant bradycardia was treated with atropine sulfate, 1 mg IV q 4 hr.

13. What is the protocol of care and what is the goal in the above case study?

The protocol of care is hypervolemic-hypertensive therapy. It is achieved by maintaining the patient in a maximally hydrated state and assessing for improvement in the neurological examination. In some cases, volume expansion alone is enough to stabilize the patient. Such patients are said to be volume responsive. Hypertensive therapy is added when the patient is unimproved or deteriorates after volume expansion. A systolic blood pressure > 240 mm Hg in the clipped patient or 160 mm Hg in the unclipped patient is not recommended. The goal of this protocol is to restore adequate blood flow to the ischemic cerebral tissue before infarction develops.

14. What are the complications of this protocol of care?

The complications of this protocol of care are pulmonary edema, dilutional hyponatremia, myocardial infarction, coagulopathy, pneumothorax, and aneurysm rebleed (unclipped patients). Patients are continually monitored for the following:

Vital signs, with special concern for systemic arterial pressure
Neurological signs
CVP, PAWP, cardiac output
ECG abnormalities
Symptoms of cerebral edema
Hemoglobin, hematocrit, creatinine, BUN, glucose, blood gases, electrolytes, and osmolalities of urine and serum

15. What other treatment methods are advocated in the literature?

Calcium-Blocking Agents (Nifedipine). These appear to act by: (*a*) inhibition of calcium influx into the cerebral artery smooth muscle and (*b*) interference with the lysis of erythrocytes and platelet aggregation. The side effects are hypotension, headache, nausea, and flushing.

Sodium thiopental has been used to decrease cerebral oxygen and metabolic demands. However, it is impossible to perform a neurological examination when the patient is receiving sodium thiopental. The patient becomes flaccid and the pupils nonreactive. It should be noted that right-to-left pupil size does not change. With sodium thiopental therapy, intracranial pressure monitoring and serial CT scans provide the only sources of information concerning neurological status. The side effects of sodium thiopental are marked respiratory depression, hypotension, and decreased cardiac output. Furthermore, sodium thiopental is cleared over a period of several days as it is released from the fat stores of the body. The return to baseline neurological status can be slow and sporadic.

Hypervolemic-Hemodilution. Some reports indicate a relationship between blood viscosity, hematocrit levels, and the amount of cerebral ischemia. An intravenous infusion of Plasmanate was used to expand intravascular volume and thin the blood, thus increasing the flow to ischemic areas. The hematocrit level was reduced to 33% with this method. The value of this approach is an augmentation of cerebral blood flow and perfusion without an increase in blood pressure. The next day, vasospasm was confirmed by angiography. Ms. Lee was maintained on hypervolemic-hypertensive therapy for 1 week. She had none of the major complications listed. Her neurological status improved so that she was again following commands with equal power. Her speech was clear. She had a negative drift. She was oriented to person and place. After 5 more days of observation, Ms. Lee was transferred to the general nursing floor. Four days after her transfer to the floor her confusion increased and she was more lethargic. Her other neurological signs were unchanged and her vital signs were stable. Blood gas analysis indicated that oxygenation was excellent.

16. **What events could cause this neurological picture after the critical phase has passed in the post-subarachnoid hemorrhage patient?**

Vasospasm. Vasospasm remains a concern for any patient for up to 1 month posthemorrhage.

SIADH. Serum sodium should be followed on a routine basis on these patients. Hemorrhage can cause excessive ADH secretion from the pituitary, fluid retention, and low serum sodium levels. ADH acts on the renal tubules to increase reabsorption of water. The body excretes highly concentrated urine in small quantities. Fluid restriction is the treatment of choice. At times it may be necessary to add diuretics or an infusion of 3% normal saline. (See Chapter 40, "SIADH.")

Hydrocephalus. The blood in the subarachnoid space posthemorrhage damages the arachnoid villi of the ventricles. This results in decreased reabsorption of cerebral spinal fluid and the development of hydrocephalus.

Ms. Lee's serum sodium is 126. She is immediately placed on a fluid restriction of 1200 ml/24hr. Her mentation and alertness improve. She is discharged 1 week later with a sodium of 134 and instructed to return to the clinic in 1 week.

17. What nursing diagnoses apply in this case?

> Altered nutrition: less than body requirements
> Potential for infection related to invasive line placement, intubation, and surgery
> Hyperthermia related to SAH
> Altered patterns of urinary elimination related to Foley catheter
> Altered cerebral perfusion related to vasospasm
> Fluid volume excess related to hypervolemic protocol
> Potential fluid volume deficit related to diuretic administration
> Impaired verbal communication related to aphasia and intubation
> Impaired physical ability related to hemiparesis
> Sleep pattern disturbance related to Neurosurgical ICU care
> Sensory/perceptual alterations related to SAH
> Altered thought processes related to SAH
> Pain related to invasive procedures and headache

SUGGESTED READINGS

Bates B. A guide to physical examination. 3rd ed. Philadelphia: JB Lippincott, 1983.

Cromwell RM. Surgical management of cerebral vascular disease. Nurs Clin North Am 1986;20(2):297–308.

Cunha BA, Tu RP. Fever in the neurosurgical patient. Heart Lung 1988;17(6):608–611.

Diamond S. Headaches that herald intracranial emergencies. Emerg Med. 1988; 20(2):20–24, 27, 31–32.

Fode NC. Subarachnoid hemorrhage from ruptured intracranial aneurysm. Am J Nurs 1988;88(5):675–680.

Gorelick PB. Cerebral vascular disease: pathophysiology and diagnosis. Nurs Clin North Am 1986;21(2):275–88.

Hickey J. Neurosurgical nursing 2nd ed. Philadelphia: JB Lippincott, 1986.

Hudak CM, Lohr TS, Gallo BM. Critical care nursing. 4th ed. Philadelphia: JB Lippincott, 1986.

Martin EM. Traumatic aneurysms. J Neurosci Nurs 1986;18(2):89–94.

McNair N. Arteriovenous malformations. Crit Care Nurs 1988;8(4):35–40.

New directions in treating aneurysmal SAH. Emerg Med 1987; 19(21):163–170.

CHAPTER 27

Closed Head Injury

Meredith King, RN, MA, CEN

Mike Parks is a 30-year-old accountant who was involved in a single-car motor vehicle accident while driving home from a bar. When the paramedics arrived, he was unresponsive, his breathing was irregular in both rate and depth, and he was bleeding from his nose. He was not wearing a seat belt. A Philadelphia collar was applied, and he was transported to the nearest hospital.

Upon arrival in the Emergency Department, Mr. Parks' vital signs were:

BP	110/70
HR	100
Resp	20
Temp	97°F

His pupils were equal and reactive to light, but sluggish. He was exhibiting decorticate posturing bilaterally, and his Glasgow Coma Scale score was 5: E1, V1, M3.

Mr. Parks was immediately intubated and placed on assist control, rate 12, tidal volume 800, FIO$_2$ 0.40. A central line was inserted in the right subclavian, and D$_5$½NS was started at 50 ml/hr. Routine laboratory work included a test for blood alcohol level and a toxicology screen. A Foley catheter was inserted and 500 ml of clear yellow urine obtained. Mr. Parks was taken to the radiology department for a CT scan, which was negative. He was admitted to the Neurosurgical ICU with a diagnosis of closed head injury. A subarachnoid screw was placed and ICP monitoring was started.

QUESTIONS AND ANSWERS

1. What are the three major categories of craniocerebral injury?

The three major categories of craniocerebral injury are focal brain injury (cerebral contusion, epidural, subdural, and intracerebral hematomas), diffuse brain injury (concussion and diffuse axonal injury), and skull fractures (linear, depressed, comminuted, and basilar).

Focal brain injuries cause local brain damage at the site of injury and produce focal, lateralizing, or localizing signs. Focal injuries occur when an object strikes the head or the head strikes an object, or when the head is forcibly moved or stopped from moving. Head injuries commonly involve both contact and movement, so it is unusual for focal injury to occur in only one area of the brain.

Diffuse brain injury is not localized to a specific region of the brain. Multiple lesions are scattered diffusely throughout the brain, causing widespread neuronal damage and generalized brain dysfunction. Diffuse brain injury is microscopic and involves damage to nerve cells deep within the white matter.

2. **What is diffuse axonal injury (DAI)?**

   Diffuse axonal injury is one of the two types of diffuse brain injury. The hallmark of diffuse axonal injury is loss of consciousness at the time of injury that continues beyond 6 hr. Coma occurs because of widespread damage to conducting white matter, which disconnects the cerebral hemispheres from the brainstem reticular activating system. DAI is microscopic in nature and can be categorized as mild, moderate, or severe depending on the patient's clinical presentation.

3. **Mr. Parks' closed head injury is ultimately categorized as severe DAI. Describe the mechanism of injury in severe DAI.**

   Severe DAI is almost always caused by a high speed motor vehicle collision. The brain is rotated and thrown forward within the skull. The greatest injury occurs at the interface between gray and white matter, as the less dense gray matter is thrown forward while the white matter lags behind. This results in severe stretching and shearing of the axonal fibers. This injury may disrupt axons throughout both cerebral hemispheres, the diencephalon, and/or the brainstem.

4. **Mr. Parks' CT scan was negative. Is this common in cases of DAI?**

   A CT scan is routinely done in head injured patients, but it may or may not be helpful in the diagnosis of DAI. The tissue and vessel tears cause small hemorrhages that may not be visible on CT scan. A CT finding that is consistent with DAI is diffuse cerebral edema. Magnetic resonance imaging is more useful than CT scanning in diagnosing DAI.

5. **A multidisciplinary approach is strongly recommended in managing the severely head injured patient. The team should be consulted when the patient is admitted. In addition to nursing and medicine, what specialists should be included on the multidisciplinary team?**

   Dietician
   Physical, occupational, speech therapists
   Social worker
   Psychologist

6. **When Mr. Parks arrived in the Emergency Department, his respiratory rate and depth were both irregular, and he was immediately intubated and mechanically ventilated. His initial postintubation arterial blood gas showed the following results:**

ABGs		Ventilator Settings	
pH	7.32	Mode	Assist control
PaCO$_2$	50	Rate	12
PaO$_2$	120	FIO$_2$	0.40
SaO$_2$	98%	Tidal volume	800
HCO$_3$	25		

Are these blood gases acceptable? What ventilator changes were indicated?

These blood gases are not acceptable for the patient who has recently sustained a closed head injury. The concern is the PaCO$_2$ of 50. Hypercarbia causes cerebral vasodilatation, increased cerebral blood flow, and increased intracranial pressure. Hypoxemia also causes cerebral vasodilatation when the PaO$_2$ falls below 50 mm Hg. Lactic acidosis can also cause vasodilatation.

When Mr. Parks arrived in the Neurosurgical ICU, he was placed on the following settings:

Mode	Assist control
Rate	14
FIO$_2$	0.40
Tidal volume	900

The results of an arterial blood gas drawn 30 min after arrival were as follows:

pH	7.50
PaCO$_2$	28
PaO$_2$	140
SaO$_2$	98%
HCO$_3$	25

The FIO$_2$ was decreased to 0.35. The goal was to maintain Mr. Parks' PaCO$_2$ in the range of 25–30 mm Hg and his PaO$_2$ at 80 mm Hg or above.

7. **Explain the relationship between hyperventilation and cerebral blood flow.**

Hyperventilation is defined as a PaCO$_2$ <35 mm Hg. Hypocarbia causes constriction of cerebral blood vessels, which decreases cerebral blood flow and therefore decreases ICP. Traditionally, the goal has been to maintain the PaCO$_2$ between 25 and 30 mm Hg; however, there is some controversy concerning hyperventilation in the head injured patient as recent research has indicated that ischemia may result from the hyperventilation-induced cerebral vasoconstriction. The $PaCO_2$ must be kept no lower than 25 mm Hg, and some authorities recommend keeping it above 30 mm Hg.

8. **Approximately 1 hr after he is intubated, Mr. Parks needs to be suctioned. What nursing measures should be taken to prevent complications in this head injured patient?**

   Endotracheal suctioning can cause hypoxia and hypercarbia, both of which can increase ICP. An increase in 1 mm Hg $PaCO_2$ causes a 2–3% increase in cerebral blood flow. To prevent these complications, the patient should be hyperventilated and hyperoxygenated with 100% O_2 for 30 sec prior to each catheter insertion. Suctioning should be limited to 10–15 sec per catheter pass. Elevations in ICP also typically accompany suctioning, and prophylactic administration of IV lidocaine or a short-acting sedative may be appropriate prior to suctioning.

   Pulmonary complications are next in line to increased intracranial pressure as the cause of death in the head injured patient. Optimal pulmonary toilet, frequent handwashing, and avoidance of contamination of ventilator circuits should be employed.

9. **Aspiration of gastric contents is a frequent occurrence in the head injured patient and may lead to ARDS. Neurogenic pulmonary edema may also occur. If refractory hypoxemia occurs, PEEP may be necessary. What possible impact can PEEP have on ICP?**

   PEEP can impede cerebral venous return and increase ICP. However, low levels of PEEP generally will not increase ICP as long as the patient's head is elevated at least 30°.

Mr. Parks' baseline neurological assessment upon arrival in the Neurosurgical ICU resulted in a Glasgow Coma Scale score of 6T. He did not open his eyes to painful stimuli (E1); there was no verbal response (V1); but he withdrew from painful stimuli (M4). His pupils were equal and sluggishly reactive to light at 4 mm.

The nursing care priorities at this time included supportive care, prevention of increased ICP, and frequent neurological assessment. Mr. Parks' IV fluid therapy consisted of D_5NS at 75 ml/hr.

10. **Would D_5W be an acceptable IV fluid for Mr. Parks?**

    No. Free water can move from the vascular space into the interstitial space and exacerbate cerebral edema. If hypernatremia occurs in the head injured patient, small amounts of D_5W can be administered with caution.

11. **When Mr. Parks arrived in the Emergency Department, he was exhibiting decorticate posturing and his Glasgow Coma Scale score was 5. A subarachnoid screw was inserted for ICP monitoring.**

    Define decorticate/decerebrate posturing. What is the clinical significance?

    Decorticate posturing consists of bringing the arms next to the body, flexing the fingers or wrists and arms, extending and internally rotating the legs, and plantar flexing the feet (Fig. 27.1).

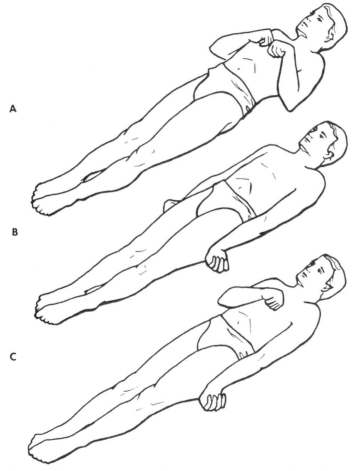

Figure 27.1. Decorticate and decerebrate responses. **A,** Decorticate response: flexion of arms, wrists, and fingers with abduction in upper extremities; extension, internal rotation, and plantar flexion in lower extremities. **B,** Decerebrate response: All four extremities in rigid extension with hyperpronation of forearms and plantar extension of feet. **C,** Decorticate response on right side of body and decerebrate response on left side of body. (Reproduced by permission from Rudy EB. Nursing care of the neurologically injured patient. In: Zschoche DA. Mosby's comprehensive review of critical care. 3rd ed. St. Louis, 1986, The C.V. Mosby Co.)

Decerebrate posturing consists of rigidly extending the arms and legs, bringing the arms close to the body and hyperpronating them, plantar flexing the feet, and sometimes arching the back.

It is not uncommon for only parts of these patterns of posturing to be seen. Posturing may occur spontaneously or with stimulation and may be either intermittent or continuous.

Decorticate and decerebrate posturing reflect significant brain dysfunction and are frequently associated with increased ICP and early herniation. Decerebrate posturing is associated with brainstem dysfunction (pons and midbrain regions) and is considered to be a worse sign than decorticate posturing, which reflects diencephalic dysfunction.

Posturing can result in flexor/extensor deformities and contractures. When decerebration is continuous, it significantly increases the metabolic rate and can cause weight loss, protein depletion, and negative nitrogen balance. Importantly, posturing can cause elevations in ICP.

12. **Mr. Parks' initial ICP is 30 mm Hg. Furosemide (Lasix), 40 mg, is given IV push, and mannitol, 100 gm, is given via rapid IV infusion.**

   How do Lasix and mannitol work, and what are the nursing implications?

   Lasix is a potent loop diuretic that decreases sodium transport into the brain, reduces body fluid volume, and inhibits CSF production. Although its effectiveness in reducing ICP is an area of controversy, Lasix causes fewer electrolyte and osmolarity disturbances than do osmotic diuretics. However, hypokalemia is a side effect and the serum potassium should be monitored.

   Mannitol is an osmotic diuretic. By causing an increase in serum osmolarity, it creates an osmotic gradient between the brain and the blood and pulls fluid from the cerebral extracellular space into the intravascular space. The brain volume is reduced and the ICP is lowered. Intravascular volume and renal blood flow are increased and diuresis occurs. Mannitol is very effective in treating increased ICP and has a rapid onset of action. It is the drug of choice for neurological emergencies and potential brain herniation. The usual dose is 0.5–1.5 gm/kg.

   Potential complications of mannitol include hyperosmolarity and acute renal dysfunction. The serum sodium and osmolarity should be monitored. The normal serum osmolarity is 275–295 mOsm/liter. In head injured patients, the osmolarity should be kept between 305 and 315 mOsm/liter. Mannitol should be administered through a central vein if possible, as extravasation causes skin sloughing.

If the blood brain barrier has sustained major damage, mannitol may cross it and actually pull fluid into the brain tissue, worsening cerebral edema. Rapid infusion is recommended to achieve the optimal effect of this drug therapy.

13. Are steroids recommended as treatment for increased ICP?

Historically, dexamethasone and methylprednisolone have been used to reduce cerebral edema and decrease ICP in the head injured patient. At present, the use of steroids in head injury is extremely controversial.

Clinicians who argue against the use of steroids point out that they may cause carbohydrate intolerance and hyperglycemia, immunosuppression and decreased resistance to infection, gastric ulceration, and sodium and water retention. Proponents argue that steroids have been proven effective in experimental models. The proposed benefits include stabilization of cell membranes and restoration of autoregulation. While some studies have shown decreased mortality with steroids, others have shown increased mortality.

14. What is the role of barbiturate therapy in the head injured patient?

Specific actions of barbiturates include reducing cerebral metabolism and cerebral blood flow while stabilizing cell membranes.

Barbiturate coma is an areflexive state caused by high doses of barbiturates. It is sometimes imposed to treat otherwise uncontrolled ICP elevation. This treatment also depresses other body systems and requires the use of mechanical ventilation, hemodynamic monitoring, and ICP monitoring. There is presently some controversy as to whether true coma with the absence of all reflexes is necessary, or if barbiturate sedation may also be effective in the treatment of elevated ICP.

On postoperative day 4, Mr. Parks spiked a fever of 103°F. His monitor showed sinus tachycardia with a rate of 120, and his skin was warm, dry, and flushed. His BP was 118/70. Cultures were obtained of his blood, urine, CSF, and sputum. Tylenol was given per orogastric tube q 4 hr for a temperature >101°F. His blood pressure was monitored every hour.

15. Why is maintenance of normothermia important in patients with head injury?

Hyperthermia has been shown to increase the cerebral metabolic rate and increase the ICP. If the body temperature rises above 100.4°F (38°C), measures to restore normothermia should be taken, including administering acetaminophen, giving tepid baths, or placing the patient on a hypothermia unit. The temperature should not be lowered so fast that shivering occurs, as shivering increases ICP. Thorazine can be given to control shivering if it occurs.

16. **Why was an orogastric tube placed instead of a nasogastric tube?**

Mr. Parks had sustained a head injury, and had blood coming from his nose. A nasogastric tube should not be inserted, as the risk of cranial intubation exists.

17. **What is the relationship between arterial blood pressure and cerebral blood flow?**

Under normal conditions, the brain receives 750 ml of blood/min or 50 ml/100 gm/min. The cerebral vasculature displays the phenomenon of autoregulation, which is the ability to maintain a constant rate of blood flow over a wide range of perfusion pressures (50–150 mm Hg) despite changes in arterial blood pressure and intracranial pressure. This autoregulation is possible because there is a mechanism present in the cerebral arterioles that causes vasoconstriction when the arterial pressure rises and vasodilatation when it falls.

Cerebral perfusion pressure (CPP) is the difference between cerebral arterial and venous blood pressures. Cerebral arterial pressure approximates mean arterial pressure (MAP), and cerebral venous pressure approximates intracranial pressure. Therefore:

$$CPP = MAP - ICP$$

$$MAP = \frac{systolic - diastolic}{3} + diastolic$$

The normal CPP is 50–150 mm Hg, with the optimal CPP being 80–90 mm Hg. CPP will be reduced by either a drop in MAP or a rise in ICP. When the ICP increases, autoregulation causes cerebral vasodilatation. This will initially increase cerebral blood flow. However, the vasodilatation also increases ICP, which compromises CPP.

The CPP should be maintained above 50 mm Hg in the head injured patient. Autoregulation fails when the CPP falls below 50 mm Hg. When autoregulation fails, the cerebral blood flow is totally dependent upon arterial blood pressure. If the arterial blood pressure is high, a large volume of blood enters the cerebral vessels, raises the ICP, and exacerbates cerebral edema. When the arterial blood pressure is low, there is inadequate cerebral blood flow and cerebral ischemia results.

18. **Mr. Parks' ICP is now 18 mm Hg, and his BP is 80/50. What is his CPP? Is this acceptable? What interventions are appropriate?**

$$CPP = MAP - ICP$$

$$MAP = \frac{\text{systolic} - \text{diastolic}}{3} + \text{diastolic} = \frac{80 - 50}{3} + 50 = 60$$

$$CPP = 60 - 18 = 42$$

Mr. Parks' CPP is less than the minimum 50 mm Hg recommended for the head injured patient. This is due to a slightly elevated ICP in conjunction with arterial hypotension. Treatment should be focused on increasing the MAP and decreasing the ICP to <15 mm Hg. Cautious fluid challenges should be used initially followed by inotropes if necessary. Diuretics cannot be used to treat the increased ICP while the patient is hypotensive, but proper positioning, hyperventilation, sedation, and oxygenation should be ensured.

19. **What is Cushing's triad? Is it a useful clinical indicator of increased ICP?**

Cushing's triad consists of arterial hypertension, bradycardia, and slow respirations. This is not a useful clinical indicator of increased ICP, as the changes in blood pressure and pulse occur late and are an ominous sign of medullary compression.

20. **What special considerations should be given to Mr. Parks' positioning?**

Patients with head trauma should be positioned with the head elevated at least 30° to facilitate cerebrovenous drainage and avoid increasing ICP. The head should not be flexed or rotated, as this can mechanically compress veins in the neck and the base of the skull. Sharp hip flexion should also be avoided, as this can increase ICP as well. Care should be taken not to bend the legs up when the patient is on his side, and he should not be positioned bolt upright in bed with his legs straight.

21. **Nursing management of the head injured patient includes steps to prevent or minimize secondary brain injury. What should this include?**

Avoidance of hypoxemia, hypercarbia, hypotension, and intracranial hypertension are essential in preventing secondary brain injury. Heavy sedation may be indicated. (See Chapter 29, "Gunshot Wound to the Head.")

22. What are the potential complications of closed head injury?

Diabetes insipidus
Syndrome of inappropriate ADH
Pulmonary edema
GI bleeding
DIC
Secondary brain injuries

23. What are the nursing diagnoses in Mr. Parks' case?

Alteration in cerebral tissue perfusion related to cerebral edema, hypotension, and decreased CPP
Altered temperature regulation related to head injury
Potential for injury related to seizure activity
Impaired physical mobility related to pharmacologic paralysis
Potential for intracranial infection related to ICP monitoring device
Ineffective airway clearance related to presence of endotracheal tube
Potential for impaired skin integrity related to paralysis
Ineffective family coping: potential related to life-threatening injury

SUGGESTED READINGS

Bourdon SE. Psychological impact of neuro trauma in the acute care setting. Nurs Clin North Am 1986;21(4):629–640.

Changaris DG, McGraw CP, Richardson JD, et al. Correlation of cerebral perfusion pressure and Glasgow Coma Scale to outcome. J Trauma 1987;27(9):1007–1013.

Cooper PR. Head injury. Baltimore: Williams & Wilkins, 1987.

Gardner DG. Acute management of the head injured adult. Nurs Clin North Am 1986; 21(4):555–562.

Hickey J. The clinical practice of neurological and neurosurgical nursing. Philadelphia: JB Lippincott, 1986.

Holloway NM. Nursing the critically ill adult. 3rd ed. Menlo Park, CA: Addison-Wesley, 1988:51–93.

McGinnis GS. Central nervous system I: head injuries. In: Cardona VD, Hurn PD, Mason PJ, Scanlon-Schilpp, Veise-Berry SW. Trauma nursing from resuscitation through rehabilitation. Philadelphia: WB Saunders, 1988:265–413.

Miller E, Williams S. Alterations in cerebral perfusion: clinical concept or nursing diagnosis. J Neurosci Nurs 1987;19(4):183–190.

Miner M, Wagner K. Neurotrauma: treatment rehabilitation and related issues. Boston: Butterworth, 1987.

Swearingen PL, Sommers MS, Miller K, eds. Manual of critical care applying nursing diagnoses to adult critical illness. St. Louis: CV Mosby, 1988:270–282.

CHAPTER 28

Epidural Hematoma

Doris M. Gates, RN, MS, CCRN

Kevin Stone is a 17-year-old who fell off his 10-speed bicycle while riding with his friend Eric. He hit his head on the pavement and was unconscious for approximately 5 min. Upon awakening, Kevin was able to ride his bicycle to Eric's house. About 30 min after the fall, Kevin began to act strangely. He was confused and belligerent and complained of headache, nausea, and vomiting. Eric became worried about Kevin and brought him to the Emergency Department approximately 90 min after the fall.

Kevin's examination in the Emergency Department revealed the following:

Vital Signs

BP	110/70
HR	64
Resp	20
Temp	37.2°C

Neurological. Oriented to person and place; speech confused. Opened eyes to verbal comands. Moved all extremities equally and purposefully to commands. No muscle weakness noted. PERRL at 4 mm, no dysconjugate gaze; EOMs intact. Moderate scalp swelling noted in the right temporoparietal area. No Battle's sign or hemotympanum. DTRs intact. Glasgow Coma Scale (GCS) score was 13: E3, V4, M6.

Cardiac. Cardiac monitor showed normal sinus rhythm at a rate of 64 beats/min. Normal heart sounds without murmur or rub. Good capillary refill; skin pink and moist. Palpable radial and dorsalis pedis pulses bilaterally.

Pulmonary. Breath sounds equal and clear to auscultation throughout lung fields. Respirations unlabored, regular, with symmetrical chest excursion.

GI. Soft, nontender, with hypoactive bowel sounds.

GU. Foley catheter inserted and returned 200 ml of clear, pale yellow urine.

Extremities. Superficial abrasions to right knee, pelvis stable.

X-ray. C-spine clear. Chest x-ray clear. Skull series showed hairline fracture of right temporal skull.

The Emergency Department physician decided to admit Kevin for observation because of his confusion, headache, and vomiting. He was admitted to the ICU for neurological observation 2 hr after his fall.

QUESTIONS AND ANSWERS

1. **Given the history of Kevin's accident and his physical examination results, which neurological parameters should be monitored?**

Level of consciousness and verbal response
Pupillary response
Eye opening and movement
Movement of extremities and sensation
Vital signs

Kevin's initial assessment in the ICU was consistent with his status in the Emergency Department. Thirty minutes after Kevin's admission to the ICU, his mental status began to deteriorate. His Glasgow Coma Scale score was 9: eye opening to pain (E2), incomprehensible verbal sounds (V2), and bilateral localizing movement to painful stimuli (M5). His pupils were 4 mm and sluggishly reactive. Kevin was given mannitol, 50 gm IV push, and was intubated and hyperventilated. Despite the mannitol and hyperventilation, Kevin's condition continued to deteriorate. Ten minutes later, his GCS score (7) showed no eye opening to pain (E1), no verbal response (intubated) (V1), and he localized to pain on the right (M5) and was extensor posturing on the left. His pupils became unequal with the right pupil fixed and dilated at 6 mm and the left at 4 mm and sluggishly reactive. A CT scan was immediately performed, which revealed a large right epidural hematoma. Kevin was then taken to the Operating Room for evacuation of the hematoma.

2. **In Kevin's initial assessment in the Emergency Department, which physical assessment findings would lead one to specifically suspect and monitor for a potential epidural hematoma? Why?**
The right temporoparietal scalp swelling and temporal hairline skull fracture should lead one to suspect and monitor for an epidural hematoma. The thickness of the skull varies according to location. The midfrontal and occipital areas are the thickest at 6 mm. The temporoparietal area is the thinnest at 2 mm and is therefore the most vulnerable to injury. The middle meningeal artery and vein lie just below the temporal bone. Fractures of the temporal bone can cause tears in the vessels, resulting in an epidural hematoma.

3. **Describe the pathophysiology of an epidural bleed.**
The dura mater is the outermost membrane that surrounds the brain and is tightly adherent to the skull. It follows the contours of the cerebral hemispheres and then superiorly dips down between the cerebral hemispheres forming a dural fold called the falx cerebri.

Laterally, the dura separates the temporal and occipital lobes from the cerebellum, forming a ledge called the tentorium cerebelli. The brainstem passes through the opening in this ledge, the tentorial notch.

The middle meningeal artery and vein lie between the dura and the skull. Trauma to the head may result in laceration of one of these vessels, causing bleeding and hematoma formation. Epidural hematoma formation is most often associated with linear skull fractures, usually of the temporal bone, but may also occur following blunt trauma to the head without the presence of a skull fracture. The source of bleeding is usually the middle meningeal artery, so the onset of symptoms is usually rapid. Early recognition of symptoms is crucial, as surgical intervention is mandatory.

As the clot quickly enlarges, it pushes the tightly adherent dura away from the skull. Lateral expansion is limited by the rigid skull, so the clot pushes medially and causes a midline and unilateral downward shift of cerebral tissue. If left untreated, the clot continues to expand and causes cerebral tissue to herniate through the tentorial notch.

4. What is meant by the term "uncal herniation"?

The uncus, or uncinate gyrus, is located on the inner basal medial edge of the temporal lobe. An expanding lesion of the lateral middle fossa may cause shifting of this area toward the midline and through the tentorial notch. With uncal herniation, the diencephalon and midbrain are compressed and displaced to the opposite side. Blood supply to the brainstem is compromised, and the third cranial nerve is compressed between the overhanging uncus and the free edge of the tentorium. Ipsilateral pupillary dilation is the result and is often the first indicator of uncal herniation.

5. What are the signs of uncal herniation?

Ipsilateral pupillary dilation
Paralysis of the muscles of eye movement (possible ptosis)
Restlessness, then deteriorating level of consciousness
Decrease or loss of sensory function
Contralateral hemiparesis or hemiplegia
Bilateral Babinski signs
Respiratory changes (Cheyne-Stokes, central hyperpnea, ataxic)
Decorticate and decerebrate posturing
Dilated, fixed pupils, flaccidity, and respiratory arrest

6. **Did Kevin present with the classical manifestations of an epidural hematoma?**

   Yes. The classical picture of a patient with an epidural hematoma involves a brief loss of consciousness at the time of injury, followed by a lucid interval of from several minutes to several hours. If the hematoma is venous in origin, the lucid interval may last several days. Subsequent signs and symptoms include deterioration in level of consciousness, headache, vomiting, hemiparesis, possible seizure, and a dilated ipsilateral pupil that becomes fixed. If the condition is not corrected, signs of uncal herniation occur. Vital signs change as a preterminal event and include bradycardia, hypertension with a widening pulse pressure, shallow, irregular respirations, and fever. If the patient continues to decompensate, the pulse becomes rapid and irregular, and hypotension occurs. This sequence of symptoms, although thought to be classic of epidural hematoma formation, has a reported incidence of only 33% (1) and no lucid period is experienced in at least 15% of all patients (2). No one may come upon the scene of the accident until after the lucid period has passed, causing the classic lucid period associated with epidural hematoma formation to go unnoticed. Therefore, failure to see the typical symptoms associated with epidural hematomas does not exclude their presence.

7. **Kevin's ipsilateral pupillary changes (right pupil fixed and dilated) and his contralateral motor changes (extensor posturing on the left) were consistent with right uncal herniation. Why are pupillary changes ipsilateral and motor changes contralateral with uncal herniation?**

   With uncal herniation, cranial nerve III is compressed on the side of the expanding temporal lobe lesion. This parasympathetic nerve controls constriction of the pupil on the ipsilateral side. When impulses from this nerve are interrupted, ipsilateral dilation occurs, followed by nonreaction of that pupil.

   In contrast, motor nerves cross in the brainstem. Therefore, compression on one side results in motor changes on the opposite (contralateral) side.

8. **What was the purpose of mannitol administration and hyperventilation when Kevin's status deteriorated?**

   These interventions were an attempt to decrease Kevin's increasing intracranial pressure by reducing the vascular volume in the cranium and the volume of the brain mass. Mannitol is an osmotic diuretic. It pulls fluid from the cerebral interstitial spaces, thus decreasing brain mass. In addition, mannitol decreases circulating blood volume via diuresis. Hyperventilation reduces carbon dioxide and thus hydrogen ion concentration in the brain, producing an alkalotic environment. Cerebral vessels respond to an alkalotic environment by constricting, thereby decreasing circulating blood volume. Because epidural bleeds are a surgical emergency, these medical interventions are only palliative and buy the patient time until he or she can be taken to the Operating Room.

When Kevin returned to the ICU from the Operating Room, he was intubated and on the Servo ventilator. His ventilator settings included assist control, rate 14, tidal volume 1000 ml, and FIO_2 0.40. His indwelling monitoring lines consisted of an intracranial (ventriculostomy) pressure line (ICP), an arterial line, a CVP line, and a Foley catheter. He was paralyzed with Pavulon, 4 mg every hour and was receiving morphine sulfate via a continuous drip at 4 mg/hr. His postoperative vital signs and laboratory results were:

Vital Signs		ABGs		Laboratory Values	
BP	108/68	pH	7.50	Na	138
HR	72	$PaCO_2$	26	K	3.8
Temp	36.8°C	PaO_2	140	Cl	105
CVP	6	HCO_3	22	CO_2	23
ICP	15			Hgb	12
				Hct	34

9. **What is the purpose of paralyzing and sedating Kevin postoperatively with Pavulon and morphine sulfate?**

    This drug regimen eliminates movement, agitation, and pain, all of which can cause increases in blood pressure and intracranial pressure. Contusion may have occurred at the time of injury, causing brain swelling and a subsequent increase in ICP. In order to minimize further cerebral damage, maintaining the ICP below 15 mm Hg is imperative. Typically, paralytic agents are avoided, because they mask neurological status and seizure activity. They may be warranted if the patient has poor ventilatory control on the ventilator or severe, uncontrollable agitation or posturing. When paralytics are used, prophylactic anticonvulsants are usually indicated. In addition, it is imperative that an ICP monitoring device be in place to monitor neurological status, because the neurological status is masked. Short-acting or easily reversible sedatives are preferred.

10. **What is usual length of time for maintaining paralysis and sedation?**

    If the patient's ICP is stable below 15 mm Hg, Pavulon and morphine may be tapered after the first 24–48 hr postoperatively. However, ICP and blood pressure parameters must be carefully monitored to avoid any sudden increases as consciousness returns.

11. **Why is the Pavulonized patient at risk for developing corneal abrasions and/or infections? What nursing interventions are necessary to decrease this risk?**

Because all skeletal muscle is paralyzed, the patient cannot blink or even close the eyes. Artificial tears or eye lubricant must be administered frequently to keep the corneas moist, and the eyes should be taped shut. If the eyes are left open, they may dry out. In addition, if the eyes are left open and the patient is unable to blink, they are vulnerable to droplet contamination, especially during suctioning. Hourly observation of the eyes should include assessment not only of the pupillary response but also of corneal moisture and any abnormal discharge. Abnormal discharge must be reported to the physician for appropriate medical intervention.

12. **Interpret Kevin's postoperative blood gases and discuss the interpretation in relation to his treatment.**

Kevin's blood gas results show a respiratory alkalosis. An alkalotic cerebral environment causes cerebral vasoconstriction, thereby reducing intracranial pressure.

Kevin's condition remained stable for the first 24 hr postoperatively, his ICP remained below 15 mm Hg, and he was still receiving paralyzing agents. The physician wrote an order to start gradually decreasing the ventilator rate in order to normalize Kevin's acid/base balance. Care must be used in decreasing ventilator support while the patient is on paralytic agents, and careful monitoring of gas exchange is imperative.

13. **Why is it important to normalize acid/base balance before weaning Kevin off of the paralyzing and sedating agents?**

As acid/base balance returns to normal, the cerebral vessels will begin to dilate. This dilatation will increase cerebral blood flow and may increase ICP. In order to differentiate between increased pressure caused by dilating vessels and increased pressure caused by movement, agitation, and pain, paralysis and sedation are continued until the acid/base balance is normalized. If an uncontrollable increase in ICP occurs with ventilator weaning, hyperventilation should be reinstituted.

Kevin's acid/base balance was returned to normal without any adverse effect. The paralyzing agent was discontinued, and his ICP pressures remained below 15 mm Hg. Finally, the morphine sulfate infusion was decreased to 2 mg/hr and discontinued without any adverse effect. Kevin's neurological assessment showed E4 (opens eyes spontaneously), V1 (intubated), M6 (obeys commands), and his ICP line was discontinued. Kevin's blood gases were: pH 7.43, $PaCO_2$ 40, PaO_2 105, HCO_3 24. Kevin was extubated and placed on 4 liters of O_2 via nasal cannula. His neurologic assessment over the next 24 hr consistently showed E4 (opens eyes spontaneously), V5 (oriented and converses), and M6 (obeys commands).

14. **Because of Kevin's classic symptomatology, he was admitted to the hospital shortly after sustaining his injury. In patients who are not hospitalized, what instructions should the family receive before the patient is sent home?**

If the patient is asymptomatic following head injury, he or she may very well be sent home. Because epidural hematomas can occur several hours following head injury, and are potentially fatal injuries, the patient must be assessed every hour for 24 hr. The patient should be awakened once an hour and assessed for orientation and ability to speak coherently.

15. **What nursing diagnoses apply in this case?**

Altered cerebral tissue perfusion related to increased intracranial pressure

Potential for infection related to craniotomy, presence of invasive devices

Pain related to surgical incision (craniotomy)

Ineffective airway clearance related to drug-induced paralysis and sedation

Impaired verbal communication related to presence of endotracheal tube

Potential for impaired tissue integrity; corneal, related to absent blink reflex

Potential for impaired skin integrity related to immobility caused by drug-induced paralysis

REFERENCES

1. McGinnis GS. Central nervous system I: head injuries. In: Cardona VD, Hurn PD, Mason PJB, Scanlon-Schilpp AM, Veise-Berry SW, eds. Trauma nursing from resuscitation through rehabilitation. Philadelphia: WB Saunders, 1988:365–418.

2. Hickey, JW. The clinical practice of neurological and neurosurgical nursing. 2nd ed. Philadelphia: JB Lippincott, 1986.

SUGGESTED READINGS

Brignall L. Extradural hematoma. Nursing Mirror 1984;158:39–41.

Manifold, SL. Craniocerebral trauma: a review of primary and secondary injury and therapeutic modalities. Focus Crit Care 1986;13(2):22–35.

Morrison CAM. Brain herniation syndromes. Crit Care Nurse 1987;7(5):34–38.

Pollack-Latham CL. Intracranial pressure monitoring: part I. physiologic principles. Crit Care Nurse 1987;7(5):40–51.

Robinet K. Increased intracranial pressure: management with an intraventricular catheter. J Neurosurg Nurs 1985;17:95–104.

Rudy EB. Advanced Neurological and Neurosurgical Nursing. St. Louis: CV Mosby, 1984.

Shpritz DW. Craniocerebral trauma. Crit Care Nurse 1983;3(2):49–61.

Wehrmaker SL, Wintermute JR. Case studies in neurological nursing. Boston: Little, Brown, 1978:229–242.

Yanko J. Head injuries. J Neurosurg Nurs 1984;16(4):173–180.

CHAPTER 29

Gunshot Wound to the Head

Meredith King, RN, MS, CEN

Daniel Brown is a 35-year-old bus driver who was brought to the Emergency Department after sustaining a gunshot wound to the back of the head. Upon initial neurological assessment, his right pupil was dilated and nonreactive to light. His left pupil was 3 mm in diameter and briskly reactive. He was unresponsive to voice but responded to noxious stimuli by moaning and decerebrate posturing. His Glasgow Coma Scale score was 5: El, V2, M2.

A central line was inserted in Mr. Brown's left subclavian vein, and 1 liter of $D_5\frac{1}{2}$ NS was started at 100 ml/hr. A CT scan was performed, which revealed an intracerebral hematoma and comminuted skull fracture. He was taken immediately to the Operating Room.

During surgery, the hematoma was evacuated and several bone fragments were removed. A .38 caliber bullet was removed and tagged as trace evidence. Chain of custody was maintained and the bullet was delivered to the proper authorities.

Following surgery, Mr. Brown was admitted to the Neurosurgical ICU. He was intubated and on the Servo ventilator. His vital signs were as follows:

BP	140/90
HR	98
Resp	20
Temp	97°F

A baseline neurological assessment was performed. Mr. Brown's pupils were both 4 mm and sluggishly reactive to light. He did not open his eyes to pain, there was no verbal response, but he withdrew his extremities from pain. His Glasgow Coma Scale score was 6T: El, Vl, M4. A subarachnoid screw was inserted and ICP monitoring was begun.

QUESTIONS AND ANSWERS

1. **What is the most important symptom of CNS dysfunction? How is this assessed and reported?**

    Alteration in the level of consciousness is the most important indicator of CNS dysfunction. It is assessed by determining the minimal stimulus (i.e., voice, shaking, peripheral pain, deep pain) required to initiate a patient response. Once a response is obtained, one can determine if the patient is oriented and behaving appropriately to better define his/her conscious state. In order to avoid confusion and ambiguity, terms such as lethargy, stupor, or obtundation are avoided. Simply stating the stimulus necessary to elicit a patient response is an easily understood mechanism of reporting. Objective reporting of assessment findings is also possible through use of the Glasgow Coma Scale. (See Appendix E.)

2. **Evaluation of pupillary response is an integral part of the neurological assessment. How should this be done?**

Pupils are assessed in terms of size, shape, and reactivity. The average pupillary size is 3 mm, but this depends on the amount of light entering the pupil. The lights should be turned off and window curtains pulled to make the room as dark as possible prior to checking the pupils. Pupil size should be checked before the light is used to check pupillary response. Variation in size is not usually significant as long as they are equal in size.

Pathological pupil signs would include inequality, asymmetry, or anisocoria (inequality of the pupils in diameter). While approximately 11–16% of the population demonstrate anisocoria of < 1 mm, a difference of ≥ 1 mm is significant and may forewarn of progressive dilation, indicating midbrain and subsequent cranial nerve III compression. This is typically seen with uncal brain herniation. (See Chapter 28, "Epidural Hematoma.")

Normal pupils are round. If a pupil changes from round to oval, it may indicate the presence of increased ICP and may forewarn of progressive dilation. An irregular or oval pupil should be reported. When pupils are checked for reactivity, both direct and consensual responses should be noted. When light is shined in one eye, both pupils should constrict. Constriction of the pupil on the opposite side of where the light is shined is the consensual response. If the direct response is absent, it indicates either midbrain compression of the third nerve or an optic nerve lesion, resulting in blindness. If the third nerve is compressed, both direct and consensual responses will be absent. In the case of unilateral blindness, the direct response will be absent, but the consensual response will be intact.

If the pupils react but in a sluggish manner, it is an abnormal finding and should be reported. This may forewarn of a pupil that will become nonreactive to light.

Pupillary abnormalities that may be useful in localizing the site of brain dysfunction are as follows:

Fixed, dilated pupils = upper brainstem (midbrain) compression
Small, reactive pupils = metabolic or hypothalamic dysfunction
Pinpoint, unreactive pupils = lower brainstem (pons) dysfunction

Pupillary abnormalities are extremely important in prognosis, and abnormalities should be reported immediately to the physician.

3. **Briefly describe the mechanism of injury in a gunshot wound to the head.**

   A gunshot wound to the head is classified as a perforating missile injury. The extent of the injury depends on the amount of energy delivered to the brain and the consequent disruption of brain tissue. The location of the missile tract(s) plays a significant role in determining the extent of the injury. A single bullet may make multiple tracts through the brain if it ricochets within the cranial cavity. Cerebral edema and subsequent increased intracranial pressure commonly occur following a gunshot wound to the head. Intracranial hematomas may also form.

4. **What factors affect survival in cases like Mr. Brown's?**

   Missile injuries to the brain are associated with a mortality rate of 30–90%. Factors that affect survival include the type of missile involved and the course of the missile through the brain. High energy, high velocity missiles are associated with a higher mortality rate than lower velocity, smaller caliber missiles. If only one lobe of the brain is involved, the mortality is significantly lower than if multiple lobes are involved or the missile crosses the midline.

   Treatment factors that increase survival include rapid transport to a trauma center, use of CT scans pre- and postoperatively, aggressive debridement of the missile tract, and close monitoring for postoperative complications, such as infection or increased ICP.

   If the patient is alert on admission to the hospital, there is a 0–20% mortality rate. If he or she is comatose on admission, the mortality rate is 100%.

5. **What is the goal of surgery in the patient with a gunshot wound to the head?**

   The goal of surgery is to debride the missile tract, including evacuation of bone fragments and hematomas, and to remove the bullet parts if accessible.

6. **Mr. Brown is to receive tobramycin and aqueous penicillin postoperatively. What is the rationale for antibiotic administration?**

   Infection, abscess formation, and sepsis are possible threats to Mr. Brown's life. Intravenous antibiotics may be prescribed prophylactically, although this treatment is not universally instituted. If the route of administration is to be IV piggyback, D_5W should not be used for dilution. This is because free water equilibrates into the interstitial space and can increase cerebral edema.

Because his injury was a perforating missile injury, Mr. Brown should receive tetanus toxoid if it was not given in the Emergency Department.

7. **In addition to infection and increased intracranial pressure, what is another complication that Mr. Brown is prone to develop?**

Seizures. Anticonvulsants such as Dilantin and phenobarbital may be prescribed in the postoperative period. However, a recent study has found that Dilantin is not effective when used prophylactically to prevent seizures after 8 days postinjury (1).

Patients who survive gunshot wounds to the head are generally put on long-term anticonvulsant therapy, especially if seizure activity is noted. Approximately 45% of the patients who survive missile injury to the head will develop epilepsy within 5 years.

8. **What nursing diagnoses would be part of your care plan while caring for Mr. Brown?**

Alteration in tissue perfusion: cerebral related to increased intracranial pressure
Potential for injury related to seizure activity
Potential for intracranial infection related to penetrating missile injury
Impaired physical mobility
Alteration in elimination: bladder and bowel
Alteration in nutrition: less than body requirements

9. **The nursing care of the patient with a gunshot wound to the head is similar to that of the patient with closed head injury. (See Chapter 27, "Closed Head Injury.") Summarize the key aspects of the nursing management of Mr. Brown.**

Maintain ventilator support and hyperventilation.
Avoid hypoxemia, hypercarbia, acidosis.
Monitor neurological signs every 15 min until stable, and then every hour. Use Glasgow Coma Scale (Appendix E). Notify physician promptly of significant changes.
Monitor vital signs and cardiac rhythm.
Monitor ICP. Goal is to keep ICP at 0–15 mm Hg.
Maintain head of bed elevation at least 30° while maintaining head and neck alignment.
Avoid sharp hip flexion.
Administer prescribed anticonvulsants. Watch for seizure activity, and employ seizure precautions.

Administer prescribed antibiotics. Monitor appropriate laboratory values.

Maintain normothermia.

Administer nutritional support.

Perform pulmonary toilet.

Monitor gas exchange (PaO_2 and $PaCO_2$) closely.

Prevent complications of immobility. (Turn every 2 hr, perform ROM exercises every 8 hr, use antiembolic stockings and pneumatic compression boots.)

Maintain IV access and administer intravenous fluids as ordered.

Monitor I & O carefully.

Follow serum osmolarity. Goal is to keep it within the range of 305–315 mOsm/liter.

Measure urine specific gravity to detect SIADH or DI.

Administer diuretics as indicated.

Limit noxious stimuli as able.

Prevent nosocomial infection (meticulous handwashing, care of invasive lines, Foley catheter care, pulmonary hygiene.)

Coordinate efforts with multidisciplinary treatment team.

Address emotional needs of patient/family.

Address religious needs of patient/family.

10. **On postoperative day 4, Mr. Brown's pupils become fixed and dilated. He is flaccid and is no longer assisting the ventilator. He does not have any spontaneous respirations or cough reflex when taken off the ventilator for suctioning. The neurologist examines Mr. Brown and tests the oculocephalic and oculovestibular reflex. What is the oculocephalic reflex?**

The oculocephalic reflex is commonly referred to as the doll's eyes phenomenon. It is essential that C-spine injury be ruled out before testing this reflex. It cannot be assessed accurately in an awake patient. The patient's eyelids are held open, and the patient's head is rotated from side to side. The normal response in the comatose patient is for both eyes to move laterally in the direction opposite the head rotation. This is labeled a positive, normal, or intact doll's eyes response. A negative doll's eyes response usually indicates that the lesion is in the brainstem. However, in the case of sedative drug intoxication, a negative doll's eyes response does not indicate brainstem involvement.

11. **What is the oculovestibular reflex?**

The oculovestibular reflex is commonly referred to as ice water calorics. The first step is to examine the ear to be certain that the tympanic membrane is intact. The patient is then positioned with the HOB elevated 30° to provide maximum stimulation of the semicircular canal. A 50-ml syringe with an IV catheter attached is then used to slowly irrigate the canal with ice cold water. Water is injected until nystagmus or ocular deviation occurs, or until 120 ml of water has been injected.

The normal response in the awake patient would be nystagmus after 20–30 sec, with slow eye movement toward the irrigated ear and rapid eye movement away. If there is a supratentorial or metabolic lesion in a comatose patient, the response would involve slow eye movements toward the irrigated ear, with eyes remaining there for 2–3 min. If the eyes deviate downward, or one eye demonstrates rotary jerking, the lesion is in the brainstem. If there is no response, there is severe brainstem involvement.

Both the doll's eyes response and ice water calorics are usually tested by the physician.

12. Both the doll's eyes response and the ice water calorics were negative in Mr. Brown. What does this indicate?

The prognosis is dismal. The brainstem is now involved, and the likelihood of recovery is nil. This is consistent with the mortality rate of 100% for patients who present in a comatose state following gunshot wound to the head.

REFERENCE

1. Temkin N, Dikeman S, Keihm J, Chabal S, Winn R. In: American Association of Neurological Surgeons Conference. Washington, DC: American Association of Neurological Surgeons, 1989.

SUGGESTED READINGS

Alspach J, Williams S. Core curriculum for critical care nursing. 3rd ed. Philadelphia: WB Saunders, 1985.

Anderson BJ. The metabolic needs of head trauma victims. J Neurosci Nurs, 1987; 19(4):211–215.

Holloway NM. Nursing the critically ill adult. 3rd ed. Menlo Park, CA: Addison-Wesley, 1988:61.

Hudak CM, Lohr TS, Gallo BM. Critical care nursing: a holistic approach. Philadelphia: JB Lippincott, 1986.

Ingersoll G, Leyden D. The Glasgow Coma Scale for patients with head injuries. Crit Care Nurse 1987;7(5):26–32.

Jennett B, Teasdale G. Management of head injuries. Philadelphia: FA Davis, 1981.

McGinnis GS. Central nervous system I: head injuries. In: Cardona VD, Hurn PD, Mason PJ, Scanlon-Schilpp, Veise-Berry SW. Trauma nursing from resuscitation through rehabiliation. Philadelphia: WB Saunders, 1988:365–418.

Rudy E. Advanced neurological and neurosurgical nursing. St. Louis: CV Mosby, 1984.

Yano M, Kobayashi S, Otsuka T. Useful ICP monitoring with subarachnoid catheter method in severe head injuries. J Trauma 1988;28(4):476–480.

CHAPTER 30

Status Epilepticus

Mary Ellen Cafiero, RN, MA, CCRN

Dan Carpenter is a 50-year-old engineer. During the past month he has been experiencing occasional headaches of moderate intensity, gait disturbances, and periods of confusion. His family noted distinct changes in his personality. He was examined by his private physician, who ordered electrolytes, CBC, ECG, and EEG. All test results were negative. Several weeks later, Mr. Carpenter experienced a headache of greater intensity than usual, accompanied by prolonged nausea and vomiting. At this time, his physician recommended hospitalization for treatment of dehydration and further diagnostic evaluation. Relevant initial assessment findings included the following:

Neuro.   Alert, oriented × 3, anxious; PERRL; appropriate reaction to stimuli. Headache less intense.

Cardiovascular.   Skin warm and dry; BP 120/80; HR 100 and irregular.

Pulmonary.   Respiratory rate 28, lungs clear; PaO_2 70 mm Hg on room air.

GI.   Nausea and vomiting subsided.

GU.   Voided 200 ml dark yellow urine.

An IV infusion of D_5W with 20 mEq KCl was started at 50 ml/hr, and oxygen was administered at 2 liters via nasal cannula. A complete neurological workup was performed, the results of which indicated a large cerebral mass.

Two days after admission Mr. Carpenter told his nurse that he felt lightheaded and could not see well. He then experienced a generalized tonic clonic (grand mal) seizure. An initial bolus of 10 mg of diazepam (Valium) was given IV push over 5 min at a rate of 2 mg/min. The seizure activity was unchanged, so the dose was repeated twice at the same rate, allowing for 10-min intervals between doses. A total dose of 30 mg was administered. In addition, a loading dose of phenytoin (Dilantin), 15 mg/kg (weight 68.2 kg), was administered IV push at a rate of 50 mg/min. Seizure activity continued but began to decrease in intensity. Approximately 30 min later, Mr. Carpenter's respiratory rhythm became irregular, followed by periods of apnea and bradycardia. He was intubated and transferred to the Neurosurgical ICU.

Treatment

Connected to volume ventilator, assist control mode, FIO_2 0.70, rate 14, tidal volume 800. FIO_2 was gradually reduced to 0.50, maintaining a PaO_2 of 70.

Arterial line inserted, BP 70–80/50. Dopamine titrated to maintain BP at 90–100/60

EEG monitoring

One hour later EEG monitoring showed significant subclinical seizure activity still present. At this time, Mr. Carpenter experienced a second generalized tonic clonic seizure. An IV loading dose of phenobarbital, 5 mg/kg, was administered at a rate of 50 mg/min, with no effect. A repeat dose was also ineffective. A medical decision was made to initiate therapy with the anesthetic barbiturate pentobarbital (Sodium Nembutal). Gradual cessation of seizure activity, muscular as well as cerebral, was achieved.

Post-Crisis Systems Assessment

Neurological. Pupils equal, dilated, sluggishly reactive.

Cardiovascular. BP 70/50, dopamine increased. Sinus tachycardia with occasional PVCs. Skin cool to touch.

Pulmonary. Crackles bilaterally, occasional spontaneous respirations.

Ventilator Settings

Mode	Assist control
Rate	12
FIO_2	0.60
Tidal volume	800

ABGs

pH	7.20
$PaCO_2$	47
PaO_2	55
SaO_2	88%
HCO_3	15

Renal

Urine output	30 ml/hr

Treatment

Maintain systolic BP of 100

Sodium bicarbonate 1 mEq/kg

Increase FIO_2 to 0.70, assist control, rate 14, PEEP 5 cm

Repeat blood gas in 30 min.

Repeat ABG Results

pH	7.33
$PaCO_2$	40
PaO_2	70
SaO_2	91%
HCO_3	20

QUESTIONS AND ANSWERS

1. **How are seizure disorders classified and how is status epilepticus defined?**

   The most frequently used system of classification at this time is the International Classification of Epileptic Seizures (1). Based on this system, seizure disorders are divided into three major categories, and then subdivided. The following is an abbreviated version:

   I. *Partial*—Hyperactive firing of neurons is noted to initiate within a localized area of the brain.
      A. *Simple or Elemental*—No loss of consciousness, focal motor or sensory, Jacksonian.
      B. *Complex*—Alteration of consciousness; manifested as altered behavior prone to repetitive, purposeless activity accompanied by brief periods of loss of consciousness. It is important to note that complex partial seizures may progress to generalized seizures.
   II. *Generalized*—Hyperactive firing of neurons spreads simultaneously to both sides of the brain. This type of seizure may or may not be associated with convulsive activity. One example of a convulsive generalized seizure is tonic-clonic or grand mal, while absence or petit mal is a nonconvulsive type.
   III. *Unclassified*—Disorders which do not fit into a particular category.

   Status epilepticus is generally defined as one seizure lasting longer than 30 min or repetitive seizures (>3) that do not allow for recovery of consciousness in between episodes (completed post-ictal phase). Exact definitions vary among authors. Although it may occur with various forms of seizure disorders, the focus of this discussion is convulsive status epilepticus. This type of status epilepticus is considered a neurological emergency because it can cause irreversible brain damage and death.

2. **Does status epilepticus usually occur in patients who have never before experienced a seizure?**

No, it is not common, but it can occur. It is most likely to occur in the patient who experiences abrupt withdrawal of antiepileptic medications.

3. **What are the common underlying causes of seizures?**

> Abrupt withdrawal of antiepileptic medications
> Infection
> Structural lesions
> Hypoglycemia
> Uncontrolled hypertension
> Hypoxia
> Metabolic imbalances
> CVA
> Head trauma
> Hyperthermia (especially in children)
> Degenerative process
> Cardiac abnormality

4. **What factors can precipitate seizures in a patient with a known seizure disorder?**

> Emotional upset
> Sleep deprivation
> Drug or alcohol intake
> Extremes—light, noise, odors
> Missed meals
> Heat

5. **Mr. Carpenter's prognosis was poor because of the size and location of his brain tumor. By what mechanisms can an intracranial neoplasm cause seizure activity?**

Brain tissue, blood, and cerebrospinal fluid are enclosed in a bony, rigid compartment with virtually no room for expansion. A change in volume in any of these three components would result in increased intracranial pressure (ICP) unless compensation occurred. This is based on the Monro-Kellie doctrine. Compensation involves displacement of cerebrospinal fluid through several mechanisms. This process eventually reaches a limit. Displacement rate becomes less than the amount of fluid that is accumulating, leading to increased ICP (normal, 0–15 mm Hg). A tumor consisting of rapidly proliferating cells will cause increased intracranial pressure by: (*a*) occupying space and (*b*) affecting surrounding tissue causing edema.

In a large percentage of patients, the increased ICP produces either a partial or a generalized tonic-clonic seizure, depending upon tumor size and location.

6. **What are the pathophysiologic processes that can induce brain damage during status epilepticus?**

Hyperactive, abnormal neuronal firing as well as intensive muscle activity are the underlying factors producing pathophysiologic changes during status epilepticus. The exact triggering mechanism remains unclear, although various theories regarding chemical and electrical activity have been proposed. Cell membrane depolarization is affected and becomes prolonged, altering transmission of impulses across the synapse. Continued seizure activity produces a tremendous increase in cerebral metabolism, necessitating more rapid use of both oxygen and glucose. Blood flow must increase 2½ times to meet increased demands. If this increased need is not met, cerebral metabolism becomes impaired and neuronal death follows. Brain damage ranges from minor loss of memory to extensive insult.

7. **What are the general management protocols used in treating status epilepticus?**

Although protocols may vary, most authorities recommend the following:

Maintain airway patency and other vital parameters. Insert an oral airway, if it can be done easily (if not, insert airway with initial dose of Valium or Ativan); do *not* use tongue blade or attempt to pry patient's teeth apart. Position the patient on his or her side to avoid aspiration.

When possible, obtain blood samples for laboratory studies as indicated (such as arterial blood gases, glucose, electrolytes, BUN, liver enzymes, toxicology screen, alcohol level, anticonvulsant levels). Start an IV line. If the patient is in the field or the Emergency Department where his or her metabolic status is unknown, or if there is a likelihood of hypoglycemia (diabetic, alcoholic) administer one ampule of $D_{50}W$ IV push and thiamine, 1 mg IV or IM.

Promote a safe environment:
    Loosen tight clothing
    Move sharp objects away from patient
    Do not restrain patient
    Keep side rails up and padded

Initially control seizure with a rapid-acting IV pharmacologic agent (usually Valium or Ativan) followed by maintenance therapy (usually Dilantin) to achieve a constant blood level.

Stay with the patient. Note duration of seizure and chart precise description of seizure.

As the patient's consciousness returns, reassure and orient him or her.

Obtain patient history review and identification of precipitating/ underlying factors.

Prevent recurrence and/or aggressively use additional drug therapy (phenobarbital IV, or general anesthesia) if seizure activity continues.

Monitor and minimize systemic response to status epilepticus.

Use cooling techniques to decrease temperature if necessary.

8. **Mr. Carpenter received specific dosages of Valium and Dilantin. What are the drug dosages used in status epilepticus? What precautions should be observed with these two medications?**

Valium should be given as an initial dose of 5–10 mg IV push (stop when therapeutic effects are visible) at a rate not to exceed 2 mg/min. Repeat doses may be administered cautiously, allowing for 10–15 min between doses. Most authorities recommend a maximum of 30 mg: however, this may vary in some institutions.

Although Valium is very effective in treating seizures, its effects are short lived and a longer acting pharmacological agent also must be given. The drug of choice is Dilantin.

A loading dose of Dilantin is given initially, followed by daily maintenance doses to achieve a therapeutic serum level (10–20 μg/ml). Recommended loading dose varies from 10 to 18 mg/kg of body weight (1000–1500 mg). Dilantin should be administered via IV injection at a rate not to exceed 50 mg/min. The cardiac monitor should be observed for bradycardia and the BP should be checked every 3–5 min. The drug should be stopped and the physician notified if bradycardia or hypotension occur.

Dilantin should be administered through a central vein if possible, as it is extremely irritating to the vein. It should be flushed with normal saline.

Nursing Implications

Diazepam (Valium)

Observe patient for hypotension, tachycardia, muscular weakness, respiratory depression, and reduction in level of consciousness. Resuscitative equipment must be on hand.

Avoid small veins.

Drowsiness, ataxia, constipation, and urinary retention may occur in the elderly, debilitated patient or with use of large doses.

Monitor intake and output.

Phenytoin (Dilantin)

Continuously monitor vital signs q3–5 min during IV infusion. Observe for respiratory depression, hypotension, and cardiac dysrhythmias.

Observe cardiac monitor for widening of the QRS, prolongation of the PR or QT intervals, and depression of the ST segment.

Doses lower than usual adult range should be given to geriatric, severely ill, or debilitated patients, as well as those with liver dysfunction.

Monitor neurological status.

Observe injection site frequently.

Do not administer hazy or precipitated solution. Warm solution at room temperature after removing from refrigerator if precipitation has occurred.

Monitor liver function, thyroid function tests, blood counts, and urinalysis.

9. **Ativan (lorazepam) is becoming increasingly used as the first line drug for seizures. Why?**

Ativan is a benzodiazepine that is similar to Valium but with a longer CNS action. Administration of Ativan, 2 mg, will give the same therapeutic effect as 10 mg of Valium. Thus, Ativan is preferred as lower doses are effective and less CNS depression results. This is especially important when the patient is receiving other CNS depressants such as Dilantin or phenobarbital.

10. **What is refractory status epilepticus and how is it managed?**

Refractory status epilepticus is considered to be prolonged convulsive activity or, in some cases, prolonged post-ictal unresponsiveness. It does not respond to conventional therapy. Treatment protocols may consist of administering phenobarbital and/or anesthesic agents plus intubation if not already done.

11. **What are the dosage ranges and precautions associated with phenobarbital and pentobarbital (Nembutal)?**

Phenobarbital may be given as an initial dose of 10 mg/kg of body weight or in divided doses of 3–5 mg/kg. Rate of injection should be maintained at 50 or 100 mg/min. Closely monitor for respiratory difficulty, hypotension, and bradycardia. The IV site should be checked frequently to avoid extravasation. Patients on long-term therapy require a daily maintenance dose and periodic blood workups.

Pentobarbital (Nembutal) is an anesthetic barbiturate with generally short-term effects. In Mr. Carpenter's case, however, blood levels were maintained through the use of a continuous infusion. Pentobarbital may have an advantage over other anesthetic barbiturates because its half-life is shorter. It also seems to depress neuronal activity through a specific mechanism of action. A bolus dose is administered based on body weight, followed by smaller doses until EEG seizure activity is suppressed. Weaning from the continuous infusion depends upon patient status, but is started as soon as possible. Bolus dose and hourly infusion rates will depend on hospital protocol. Pentobarbital can cause severe respiratory depression and hypotension.

12. **Why was continuous EEG monitoring initiated for Mr. Carpenter?**
Continuous EEG monitoring is an adjunct to the use of various anesthetic agents in treating refractory status epilepticus. As a bolus dose is administered, the EEG is observed for cessation of seizure activity. This is referred to as burst suppression, or the point at which the characteristic erratic sharp waveforms return to baseline. Continuous monitoring also ensures more timely therapy because it can be used to determine whether persistent unresponsiveness is due to a prolonged post-ictal state alone or in combination with cerebral seizure activity. The latter requires treatment.

13. **Mr. Carpenter's post-crisis assessment showed evidence of some abnormalities. What are the possible systemic complications of status epilepticus?**
The major systemic complications are as follows:
Respiratory

Hypoxia
Alveolar hypoventilation (increased $PaCO_2$)
Neurogenic pulmonary edema
Aspiration pneumonia

Cardiac

Hypotension
Dysrhythmias

Metabolic

Increased blood lactate levels (acidosis)
Electrolyte imbalance

Renal

Acute renal failure (rhabdomyolysis)

Muscle tissue damage
Hyperthermia
Blood dyscrasias

It is clear that Mr. Carpenter experienced cardiopulmonary changes, as well as metabolic acidosis (HCO_3, 15). Bicarbonate replacement should be given according to body weight and blood gas results. PEEP was added as a component of respiratory management. It is thought to improve oxygenation in both cardiogenic and noncardiogenic pulmonary edema by increasing the functional residual capacity and decreasing the shunt. This modality must be used cautiously because it can impair venous return. All hemodynamic as well as neurological factors must be taken into consideration in order to avoid an increase in ICP.

14. Which nursing diagnoses would be applicable to this patient's plan of care?

Impaired gas exchange and ineffective breathing pattern related to compromised neurological status.

Altered tissue perfusion (cerebral) related to increased ICP and physiological changes associated with seizure activity.

Potential for injury related to episodic generalized tonic-clonic movement

Sensory/perceptual alteration related to effects of neoplasm on brain tissue.

Altered nutrition: potential for greater than body requirements related to increased caloric need associated with critical illness.

REFERENCE

1. Gaustaut H: Clinical and electroencephalographic classification of epileptic seizures. Epilepsia 1970:11:102.

SUGGESTED READINGS

Callahan M. Epilepsy: putting the patient back in control. RN 1988;51(2):48–55.

Govoni L, Hayes J. Drugs and nursing implications. 6th ed. East Norwalk, CT: Appleton Lange, 1988:389–390, 939–940.

Hickey JV. The clinical practice of neurological and neurosurgical nursing. 2nd ed. Philadelphia: JB Lippincott, 1986.

Mikati MA, Browne T. Tonic-clonic seizures. Hosp Med 1987; 23(3):19–21, 25–27, 31–32.

Neurologic Disorders Nurse's Clinical Library. Springhouse, PA: Springhouse, 1984.

Orlowski J, Erenberg G, Leuders H, Cruise R. Hypothermia and barbiturate coma for refractory status epilepticus. Crit Care Med 1984;12(4):367–372.

Rashkin M, Youngs C, Penovich P. Pentobarbital treatment of refractory status epilepticus. Crit Care Clin 1985;1(2):339–353.

CHAPTER 31

Subdural Hematoma

Doris M. Gates, RN, MS, CCRN

George Lowe is a 19-year-old construction worker. While working on a second floor balcony, George fell 10 feet. He landed directly on his head on the cement. George suffered an immediate loss of consciousness. The paramedic's assessment at the scene showed George's pupils to be 4 mm, briskly reactive. His Glasgow Coma Scale (GCS) score showed eye opening to painful stimuli (E2), incomprehensible sounds (V2), and withdrawal to painful stimuli (M4) with all four extremities. En route to the hospital, George became more responsive and his GCS showed eye opening to painful stimuli (E2), incomprehensible sounds (V2), and localizing to pain (M5). On arrival in the Emergency Department, his initial assessment showed:

Vital Signs
BP	110/72
HR	65
Resp	18
Temp	37°C

Neurological.   GCS 11: eye opening to verbal stimuli (E3), inappropriate words (V3), and localizing equally and bilaterally to painful stimuli (M5). PERRL at 4 mm, brisk. Negative racoon eyes, Battle's sign, hemotympanum. Right temporal scalp swelling; swelling around occiput. Hard cervical collar in place, arrived on backboard.

Cardiac.   Cardiac monitor showed normal sinus rhythm without ectopy at a rate of 65 beats/min. Normal heart sounds without murmur or rub. Good capillary refill, skin pink and moist. Palpable radial and dorsalis pedis pulses bilaterally.

Pulmonary.   40% face mask. Respiratory rate 18 breaths/min, unlabored, regular, with symmetrical chest excursion. Breath sounds equal and clear throughout lung fields.

GI.   Abdomen soft, nontender with normoactive bowel sounds.

GU.   Foley catheter inserted. 250 ml clear, yellow urine.

Extremities.   Scattered abrasions on hands, arms, and legs. No extremity fractures. Pelvis stable.

X-ray.   Chest x-ray normal. Spinal x-rays normal, no cervical or lumbar fractures. Skull x-rays revealed stellate occipital skull fracture.

George was intubated and hyperventilated soon after arrival in the Emergency Department and was given mannitol, 50 gm IV push. A CT scan revealed moderate generalized cerebral edema. He was then admitted to the Neurosurgical Intensive Care Unit.

QUESTIONS AND ANSWERS

1. **Why was George intubated and hyperventilated in the Emergency Department if his pulmonary status was stable? What was the purpose of the mannitol administration?**

   George was intubated and hyperventilated in the Emergency Department because of the high risk of developing increased ICP with this type of injury. Hyperventilation is an immediate measure to aid in decreasing ICP. Intracranial pressure is regulated by the relationship between brain mass, CSF volume, and blood volume.

   Hyperventilation causes cerebral vasoconstriction, which reduces the blood volume in the cranial vault, resulting in a decrease in ICP. Mannitol is also administered to immediately aid in decreasing ICP. As an osmotic diuretic, mannitol pulls fluid from the brain mass, and the excess fluid is excreted in the urine.

Over the next 6 hr, George's physical status remained unchanged. His ventilator settings, arterial blood gases, and laboratory results were:

Mode	Assist control	pH	7.50	Na	142
Rate	12	$PaCO_2$	28	K	3.6
FIO_2	0.40	PaO_2	176	Cl	114
Tidal volume	1000	SaO_2	98%	CO_2	21
PT	14.6/12.2	HCO_3	21	Hgb	12
PTT	26.8/24.5			Hct	30

2. **Discuss the importance of monitoring serum potassium and chloride levels in the hyperventilated patient.**

   Hyperventilation produces a respiratory alkalosis by rapid excretion of carbon dioxide. Body mechanisms are constantly trying to maintain a normal arterial pH of 7.35–7.45. In an alkalotic state, protein and phosphate buffers in the cells "soak up" excess bicarbonate (base) molecules. In addition, there is a cellular exchange between hydrogen and potassium molecules. When the blood is alkalotic, hydrogen leaves the cell and moves into the blood in an effort to normalize the arterial pH. As a positive ion moves into the blood, a positive ion must move into the cells to maintain electrochemical neutrality. Potassium, a positive ion, moves into the cells for this purpose; thus, the blood becomes hypokalemic. Furthermore, the kidneys preferentially retain hydrogen ions and excrete potassium ions into the urine, adding to the serum potassium loss.

   Bicarbonate and chloride compete for reabsorption with sodium ions in the kidneys. In an alkalotic state, the kidneys excrete bicarbonate and retain chloride. This results in elevated serum chloride levels.

Thus, potassium and chloride levels must be carefully monitored when altering a patient's acid/base balance. Hyperventilation and the resulting respiratory alkalosis can cause severe hypokalemia, leading to dysrhythmias, weak muscles, and hypoactive or absent bowel sounds (ileus).

Over the next 2 hr, George became more difficult to arouse. The nurse needed to exert more intense stimuli to elicit a response from him. His GCS deteriorated to E2, V1 (intubated), and M4. His right pupil was sluggishly reactive at 4 mm and his left pupil was briskly reactive at 4 mm. The physician was notified, and George was taken for a repeat CT scan. The CT scan showed a right subdural hematoma. George was taken to the Operating Room for evacuation of the subdural hematoma.

3. **What is the usual origin of a subdural hematoma?**

   Subdural hematomas collect in the space between the cerebral tissue and dura mater. Subdural hematomas arise from two primary mechanisms: (*a*) tearing of cortical veins within the subdural space and (*b*) lacerations or contusions of the brain tissue itself. A subdural hematoma is usually formed from a venous bleeding source.

4. **When might an arterial subdural hematoma occur?**

   Occasionally an arterial subdural hematoma may occur if the middle meningeal artery is lacerated in conjunction with a dural tear. The arterial blood leaks into the subdural space and forms a hematoma, instead of collecting in the epidural space as expected. As with an epidural hematoma formation, an arterial subdural hematoma is a surgical emergency.

5. **What are the classic signs and symptoms of an acute subdural hematoma?**

   Because of the gradual accumulation of blood from a venous source, symptoms of an acute subdural hematoma usually develop slowly within 24 hr of injury. The signs and symptoms are those of expanding space-occupying lesions and/or increased ICP. The expanding hematoma results in progressive deterioration in level of consciousness as brain tissue is compressed. Without intervention, further expansion causes a displacement of brain tissue and eventual uncal herniation. Symptoms of uncal herniation include unequal pupillary response (ipsilateral pupillary changes) and motor response (contralateral changes). (See Chapter 28, "Epidural Hematoma," for a complete description of the uncal herniation syndrome.) If left untreated, brainstem herniation and death may occur. Even after evacuation of a subdural hematoma, the patient may continue to show signs of increased ICP, especially if the bleeding source was severely contused or lacerated cerebral tissue.

George returned from the Operating Room 4 hr later. His invasive monitoring lines included a ventriculostomy (ICP), arterial line, CVP catheter, and a Foley catheter. He was intubated and his ventilator settings were: assist control rate 13, FIO_2 0.30, tidal volume 1000 ml. He was paralyzed and sedated with Pavulon, 6 mg every hr and a morphine sulfate continuous drip at 6 mg/hr. His pupils were equal and briskly reactive at 4 mm. His maintenance IV fluid was Ringer's lactate at 100 ml/hr. His postoperative data were:

Vital Signs		ABGs	
BP	100/60	pH	7.48
HR	78	$PaCO_2$	30
Resp	13	PaO_2	124
Temp	37.8°C	SaO_2	98%
ICP	20	HCO_3	23
Cerebral perfusion pressure	53		

Laboratory Values	
Na	139
K	3.8
Cl	110
CO_2	22
Gluc	112
Serum osmolarity	305

(See Chapter 27, "Closed Head Injury," for a discussion of cerebral perfusion pressure.)

Over the next 3 days, George's ICP remained elevated. He required frequent draining of the CSF through his ventriculostomy, continued hyperventilation, fluid restriction of 2000 ml/24 hr, periodic mannitol administration, and increased sedative and paralyzing agents.

6. **Why does George continue to exhibit signs of increased ICP even though his subdural hematoma was evacuated?**

George is suffering from cerebral edema. Subdural hematomas are a complication of severe head trauma and are usually associated with cerebral lacerations and contusions. In addition, subdural bleeding is not confined and may spread over the entire frontotemporoparietal region. This generalized pressure may injure the underlying brain tissue. Thus, moderate to severe cerebral edema will result from the contused and traumatized brain tissue.

By postoperative day 8, George's ICP became stable and remained below 20 mm Hg without draining or mannitol administration. The physician wrote orders to begin to wean George from the ventilator and normalize his $PaCO_2$; however, when his $PaCO_2$ reached 42, George's ICP began to elevate above 20 mm Hg. His ventilator was returned to its previous settings (assist control rate 14), and George's ICP fell below 20 mm Hg. The next day, George's $PaCO_2$ was successfully normalized at an assist control rate of 10 without an increase in his ICP. On postoperative day 10, the paralyzing agent was discontinued, and the morphine sulfate infusion was decreased from 6 to 3 mg/hr. Four hours later, George's neurological examination showed eye opening to painful stimuli (E2), no verbal response (intubated) (V1), and withdrawal to painful stimuli with all four extremities (M4). Over the next 24 hr, the morphine sulfate infusion was weaned off and the ventriculostomy was discontinued. George was then weaned from the ventilator and extubated. On postoperative day 14, George's neurological examination revealed spontaneous eye opening (E4), inappropriate conversation (V3), and localizing movement of all extremities (M5). His vital signs were stable, and he was transferred to the floor. He was later transferred to a rehabilitation center.

7. **What is the expected outcome following a subdural hematoma complicated with cerebral edema?**

    Acute subdural hematomas carry a high mortality rate of >40%. Those patient's surviving the injury often have long-term cognitive, emotional, and personality disturbances that require extensive rehabilitation. They may also suffer from seizures and other neurological impairments.

8. **Describe the major differences between an epidural hematoma and acute subdural hematoma.**

    Epidural hematomas may form after minor head trauma, are arterial in origin, develop rapidly, and are usually associated with temporoparietal skull fractures. The patient may have a brief period of unconsciousness followed by a lucid interval. Once symptoms begin to show, the patient exhibits a quickly deteriorating LOC followed by signs of uncal herniation. If left untreated, brainstem herniation occurs, resulting in death. If promptly treated, the outcome is good.

Acute subdural hematomas are associated with severe head trauma and cerebral laceration and/or contusions, are venous in origin, develop slowly, and are not usually associated with skull fractures. The patient may or may not lose consciousness at the time of injury. The hematoma formation and symptoms develop over 24 hr. Symptoms include gradual decrease in LOC followed by signs of uncal herniation if left untreated. Cerebral edema continues to be problematic after the clot is removed. Acute subdural hematomas have a poor prognosis, and long-term rehabilitation is necessary for many patients surviving the injury.

9. Describe the three classifications of subdural hematomas.

Subdural hematomas are classified as acute, subacute, and chronic. Acute subdural hematomas develop within 24 hr of injury, are associated with moderate to severe contusion, require surgical intervention, and have a poor prognosis. Subacute subdural hematomas develop over 2–10 days following the injury. The associated contusion is usually minimal to mild, thus improving the prognosis. The need for surgical evacuation of the clot depends upon the patient's presenting symptoms and the location and size of the clot. Chronic subdural hematomas develop very slowly over weeks to months. They occur most commonly in the elderly and in alcoholics. The initiating injury is usually minor, and many patients do not remember it. Symptoms include vague complaints of headache, drowsiness, mood changes, mental changes, irritability, or seizures. As with subacute subdural hemorrhages, the need for surgical intervention depends upon the patient's symptoms and the size and location of the clot.

10. What nursing diagnoses apply in George Lowe's case?

Altered cerebral tissue perfusion related to increased intracranial pressure

Pain related to surgical incision (craniotomy)

Potential for infection related to presence of invasive lines

Ineffective airway clearance related to drug-induced paralysis and sedation

Potential impaired skin integrity related to drug-induced paralysis and immobilization

Altered nutritional status: less than body requirements related to long-term intubation and inability to ingest food

Potential impaired home maintenance management related to moderate to severe cerebral trauma/injury

SUGGESTED READINGS

Hickey JW. The clinical practice of neurological and neurosurgical nursing. 2nd ed. Philadelphia: JB Lippincott, 1986.

Manifold SL. Craniocerebral trauma: a review of primary and secondary injury and therapeutic modalities. Focus on Crit Care 1986;13(2):22–35.

Morrison CAM. Brain herniation syndromes. Crit Care Nurse 1987;7(5):34–38.

Robinet K. Increased intracranial pressure: management with an intraventricular catheter. J Neurosurg Nurs 1985;17(2):95–104.

Shpritz DW. Craniocerebral trauma. Crit Care Nurse 1983;3(2):49–61.

Stalking the subdural hematoma. Emerg Med 1983;15:116–117.

Wehrmaker SL, Wintermute JR. Case studies in neurological nursing. Boston: Little, Brown, 1978:229–242.

Yanko J. Head injuries. J Neurosurg Nurs 1984;16(4):173–180.

Part IV

Renal System

CHAPTER 32

Acute Tubular Necrosis

Kathleen H. Toto, RN, MSN, CCRN

Jack Miller, a 55-year-old retired cab driver, presented to the Emergency Department with a 6-day history of chest discomfort, paroxysmal nocturnal dyspnea (PND), and orthopnea. He denied palpitations but acknowledged profound diaphoresis with his chest discomfort. He stated he had had multiple episodes of these symptoms every day for the past 6 days and that they had recently become more severe. He came to the hospital at 1 AM because of severe orthopnea and an inability to sleep.

Physical examination at the time of admission revealed the following vital signs:

BP	126/80	Resp	32
HR	108	Temp	99°F

Mr. Miller was alert and oriented. His cardiac monitor displayed sinus tachycardia without ectopy. Cardiac auscultation revealed S_4, S_1, S_2, S_3, and no murmur. His skin was cool and dry. He was visibly short of breath, and rales were auscultated halfway up both lung fields bilaterally. A Foley catheter was placed and 60 ml of dark amber urine was obtained and a specimen was sent to the laboratory for urinalysis. Blood was drawn and sent to the laboratory for analysis of cardiac enzymes, serum electrolytes, arterial blood gases, and CBC. A 12-lead electrocardiogram demonstrated ST elevation and Q waves in leads V_1, V_2, V_3, and V_4. Laboratory results were as follows:

ABGs		Serum Electrolytes		Cardiac Enzymes	
pH	7.49	Na	136	CK	161
$PaCO_2$	25	K	5.0	LDH	1495
PaO_2	56	Cl	99	AST	37
SaO_2	88%	CO_2	21		
HCO_3	21	Gluc	304		
		Creat	1.2		
		BUN	15		

291

The CBC and urinalysis results were within normal limits. Mr. Miller was placed on O_2 via nasal cannula. Intermittent doses of regular insulin IV push were given for hyperglycemia. The patient was also given Lasix, 40 mg IV push, and then was transferred to the CCU.

The nurse assessed Mr. Miller to be anxious and at times restless. His respirations were labored and irregular at 32–40/min. He also began having 10–15 PVCs/min. These were treated with a lidocaine bolus followed by an infusion at 2 mg/min. Another ABG sample was drawn and sent to the laboratory and revealed a $PaCO_2$ of 48 and a PaO_2 of 70 on an FIO_2 of 1.0. Mr. Miller was sedated with Versed and orally intubated for progressive respiratory distress due to pulmonary edema. He was given another dose of Lasix, 40 mg IV push. At 6 AM, total urine output since admission was 860 ml. A radial arterial line and a pulmonary artery catheter were also placed with the following readings:

CVP	15
PAWP	29
CO	4.2
SVR	1238
BP	100/70

Throughout the day, Mr. Miller's condition worsened. Despite Lasix administration, his PAWP remained high and his urine output slowly decreased. He was started on dobutamine at 10 μg/kg/min and dopamine at 3.2 μg/kg/min. He also developed an elevation in his temperature to 101°F and was started on tobramycin and cefotaxime. Mr. Miller remained on an FIO_2 of 1.0 and his PaO_2 stabilized at 80–90.

At 3:15 AM the day after admission, Mr. Miller developed ventricular tachycardia requiring defibrillation. He was defibrillated three times before converting to sinus tachycardia with a systolic BP of 60 mm Hg. He was switched to IV procainamide and the lidocaine was discontinued.

Mr. Miller remained unresponsive after the arrest and required high doses of dopamine to maintain his systolic BP above 90. When a dose of 30 μg/kg/min was reached, he was switched to Levophed. His BP stabilized at a systolic of 94 on 9 μg/min of Levophed. He received Lasix, 200 mg IVP push q 4 hr and maintained a urine output of 40–50 ml/hr.

On hospital day 3, Mr. Miller remained in cardiogenic shock with a systolic BP of 90 mm Hg on 3 μg/min of Levophed and 10 μg/kg/min of dobutamine. His pulmonary artery wedge pressure was 22 mm Hg and his urine output remained low despite high doses of Lasix IV push. His breath sounds had coarse rales and rhonchi throughout. He had gained 3 kg since admission.

Laboratory data on day 3 were as follows:

Serum Electrolytes		Urine Chemistries		Urinalysis	
Na	130	Na	63	Color	Dark amber
K	4.6	Osmolality	372	S.G.	1.008
Cl	90	Creat	50	Protein	1+
CO_2	21	FENa	5.2%	Glucose	Neg
Creat	5.4				
Ca	8.8			**Sediment**	
Mg	1.8			WBC	2–4/HPF
PO_4	4.0			RBC	2–3/HPF
BUN	58			Casts	Granular
				Cells	Tubular epithelial

Femoral lines were placed and continuous arteriovenous hemofiltration (CAVH) was carried out in an attempt to remove excess plasma volume. Mr. Miller tolerated the procedure well. Two liters of fluid were removed over the next 24 hr and the patient's PAWP was 14 mm Hg. The doses of tobramycin and cefotaxime were adjusted in accordance with his rising creatinine, and peak and trough levels were obtained.

On hospital day 4, Mr. Miller was on an FIO_2 of 0.60 with adequate arterial blood gases. He continued to have diffuse rales and rhonchi. He was receiving dobutamine at 15 μg/kg/min. The Levophed had been discontinued, and Mr. Miller was changed to dopamine, 6.2 μg/kg/min, with a BP of 102/59. His cardiac output was 3.6 liters/min and PAWP was 19 mm Hg. His urine output averaged 30 ml/hr.

On hospital day 5 his PAWP had increased to 26 mm Hg and serum electrolytes were as follows:

Na	131
K	6.0
Cl	91
CO_2	18
Creat	6.2
Ca	8.0
Mg	2.0
PO_4	6.0
BUN	70

CAVH was discontinued and Mr. Miller was hemodialyzed for volume overload, azotemia, and hyperkalemia. He tolerated the procedure well. The evening of hospital day 5, he suddenly developed ventricular tachycardia, which quickly deteriorated to ventricular fibrillation. Advanced cardiac life support was initiated and, despite treatment, he was pronounced dead 45 min later.

QUESTIONS AND ANSWERS

1. **Define acute renal failure and discuss its etiology in the case of Mr. Miller.**

   Acute renal failure (ARF) is defined as a rapid deterioration in renal function characterized by progressive azotemia (a high blood urea nitrogen concentration) and oliguria. The etiology of ARF is divided into three major categories according to the location of the cause: prerenal, intrarenal, and postrenal. Mr. Miller developed a form of intrarenal failure.

   Intrarenal failure occurs when there is intrinsic damage to the renal vasculature, glomerular capillaries, interstitium of the kidney, or the renal tubules. Acute tubular necrosis (ATN) is the most common form of intrarenal failure. It occurs due to damage of the renal tubular epithelia. ATN accounts for approximately 75% of all cases of ARF.

   There are two subclassifications of ATN; ischemic and nephrotoxic. Ischemic ATN occurs when perfusion to the kidney is severely reduced or obliterated. It can occur due to trauma, shock, sepsis, aortic cross-clamping, open heart surgery, and any of the causes of prerenal failure. (See Chapter 34, "Prerenal Azotemia.") Nephrotoxic agents can also cause ATN. There are a number of agents that are toxic to the renal tubules including aminoglycoside antibiotics, cephalosporin antibiotics, radiographic contrast dye, nonsteroidal anti-inflammatory drugs, hemoglobin, myoglobin, and many others.

   Mr. Miller developed ischemic ATN due to renal hypoperfusion secondary to cardiogenic shock. He had an anterior myocardial infarction 6 days before coming to the hospital (as evidenced by low admission CK and high LDH as well as patient history). However, on admission his creatinine and BUN were within normal limits, suggesting adequate renal blood flow. As his hospital course progressed, Mr. Miller's left ventricular function deteriorated, resulting in cardiogenic shock, hypotension, and poor renal perfusion. Consequently, his creatinine and BUN began to elevate and by the third hospital day his creatinine was 5.4 mg/dl and BUN 58 mg/dl.

   Aside from cardiogenic shock, high doses of dopamine and Levophed also contributed to the development of ATN in Mr. Miller. High doses of these drugs stimulate α-adrenergic receptors, causing vasoconstriction. This further contributed to the reduction in renal blood flow and ischemia to the renal tubules.

2. **What laboratory tests are helpful in the evaluation of acute renal failure?**

   Serum chemistry panel
   Urine chemistries/urinalysis
   Fractional excretion of sodium (FENa)

Mr. Miller's admission laboratory tests (electrolytes, urinalysis) were not indicative of renal failure. The laboratory values from hospital days 3 and 5 are, however, abnormal. It is possible that Mr. Miller could have had prerenal azotemia rather than intrarenal failure as shock can cause a prerenal state initially and then progress to ischemic ATN. The laboratory tests listed above are helpful in differentiating prerenal from intrarenal failure. (For a discussion of these tests in prerenal failure, see Chapter 34, "Prerenal Azotemia.")

Serum Chemistry Panel

The normal BUN to creatinine ratio is 10 : 1 to 15 : 1. In intrarenal failure, this ratio is normal. Both the BUN and creatinine will increase but their relationship stays the same, unlike prerenal azotemia where the BUN : creatinine ratio can go as high as 40 : 1. On hospital day 4, Mr. Miller's BUN was 58 mg/dl, and creatinine was 5.4 mg/dl with a ratio of 10 : 1. On hospital day 5, the BUN was 70 mg/dl, and creatinine was 6.2 mg/dl with a ratio of 11 : 1.

Sodium and water imbalances are common in intrarenal failure. Tubular function is grossly impaired and sodium and water can no longer be regulated efficiently. This results in volume overload and a dilutional hyponatremia. Metabolic acidosis is also common due to an inability of the renal tubules to secrete hydrogen (H^+) and reabsorb bicarbonate. Hyperkalemia may also be present in the oliguric phase of ATN. If urine output can be maintained, serum K^+ levels can often be controlled without dialysis. If oliguria develops, hyperkalemia will usually follow. Mr. Miller exhibited all of the imbalances discussed above as evidenced by hospital day 5 laboratory data. He was hyponatremic (Na^+ = 131 mEq/liter), hyperkalemic (K^+ = 6.0 mEq/liter), and had a metabolic acidosis (CO_2 = 18 mEq/liter).

Hyperphosphatemia may also develop as the filtered load of phosphorus is sharply reduced. Consequently, serum calcium falls due to both the rise in serum phosphorus and as a result of vitamin D deficiency (owing to the kidney's inability to synthesize vitamin D). On hospital day 5, Mr. Miller's serum calcium level was 8.0 mg/dl (normal, 8.4–10.2), and his phosphorus was 6.0 mg/dl (normal, 2.7–4.5).

Urine Chemistries/Urinalysis

The urine sodium can be helpful in differentiating prerenal from intrarenal failure. In intrarenal failure, the renal tubular sodium reabsorption is impaired. As a result, the urine Na^+ concentration will be elevated (>20–40 mEq/liter). In prerenal failure, tubular function is normal and urine Na^+ is low (<20–40 mEq/liter) as the renal tubules avidly reabsorb Na^+ in the hypoperfused state. It is important to remember that the administration of diuretics prior to obtaining urine for electrolytes can skew the results by transiently increasing urine

Na^+. Mr. Miller had not received Lasix for 8 hr prior to the obtaining of urine chemistries. His urine Na^+ is high (63 mEq/liter) in the setting of ARF, suggesting an intrarenal etiology as opposed to a prerenal etiology.

The urine osmolality and specific gravity are indicative of the kidney's ability to concentrate the urine. A low urine osmolality and a low specific gravity (S.G.) are indicative of a dilute urine, whereas high values are seen with concentrated urine. Normal urine osmolality is 50–1400 mOsm/kg; specific gravity is 1.002–1.030. In renal failure, the urine osmolality and S.G. can provide supportive information in determining the etiology of renal failure. In intrarenal failure, these values will be low because the kidneys have lost their ability to concentrate the urine (despite the dark and concentrated appearance of the urine). Mr. Miller had dilute urine with a urine osmolality of 372 mOsm/kg and a S.G. of 1.008. His urine appeared dark due to the discoloration from large amounts of pigment and granular casts, which represent dead sloughed tubular cells. Mr. Miller's urinalysis revealed dark amber, dilute urine with sediment such as red blood cells, white blood cells, granular casts, and tubular epithelial cells. His urinalysis is consistent with intrarenal failure, as casts and cells are rarely seen in the urine in prerenal failure. This is an important distinction for the differential diagnosis of ARF. Furthermore, in prerenal states the urine osmolality and S.G. are elevated as the functional kidneys create a concentrated urine.

Fractional Excretion of Sodium

The FENa assists in the evaluation of renal tubular function. (For a more complete discussion, see Chapter 34, "Prerenal Azotemia.") The FENa is calculated as follows:

$$FENa = \frac{U_{Na} \times P_{cr}}{U_{cr} \times P_{Na}} \times 100$$

where U_{Na} = urine sodium; P_{cr} = plasma creatinine; U_{cr} = urine creatinine; and P_{Na} = plasma sodium.

A FENa $\leq 1\%$ is indicative of normal renal tubular function and is also seen in prerenal states. A FENa $> 1\%$ is consistent with intrarenal failure. Mr. Miller's FENa is calculated using the laboratory results from hospital day 3, as follows:

$$\frac{63 \times 5.4}{50 \times 150} \times 100 = 5.2\%$$

Mr. Miller's FENa is consistent with intrarenal failure.

3. **Describe the clinical course of a patient with ATN.**
   There are three phases of ATN:

   > Oliguric/nonoliguric
   > Diuretic
   > Recovery

   Oliguric/Nonoliguric Phase

   A patient with ATN may be oliguric or nonoliguric. Oliguria is defined as a urine output of <400 ml/24 hr. The oliguric phase begins a short time after the causative event and lasts an average of 1–2 weeks. It is during the period of oliguria that the patient is most likely to develop complications such as volume overload, electrolyte imbalances (hyperkalemia, hyponatremia, hyperphosphatemia, hypocalcemia), metabolic acidosis, and uremia.

   Nonoliguric ATN is characterized by a urine output of >400 ml/24 (usually 1–2 liters/24 hr) in the setting of elevated BUN and creatinine levels. Nonoliguric ATN is more commonly associated with nephrotoxic agents, whereas oliguric ATN is seen more commonly in patients with ischemic ATN. Both morbidity and mortality rates are lower in patients with nonoliguric ATN as compared to patients with oliguric ATN. This is most likely due to the maintenance of an adequate urine output promoting the excretion of water, sodium, potassium, and other electrolytes and drugs that would otherwise accumulate in the plasma.

   Diuretic Phase

   The diuretic phase of ATN usually lasts about 5–7 days. The first sign of improvement from oliguric ATN is an increase in urine output. Renal tubular function, although improving, is still impaired in this phase. The renal tubules remain unable to regulate sodium and water balance and are not as responsive to antidiuretic hormone (ADH). Therefore, excessive diuresis, even to the point of volume depletion, can occur, if fluid and electrolyte replacement is inadequate. Nonoliguric ATN does not progress through as clinically distinct phases as oliguric ATN. The nonoliguric patient with ATN will have a sharp increase in urine output and a decline in BUN and creatinine during the diuretic phase. Twenty-five percent of deaths in ARF occur during the diuretic phase.

   Recovery Phase

   The recovery phase of ATN lasts from 2 to 4 weeks. The patient's urine output and electrolyte concentrations gradually return to normal or near normal. Stable BUN and creatinine levels indicate maximum recovery of function. The completeness of recovery from ATN is variable. Some patients, especially those with preexisting medical problems or renal insufficiency, may never regain function, although this is uncommon.

Mr. Miller developed the nonoliguric form of ATN. His urine output never fell below 30–40 ml/hr or approximately 850 ml/24 hr. He did not demonstrate the diuretic or recovery phases of ATN due to his death in the nonoliguric phase. Morbidity and mortality rates are highest (50–60%) in the initial (oliguric) phase of ATN, as compared with the diuretic and recovery phases.

4. Discuss the complications and treatment of acute renal failure.

> Fluid and electrolyte imbalances
> > Volume overload
> > Hyperkalemia
> > Hyponatremia
> > Hyperphosphatemia
> > Hypocalcemia
> > Hypermagnesemia
> > Metabolic acidosis
> > Altered drug elimination
> > Uremia

The complications of ARF depend on the extent and duration of renal injury, volume of urine produced, etiology of renal failure, and concurrent involvement of other body systems. For example, a patient with nonoliguric ATN secondary to aminoglycosides who has no other systemic involvement is likely to have few complications and a good chance for full recovery. On the other hand, a patient, such as Mr. Miller, who developed ischemic ATN secondary to cardiogenic shock and also had pulmonary edema, poor oxygenation, and diabetes mellitus would be much more likely to develop the complications listed above and will have a higher mortality rate.

Fluid and Electrolyte Imbalances

Fluid and electrolyte imbalances are common in ARF. The kidneys are the primary regulators of volume and electrolyte homeostasis. Abnormalities of water and sodium balance occur as a result of inadequate excretion via the kidneys. Although there is sodium retention by the kidneys, the serum sodium level appears low because of a dilutional effect from excess plasma water and volume overload. Manifestations of volume overload include edema, hypertension, congestive heart failure, and pulmonary edema. Volume overload is treated with the administration of diuretics such as Lasix and mannitol. Both of these agents increase renal blood flow and renal tubular flow rates. If urine output can be maintained (convert oliguric to nonoliguric ATN), it will lessen the extent of complications. Mr. Miller received Lasix and responded fairly well initially even though he required 200-mg doses (normal dose range, 20–400 mg). He did not receive mannitol, as this was contraindicated due to heart failure and pulmonary edema. Mannitol is an osmotic diuretic that causes the shifting of volume from the intracellular to the extracellular (plasma) compartment. This can result in increased intravascular volume and lead to congestive heart failure. Mr. Miller's PAWP pressure was already significantly elevated due to heart failure. Administration of mannitol could have made this worse.

If the patient does not respond to diuretics, ultrafiltration or dialysis may be necessary for volume removal. Ultrafiltration is primarily the removal of plasma water. Dialysis (peritoneal or hemodialysis) works by diffusion and establishes a concentration gradient between plasma and dialysate. Dialysis is capable of removing plasma volume, regulating electrolyte and acid-base homeostasis, and controlling uremia and/or azotemia. It is during the oliguric phase that the patient is most likely to require ultrafiltration or dialysis. Dialysis is initiated for the following complications of ARF:

Hyperkalemia
Volume overload
Pericarditis (due to uremia)
Severe metabolic acidosis
Seizures or coma (due to uremia)
Hyperphosphatemia

Mr. Miller required hemodialysis for azotemia and progressive elevation in his serum potassium. Mr. Miller had been on CAVH for volume removal but this form of treatment is not as efficient or effective as hemodialysis for controlling BUN and electrolyte concentrations. (For a more complete discussion on dialysis, see Chapter 33, "Chronic Renal Failure.")

Hyperphosphatemia usually can be controlled with phosphate binding agents such as Basaljel, Amphojel, calcium carbonate, and calcium citrate. Calcium supplements such as Os-Cal or calcium carbonate may be given to raise serum calcium levels as well. Hypocalcemia is also treated, in part, by lowering the serum phosphorus.

In ARF, the renal elimination of magnesium is impaired, resulting in hypermagnesemia. This rarely causes clinical problems and can be controlled by restricting magnesium intake. Therefore, the patient with renal failure should not receive magnesium-containing substances such as Maalox, magnesium sulfate, or the cathartic magnesium citrate.

Metabolic Acidosis

Metabolic acidosis is common in ARF. It occurs due to an inability of the renal tubules to secrete hydrogen and reabsorb bicarbonate. This may be treated by the administration of a PO base such as Shohl's solution. If severe, hemodialysis using a bicarbonate dialysate bath may be required. Mr. Miller developed a metabolic acidosis as evidenced by a total CO_2 of 18 on the serum chemistries obtained on hospital day 5.

Altered Drug Elimination

Among its many other functions, the kidney also serves as a major route for the elimination of medications. Many drugs are eliminated primarily by urinary excretion. In renal dysfunction, significant alterations in drug dosing regimens are required to avoid toxicity. This can be done by reducing the dose or the frequency of the administered drug. Space does not permit adequate discussion of the variables to be considered or the specific formulas that can be used to alter the dosing regimen. In general, the higher the creatinine is, the greater the degree of impaired renal drug elimination. Peak and trough blood drug levels should be monitored whenever possible to evaluate the efficacy and safety of a given dosing schedule. It must also be remembered that several drugs frequently used in patients with renal failure may be partially or completely removed via dialysis (hemodialysis or peritoneal dialysis). This will result in subtherapeutic drug levels. Therefore, supplemental doses of certain medications must be given at the conclusion of dialysis to maintain therapeutic drug levels. Mr. Miller required antibiotic dosing adjustments for his rising creatinine as both tobramycin and cefotaxime are renally eliminated. Furthermore, these drugs are also nephrotoxic. If the dose had not been adjusted in the setting of ATN, Mr. Miller could have worsened his renal failure with the iatrogenic development of nephrotoxic ATN. The peak and trough levels were obtained on Mr. Miller during CAVH to assess for therapeutic drug levels.

The following are some general nursing guidelines to be considered in the administration of drugs to the patient with renal failure:

> Avoid administering agents that may cause hypotension prior to hemodialysis including:
> Antihypertensives
> Antiemetics
> Narcotics
> β-Blockers
> Calcium channel blockers
> Avoid administering dialyzable drugs immediately prior to hemodialysis whenever possible.

For example:
    Drug regimen: penicillin 2 million units IV piggyback q 12 hr
    Scheduled at 8:00 AM and 8:00 PM
    Patient is dialyzed from 9:00 AM to 12:00 PM
    Reschedule penicillin for 12:00 PM and 12:00 AM
Check serum creatinine on admission and monitor frequently for patients with renal failure or those at risk for renal failure (receiving nephrotoxic drugs, volume depleted, heart failure, etc.)
Be aware of drugs eliminated by the kidney in patients with renal insufficiency and check doses and intervals for adjustments prior to administration.

Uremia

Uremia literally means "urine in the blood." Clinically the term refers to the symptoms and signs of toxicity resulting from retention of metabolic waste products normally excreted in the urine. (See Chapter 33, "Chronic Renal Failure," for a discussion of the clinical manifestations and treatment of uremia.)

5. **What are the indications for continuous arteriovenous hemofiltration?**
    CAVH, also termed slow continuous ultrafiltration (SCUF) and continuous arteriovenous ultrafiltration (CAVU), is a procedure of slow ultrafiltration using a hemofilter capable of rapid fluid removal. This procedure allows for uninterrupted blood flow from an artery to a vein through an extracorporeal filter. Ultrafiltration is the removal of plasma water as well as some electrolytes and minimal removal of BUN. CAVH is an alternative or adjunct to dialysis, indicated for the diuretic-resistant, volume-overloaded patient. In hemodialysis, fluid is removed rapidly over 2–4 hr. Many hemodynamically unstable patients cannot tolerate the rapid volume shifts. CAVH, on the other hand, is a more gentle method of fluid removal, performed continuously, over a 24-hr period. Clinical conditions amenable to CAVH include congestive heart failure, pulmonary edema, postoperative volume overload (especially in the cardiothoracic patient), hepatorenal syndrome, acute renal failure, and a combination of any of the above.
    On hospital day 3, Mr. Miller was exhibiting signs of volume overload. His PAWP was 22 mm Hg, he had rales and rhonchi throughout both lung fields, and he had gained 3 kg (equal to approximately 3 liters total body fluid excess). However, his electrolytes were fairly stable and he was not exhibiting signs or symptoms of uremia. Mr. Miller was also hemodynamically unstable requiring Levophed for blood pressure support. Considering all the information stated above, CAVH was initiated and was successful as evidenced by a PAWP of 19 mm Hg after 24 hr. However, on hospital day 5, Mr. Miller's PAWP had

increased to 26 mm Hg, his BUN was 70 mg/dl, his potassium was 6.0 mEq/liter, and he had a metabolic acidosis (CO_2 = 18 mEq/liter). He was also off Levophed but was requiring low doses of dopamine for blood pressure support. Hemodialysis was initiated rather than CAVH due to uremia, metabolic acidosis, and hyperkalemia, as CAVH is primarily indicated for volume removal.

6. What nursing diagnoses apply in this case?

Decreased cardiac output related to acute myocardial infarction

Altered renal tissue perfusion related to acute myocardial infarction

Fluid volume excess related to acute myocardial infarction and acute renal failure

Impaired gas exchange related to pulmonary edema

Electrolyte imbalances related to acute renal failure

Altered family processes related to unexpected death of family member

SUGGESTED READINGS

Allaire M. Implications of administering drugs in renal insufficiency. Focus Crit Care 1986;13(1):46–49.

Brenner BM, Coe FL, Rector FC. Clinical nephrology. Philadelphia: WB Saunders, 1987.

Lancaster LE. Core curriculum for nephrology nursing. Pitman, NJ: Anthony J. Janetti, 1987.

Mars DR, Treloar D. Acute tubular necrosis—pathophysiology and treatment. Heart Lung 1984;13(2):194–201.

Maxwell MH, Kleeman CK. Clinical disorders of fluid and electrolyte metabolism. New York: McGraw-Hill, 1980.

Price CA. Continuous arteriovenous ultrafiltration: a monitoring guide for ICU nurses. Crit Care Nurse 1989;9(1):12–19.

Richard CJ. Comprehensible nephrology nursing. Boston: Little, Brown, 1986.

Vander AJ. Renal physiology. New York: McGraw-Hill, 1985.

CHAPTER 33

Chronic Renal Failure

Susan Nussle, RN, BSN, CCRN

James Brubaker is a 55-year-old man who was diagnosed 2 years ago with end-stage renal disease secondary to hypertension, necessitating treatment with hemodialysis. He is dialyzed at an outpatient clinic three times per week and is restricted to 1000 ml of fluid/day. His medications include:

> Basaljel, two tablets PO TID
> Iberet Folate, 500 mg PO q AM
> Os-Cal, 250 mg two tablets PO TID with meals
> nifedipine, 30 mg TID

During the past week, Mr. Brubaker had been feeling ill and was not able to come for his dialysis appointments. In addition to his noncompliance in meeting his scheduled dialysis appointments, Mr. Brubaker omitted his medications on several occasions.

Today, Mr. Brubaker arrives in the Emergency Department extremely dyspneic. Initial vital signs reflect the following:

BP	210/120
HR	108
Resp	36
Temp	37.8°C
Weight	178 pounds

He is immediately transferred to the Medical ICU. Upon arrival, you assess Mr. Brubaker and find he is lethargic, slightly confused, nauseated, and vomiting. He complains of chest pain, described as moderate in intensity, diffusely located over the precordium and worsened by deep inspiration. Neck vein distention is present. He has rapid, shallow respirations at 36 breaths/min. Auscultation of his lungs reveals crackles scattered throughout the lower 2/3 of his lung fields. A pericardial friction rub is auscultated in addition to an S_3 gallop. Pitting peripheral edema is noted bilaterally in the lower extremities. The ECG monitor shows sinus tachycardia with occasional PVCs. The outpatient dialysis clinic states Mr. Brubaker's dry (ideal) weight is 160 pounds.

Laboratory data reflect the following:

Na	132	Hgb	6.5	ABGs (Room Air)	
K	7.5	Hct	20	pH	7.20
Cl	100	RBC	2.9	$PaCO_2$	16
CO_2	10	WBC	12,000	PaO_2	53
Gluc	100	Plat	200,000	SaO_2	85%
Creat	20			HCO_3	10
Ca	7				
Mg	1.5				
PO_4	12				
BUN	170				

The physician's orders include placement of a 40% face mask. Hemodialysis is initiated immediately via a permanent AV fistula in the left forearm. After 4 hr of intense dialysis, therapy is discontinued and scheduled again for the next morning. Mr. Brubaker is now less restless and more alert with a respiratory rate of 26 breaths/min, BP 140/90, and a postdialysis weight of 166 pounds. After dialysis the next morning, the friction rub is still present. However, Mr. Brubaker's postdialysis weight is 160 pounds, BP is 118/80, and he denies any discomfort except for the mild pain in his chest with inspiration. Thirty-six hours after admission to the ICU, Mr. Brubaker is transferred to the telemetry floor with daily hemodialysis treatments scheduled.

QUESTIONS AND ANSWERS

1. What are the main functions of the kidney?

The kidneys are paired organs located in the dorsal abdominal cavity in the retroperitoneal space on either side of the vertebral column. They regulate the body's internal environment by maintaining the proper fluid and electrolyte balance and removing metabolic waste products from the body. Regulation of body water is achieved by the kidney's ability to concentrate or dilute urine. Electrolyte regulation involves appropriate reabsorption and secretion of electrolytes in the tubular system of the nephron. Urea, a nitrogenous waste product of protein metabolism, and creatinine, a waste product of muscle metabolism, are the two most common waste products measured for interpretation of renal function.

In addition, the kidneys participate with the lungs in maintenance of acid-base balance by generation of new bicarbonate and appropriate retention or excretion of hydrogen ions and bicarbonate. The kidneys are also involved with the production of several renal hormones, most importantly: vitamin D, erythropoietin, and renin. Vitamin D is transformed into its active form, 1,25-DHCC, by the kidney before it can be used by the body. Erythropoietin, produced and then secreted by the kidney, stimulates RBC production in the bone marrow and prolongs the life of the erythrocyte. Renin, produced by the juxtaglomerular cells in the kidney, is a critical element in the renin-angiotensin system, which contributes to blood pressure regulation. After entering the systemic circulation, renin eventually leads to the production of angiotensin II. Angiotensin II, a potent vasoconstrictor, also enhances the release of aldosterone from the adrenal cortex, which promotes renal absorption of sodium and water, thereby increasing intravascular volume and arterial blood pressure.

2. What is chronic renal failure?

Chronic renal failure, or end-stage renal disease (ESRD), is present when irreversible kidney damage has occurred and renal function has deteriorated to less than 10–15%. Chronic abnormalities occur in relation to fluid and electrolyte imbalances, abnormal regulatory functions, and an accumulation of metabolic waste products, which affects all body systems. Initially, as kidney function deteriorates and the glomerular filtration rate (GFR) decreases, a patient can be managed with medications, diet restriction, and fluid control. However, when chronic renal failure can no longer be controlled by these conservative measures, hemodialysis, peritoneal dialysis, or kidney transplantation is necessary to maintain the body's internal environment. The indication for chronic dialysis is uremic manifestations, including the associated volume overload, electrolyte abnormalities, and acid-base disturbances refractory to conservative therapy. This usually occurs when the GFR has decreased to less than 5 ml/min (normal GFR, 125 ml/min). Uremia is the collection of signs and symptoms associated with renal failure that commonly occur in the presence of elevated blood levels of urea and creatinine.

Manifestations of Uremia

Skin changes
    Yellow, grey tinged skin
    Dry and scaly skin
    Pruritus
    Potential uremic frost
Cardiovascular changes
    Uremic pericarditis
    Pulmonary edema
    Hypertension
    Arteriosclerosis
Neurologic changes
    Encephalopathy
    Fatigue
    Memory loss

Neuromuscular irritability
Peripheral neuropathy
Diminished muscle strength
Hematologic changes
  Anemia
  Thrombocytopenia
Gastrointestinal changes
  Fetor uremicus
  Gum ulceration
  Anorexia
  Nausea and vomiting
  Gastritis
  Ulcers
Skeletal changes
  Bone demineralization
  Osteodystrophy
  Metastatic calcifications

3. Why was hemodialysis initiated so emergently upon Mr. Brubaker's arrival?

The main goals of hemodialysis are to alleviate uremic symptoms, correct the associated electrolyte derangements, and remove metabolic waste products in a patient without a functioning kidney. Mr. Brubaker was admitted with overt uremia, severe volume overload, and marked electrolyte and acid-base disturbances resulting from noncompliance with dialysis therapy. Therefore, hemodialysis was essential to correct the uremia and associated fluid and electrolyte imbalances.

4. Mr. Brubaker had a primary AV fistula in his left forearm. What are important concepts related to a dialysis access?

A primary arteriovenous fistula is an anastomosis between an artery and a vein that allows arterial blood to flow into the vein, thus

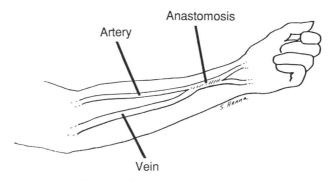

Figure 33.1. Arteriovenous fistula.

causing venous engorgement and enlargement (Fig.33.1). This vein is then used as an access to the bloodstream for hemodialysis. Patency of the access should be assessed several times each day and can be determined by palpating for a thrill (buzzing sensation) or auscultating with a stethoscope for a bruit (buzzing sound). The area should be assessed daily for signs of infection, such as redness, pain, or swelling along the fistula site. This access is the patient's lifeline and must be protected; therefore, no blood pressures, intravenous lines, or needle sticks should be performed on the access arm.

5. **What are typical laboratory findings in a chronic renal failure patient?**

   Pertinent laboratory tests include a complete blood count, electrolytes, serum creatinine, BUN, and a baseline arterial blood gas. While a normal hematocrit range is 40–54% for men and 37–47% for women, a renal patient is chronically anemic and will adapt to hematocrits of 20–25%. Because of multiple blood transfusions given to treat the chronic anemia in some ESRD patients, there is an increased risk of hepatitis B among these patients. Hyperkalemia and hyponatremia are also frequent occurrences in dialysis patients. While a normal BUN range is 7–18 mg/dl and normal creatinine range is 0.6–1.2 mg/dl, the corresponding values in dialysis patients are markedly higher. A normal bicarbonate level is 22–26 mEq/liter but ESRD patients, unable to generate new bicarbonate from a nonfunctioning kidney, typically demonstrate a chronic metabolic acidosis. Dialysis, medications, diet, and fluid restriction are essential for an ESRD patient. Mr. Brubaker's extreme alterations in laboratory values resulted from his noncompliance with his prescribed therapy.

6. **What is the relationship between calcium and phosphate and how is this relationship altered in chronic renal failure?**

   Plasma calcium and phosphate exist in a reciprocal relationship. If the calcium level decreases, the phosphate level increases. The body maintains the calcium phosphate product (Ca $\times$ PO_4) at 30–40 mg/dl. Approximately 98% of the total body calcium is found in bones, with the remaining 2% in the plasma. The ionized plasma calcium level controls the amount of calcium absorbed from the gastrointestinal tract. Vitamin D facilitates the absorption; however, vitamin D must be metabolized by the kidney into its active form, 1,25-DHCC, before it can be used.

   While the serum calcium level is maintained at 8.4–10.2 mg/dl, the phosphate level is maintained at 2.7–4.5 mg/dl. The majority of dietary phosphate is excreted via the kidney to maintain a normal serum phosphate level. Phosphate excretion by the kidney is directly proportional to the serum phosphate level. An increased plasma phosphate level will result in an increased phosphate excretion; thus, a normal serum phosphate level is maintained. The parathyroid hormone plays a major role in maintaining calcium phosphate balance. When the serum calcium level decreases, the parathyroid glands are stimulated to release parathyroid hormone, which causes calcium release from bone, leading to an increased plasma calcium level. Parathyroid hormone also enhances phosphate excretion via the kidney, thereby decreasing the plasma phosphate level and promoting a normal calcium phosphate balance.

The kidneys play a critical role in this complex interrelationship between calcium and phosphate. This relationship is severely altered in chronic renal failure. Because the kidney is the primary route of phosphate excretion, an elevation of the plasma phosphorus occurs in ESRD. Plasma calcium decreases in response to the hyperphosphatemia. Furthermore, in the presence of advanced renal disease, conversion of vitamin D into its active metabolite is severely impaired. Therefore, there is reduced calcium absorption from the gastrointestinal tract and impaired calcium mobilization from bone, worsening the hypocalcemia. The parathyroid glands respond to the hypocalcemia by secreting parathyroid hormone. This enhances calcium resorption from bone, thereby increasing the serum calcium level. With a rising calcium and phosphate level, the calcium phosphate balance is not maintained. When the calcium phosphate product (Ca $\times$ PO$_4$) exceeds 70 mg/dl (solubility product) calcium phosphate crystals may form and precipitate in the body. These metastatic calcifications can be found in the brain, eyes, myocardium, lungs, joints, blood vessels, and skin. As the calcium binds to the phosphate, forming metastatic calcifications, the serum calcium level falls, stimulating the parathyroid glands to release more parathyroid hormone. A secondary hyperparathyroidism may develop, promoting bone demineralization. While skeletal disturbances may not be clinically seen during the first years of ESRD, extensive bone dissolution can be seen in later years and is manifested as bone pain and fractures.

It is essential to maintain a proper calcium phosphate balance, thereby preventing metastatic calcifications and renal osteodystrophy. Lowering the serum phosphate is of utmost importance. Ideally, a low phosphate diet will prevent hyperphosphatemia. However, in some patients, phosphate binding agents are required. Calcium salts, such as a calcium carbonate (i.e., Os-Cal), or aluminum-containing antacids, such as Amphojel or Basaljel, are commonly used for this purpose. These medications bind with the phosphate in the gastrointestinal tract and are excreted in the feces, thus preventing absorption of the phosphate from the GI tract. Once the plasma phosphate is within a normal range, vitamin D supplements or oral calcium supplements may be prescribed for hypocalcemia. Serum phosphate should be maintained within acceptable limits, however, or metastatic calcifications can occur from an elevated calcium phosphate product.

7. **What is aluminum toxicity and how is it associated with ESRD?**

Aluminum, a cation normally excreted by the kidney, accumulates in some patients with ESRD, resulting in CNS, hematologic, and bone toxicity. Currently, the main sources of aluminum for renal patients are aluminum-containing phosphate-binding antacids, such as Basaljel and Amphojel. Aluminum accumulation can result in encephalopathy, manifested by speech disturbances, seizures, and a deteriorating mental status. Aluminum toxicity can also contribute to the anemia seen in ESRD. Finally, aluminum can play a major role in the development of renal osteodystrophy by interfering with effective bone mineralization. Based on the above considerations, avoidance of aluminum-containing antacids, if possible, by substitution with calcium salts as phosphate binders may help to prevent the development of aluminum toxicity and its manifestations. However, calcium salts are not as effective in phosphate binding as aluminum-containing antacids and a serious side effect is hypercalcemia. Therefore, control of serum phosphorus without aluminum toxicity is a difficult aspect of care and continues to be researched.

8. **How are pericarditis and chronic renal failure related?**

Pericarditis is a common complication that occurs in patients with chronic renal failure and results from an accumulation of uremic toxins. The visceral and parietal layers of the pericardium become inflamed and irritated and "rub" instead of gliding across each other. Manifestations include chest pain, usually relieved by leaning forward, low grade fever, possible hypotension, and a pericardial friction rub (a scratchy "leathery" sound heard best with the stethoscope's diaphragm placed over the left mid to lower sternal border). Treatment for pericarditis in an ESRD patient consists of intense daily dialysis until the condition improves.

9. **What are some complications of pericarditis?**

Complications of pericarditis include myocarditis, dysrhythmias, constrictive pericarditis, and pericardial effusion. The most life-threatening complication is cardiac tamponade, a compression of the heart by an enlarging pericardial effusion. Signs of tamponade include hypotension, pulsus parodoxus, jugular venous distention, muffled heart sounds, and decreasing consciousness. Acute treatment for tamponade includes IV fluids to increase the circulating blood volume and pericardiocentesis.

10. What is the likely cause of Mr. Brubaker's fever?

Mild temperature elevation is sometimes associated with pericarditis, which is a likely cause of the fever. However, because renal patients are more susceptible to infections in general, strict aseptic nursing technique is essential. Indwelling catheters and invasive monitoring techniques should be avoided unless essential. Fever should be reported promptly to the physician and pertinent cultures should be obtained.

11. Mr. Brubaker's treatment modality for ESRD was hemodialysis. What are the main differences between hemodialysis and peritoneal dialysis?

The principles governing hemodialysis and peritoneal dialysis are the same. Diffusion, osmosis, and filtration via a semipermeable membrane remove excess electrolytes, fluid, and metabolic waste products to maintain the patient at a near-normal fluid and electrolyte balance. However, hemodialysis involves an extracorporeal technique using an artificial membrane outside the body to accomplish these objectives, while peritoneal dialysis uses the peritoneal membrane in the abdominal cavity.

In acute renal failure, peritoneal dialysis is a popular choice of treatment, as it is a more gentle treatment modality than hemodialysis and is generally well tolerated by most patients. It is inexpensive, the technique is relatively simple, and it can be performed at small or remote hospitals on an emergency basis. On the other hand, hemodialysis is faster and is preferred when dramatic results are needed quickly. However, hemodialysis requires trained personnel, is much more expensive, and requires a more stable patient (systolic blood pressure above 90 mm Hg) to be performed.

Chronic renal failure develops more gradually than acute failure and may involve partial or complete destruction of the kidney. Chronic glomerulonephritis and chronic hypertension are the most common causes of kidney damage in the United States. Diabetic nephropathy, chronic pyelonephritis, and systemic lupus erythematosus are other causes of kidney damage. When maintenance dialysis is required, all aspects of hemodialysis and peritoneal dialysis are considered in selecting the therapeutic modality best suited for the ESRD patient. Kidney transplantation is the other treatment option for ESRD.

12. What complications did Mr. Brubaker manifest?

It is essential for ESRD patients to comply with their dialysis treatments, prescribed medications, and fluid and dietary restrictions. Mr. Brubaker's noncompliance in these areas resulted in several complications, some of which were life-threatening. His complications included:

Uremic manifestations: pericarditis, nausea, vomiting, confusion, lethargy

Extreme volume overload, resulting in pulmonary edema and hypertension

Hyperkalemia

Dysrhythmias

Anemia

Metabolic acidosis

Hyponatremia

Hyperphosphatemia

Hypocalcemia

13. What nursing diagnoses apply in this case?

Fluid volume excess related to noncompliance with scheduled hemodialysis appointments

Noncompliance with the treatment of ESRD related to denial and/or unacceptance of chronic renal failure limitations

Potential for alteration in cardiac output related to uremic pericarditis secondary to inadequate dialysis therapy

Impaired gas exchange related to pulmonary edema secondary to noncompliance with scheduled dialysis appointments

Alterations in nutrition: less than body requirements related to nausea and vomiting

Alterations in mentation related to uremia

Potential for infection related to decreased defense barriers associated with chronic renal failure

SUGGESTED READINGS

Lancaster LE, ed. Core curriculum for nephrology nursing. 1st ed. Pitman, NJ: Anthony J. Jannetti, 1987.

Lancaster LE, ed. The patient with end stage renal disease. 2nd ed. New York: John Wiley & Sons, 1984.

Richard CT. Comprehensive nephrology nursing. 1st ed. Boston: Little, Brown, 1986.

Stark JL. The renal system. In: Alspach JG, Williams SM, eds. Core curriculum for critical care nursing. 3rd ed. Philadelphia: WB Saunders, 1985:347–450.

CHAPTER 34

Prerenal Azotemia

Kathleen H. Toto, RN, MSN, CCRN

Linda Hererra, a 45-year-old businesswoman with a history of peptic ulcer disease, presents to the Emergency Department with a 10-day history of intractable vomiting and abdominal pain. She has been unable to keep solid foods down but has been drinking small amounts of water at frequent intervals. She has become progressively weaker and now complains of dizziness upon assuming an upright position. On physical examination, Ms. Hererra appears acutely ill and pale.

Vital Signs (Supine)		Vital Signs (Sitting)	
BP	96/50	BP	72/38
HR	110	HR	140
Resp	20		
Temp	99°F		

Physical examination is remarkable for tenting of the skin, sunken eyes, dry mucous membranes, flat jugular veins, absence of axillary sweat, and epigastric tenderness.

Pertinent laboratory data includes:

Serum Electrolytes		ABGs		Hematology Values	
Na	134	pH	7.55	Hct	51
K	2.6	$PaCO_2$	50	Hgb	17
Cl	70	PaO_2	90	WBC	10,000
CO_2	41	SaO_2	95%		
Gluc	80	HCO_3	40		
Creat	4.5				
BUN	112				

Urine Chemistries		Urinalysis		Sediment	
Na	15	Color	Dark amber	WBC	0–1/HPF
K	40	pH	5.0	RBC	0–1/HPF
Cl	<10	S.G.	1.020	Casts	None
Creat	200	Ketones	+	Crystals	none
Urea	2000	Protein	−		
Osmolality	700	Blood	−		

A central line is placed and reveals a central venous pressure (CVP) of 2 cm H_2O. Volume replacement is initiated with normal saline, and Ms. Hererra receives a total of 6 liters over 36 hr. Six hours after initiation of IV therapy, the BUN and creatinine levels begin to fall. Forty-eight hours after admission her BUN is 12 mg/dl and her creatinine is 1.0 mg/dl.

QUESTIONS AND ANSWERS

1. **Explain Ms. Hererra's physical findings.**

   Ms. Hererra has a history of ulcer disease, has had prolonged vomiting, and has been drinking only water. She is markedly volume depleted as evidenced by severe orthostatic hypotension and other physical signs of volume depletion (tented skin, dry mucous membranes, sunken eyes, flat jugular veins, and a CVP of 2 cm H_2O).

2. **Define prerenal azotemia and discuss its etiology and pathogenesis.**

   Prerenal azotemia is an elevation in the BUN due to renal hypoperfusion. If not corrected, prerenal azotemia can develop into acute or chronic renal failure. The most common causes of prerenal azotemia are intravascular volume depletion, inadequate cardiac output, or decreased systemic vascular resistance. These all result in a decrease in effective arterial blood volume (EABV). EABV is not a true body compartment but rather a concept that allows a meaningful explanation of renal physiology. For example, in congestive heart failure, there is total body volume overload but EABV is reduced as evidenced by poor renal perfusion secondary to a low cardiac output. In Ms. Hererra's case, EABV was reduced due to volume depletion caused by severe vomiting. Table 34.1 lists causes of prerenal azotemia classified according to hemodynamic abnormalities.

   Prerenal azotemia results from inadequate renal perfusion. The nephrons (glomeruli and renal tubules) are functionally intact in prerenal states. If renal hypoperfusion is severe enough, renal blood flow (RBF) and glomerular filtration rate (GFR) will be markedly reduced.

Table 34.1. Causes of prerenal failure hemodynamically classified

Impaired Cardiac Performance	Vasodilation	Intravascular Volume Depletion
Congestive heart failure	Distributive shock	Hypovolemic shock
Myocardial infarction	Sepsis	Volume depletion
Cardiogenic shock	Septic shock	Hemorrhage
Pericardial tamponade	Anaphylaxis	GI losses
Dysrhythmias	Drugs	Diarrhea
		Vomiting
		Renal losses
		Osmotic diuresis
		Excessive diuretics
		Volume shifts
		Burns
		Peritonitis
		Pancreatitis
		Ileus

Furthermore, renal vasoconstriction occurs due to neural and humoral factors activated during the prerenal state. These include sympathetic nervous system stimulation by catecholamines and activation of the renin-angiotensin system. With reduction in RBF (CHF, sepsis, volume depletion, etc.), the kidneys perceive a state of volume depletion, and intrarenal mechanisms are activated to conserve sodium and water. In addition, the reduced GFR results in reduced renal excretion of BUN and creatinine. In this form of acute renal failure, the kidney exhibits the "normal" response to what it interprets as a life-threatening fall in body fluid volume. In attempting to restore EABV, the kidneys fail to carry out their usual task of eliminating excesses (K^+, H^+, H_2O, etc.) and wastes (BUN, creatinine, etc.). These responses are compensatory and not pathologic. Hence, the term prerenal is used as compared to intrarenal failure, where there is intrinsic renal damage.

3. **What laboratory tests may be useful in diagnosing prerenal azotemia?**
   The distinction between a patient with prerenal azotemia and one with early acute intrinsic renal failure may be difficult. Measurement of the BUN:creatinine ratio, urinary specific gravity and osmolality, urine electrolytes, the fractional excretion of sodium (FENa), and examination of urinary sediment may be useful. The following laboratory tests may be ordered:

   > Serum electrolytes
   > Urine chemistries
   > Urinalysis
   > Fractional excretion of sodium (FENa)

   Serum Electrolytes
   Both the BUN and creatinine are elevated. (Normal BUN is 7–18 mg/dl: normal serum creatinine is 0.5–1.1 mg/dl in females.) However, the BUN is elevated to a greater degree than the creatinine. In prerenal states, renal tubular flow rates are slow and there is avid reabsorption of filtered urea. This results in a high BUN. The serum creatinine is elevated because of a fall in GFR, which is the main mechanism for excretion of creatinine. Unlike urea, creatinine is not reabsorbed in the renal tubules. Avid reabsorption of urea with volume contraction accounts for this marked and disproportionate increase in BUN. Ms. Hererra's BUN:creatinine ratio was 25:1. The normal BUN:creatinine ratio is 10:1 to 15:1. In prerenal states this ratio can be as high as 40:1.
   Ms. Hererra's serum sodium is slightly low. The development of hyponatremia occurred as a result of impaired renal free water excre-

tion because the kidney is avidly reabsorbing water. In Ms. Hererra's case, free water intake was maintained, which further diluted the serum sodium.

Hypokalemia may be present due to renal losses of K^+ in part due to hyperaldosteronism. The adrenal cortex releases aldosterone in response to hypovolemia, causing renal reabsorption of Na^+ and water and loss of K^+. Aside from volume depletion and hyperaldosteronism, Ms. Hererra was also hypokalemic due to impaired dietary K^+ intake (she could only drink water). Ms. Hererra also presented with hypochloremia. This can be explained for two reasons: (*a*) external loss of Cl^- due to vomiting and (*b*) a dilutional effect due to free water ingestion (as was the primary cause of hyponatremia). Ms. Hererra also presented with a metabolic alkalosis (CO_2 = 41 mEq/liter). The CO_2 is elevated because of a loss of hydrochloric acid from excessive vomiting.

Urine Chemistries/Urinalysis
In prerenal states, the urine sodium and chloride concentrations are reduced due to the avid tubular reabsorption of Na^+ and Cl^-. In a prerenal state the urine sodium is usually <20–40 mEq/liter. Ms. Hererra's urine sodium was 15 mEq/liter.

The urine osmolality and specific gravity (S.G.) will be elevated in a prerenal state. The osmolality and S.G. reflect the kidney's ability to concentrate the urine. Normal urine osmolality may vary from 50 to 1400 mOsm/kg, depending upon the hydration status of the individual. A urine osmolality of 50 mOsm/kg would be very dilute urine and an osmolality of 1400 mOsm/kg is consistent with a very concentrated urine. Normal S.G. is 1.002–1.030 (1.002 is dilute urine and 1.030 is concentrated urine). Ms. Hererra's urine S.G. was 1.020 and her urine osmolality was 700 mOsm/kg, which is consistent with the prerenal state. The kidneys create a concentrated urine in prerenal states due to the avid reabsorption of water from the renal tubules in an attempt to restore intravascular volume.

The urinary sediment in prerenal states is normal, indicating that the renal parenchyma is intact. In intrarenal failure, the sediment is abnormal and cells, tubular debris, and casts become prominent.

Fractional Excretion of Sodium (FENa)
FENa is used to assess renal tubular function. The FENa is the ratio of the amount of sodium excreted to the amount of sodium filtered by the kidney. The normal FENa is ≤1%. In prerenal states, renal tubular function is not impaired, therefore, FENa is normal (≤1%), indicating normal tubular function. To determine FENa, a spot urine sample for sodium and creatinine is obtained simultaneously with a serum sample for sodium and creatinine. The FENa is calculated as follows:

$$FENa = \frac{U_{Na} \times P_{cr}}{U_{cr} \times P_{Na}} \times 100$$

where U_{na} = urine sodium; U_{cr} = urine creatinine; P_{na} = plasma sodium; P_{cr} = plasma creatinine.

Ms. Hererra's FENa was calculated as follows:

$$\frac{15 \times 4.5}{200 \times 134} \times 100 = 0.25\%$$

This is a normal FENa occurring in the setting of azotemia consistent with prerenal failure rather than intrarenal failure. If Ms. Hererra had intrarenal failure, the FENa would be abnormal (>1%).

4. Discuss the treatment of prerenal azotemia.

Management will be directed toward restoring normal hemodynamic status and will vary greatly depending on the cause of renal hypoperfusion. Volume-depleted patients should have their intravascular volume restored with the administration of intravenous crystalloids (saline, lactated Ringer's) and/or colloids (albumin, plasma, or blood). In the patient with prerenal azotemia resulting from decreased systemic vascular resistance, volume and vasoconstrictors may be administered to restore renal perfusion. Treatment of prerenal azotemia in the patient with impaired cardiac function is aimed at maximizing cardiac output. This may include optimizing cardiac filling pressures (PAWP) and administration of positive inotropic agents and/or vasodilating agents.

Failure to correct the prerenal state may result in intrarenal failure. The therapeutic goal in prerenal azotemia is to restore effective arterial blood volume and improve renal perfusion before acute tubular necrosis supervenes. (See Chapter 32, "Acute Tubular Necrosis.") It is impossible to say how long it will take the prerenal kidney to develop intrarenal failure in any given individual. It is highly variable depending upon the extent of the reduction in renal blood flow and preexisting disease states. Ms. Hererra's prerenal state was corrected by the administration of 6 liters of normal saline over 36 hr. Her improved renal function was evidenced by the normalization of BUN and creatinine within 48 hr after admission (BUN, 12 mg/dl; creatinine, 1.0 mg/dl).

5. What nursing diagnoses apply in this case?

Altered renal perfusion related to reduction in effective arterial blood volume

Fluid volume deficit related to protracted vomiting

Electrolyte disturbances related to protracted vomiting with free water replacement

Electrolyte disturbances related to prerenal state

Potential for uremia related to inadequate renal elimination of nitrogenous waste products

SUGGESTED READINGS

Brenner BM, Coe FL, Rector FC. Clinical nephrology. Philadelphia: WB Saunders, 1987.

Lancaster LE. Core curriculum for nephrology nursing. Pitman, NJ: Anthony J. Janetti, 1987.

Richard CJ. Comprehensive nephrology nursing. Boston: Little, Brown, 1986.

Whittaker AH. Acute renal dysfunction: assessment of patients at risk. Focus Crit Care 1986;12(3):12–17.

CHAPTER 35

Renal Transplantation

Connie Glass, RN, MSN, CCRN

Andy Holland is a 49-year-old retired plumber who lives with his wife and son. After experiencing renal insufficiency with proteinuria and a gradual increase in blood urea nitrogen and creatinine over several years, Mr. Holland was diagnosed with chronic focal glomerulonephritis in 1985. He was discharged from the hospital on a low protein, low sodium, and low potassium diet with a BUN of 58 and a creatinine of 6.6.

Two years later, Mr. Holland's disease had progressed to end-stage renal disease (ESRD) with hypertension and anemia. He was admitted to the hospital for evaluation and treatment in March 1987. With hemodialysis he was able to be weaned from his metaprolol but continued on a calcium channel blocker for hypertension control. At this time he was extensively evaluated and found to be a good candidate for transplantation. He was discharged after 10 days with an AV fistula for dialysis access. Relevant laboratory values included:

BUN	83 (down from 121)
Creat	9.8 (down from 11.3)
Hgb	9.1
Hct	28.1

Mr. Holland was dialyzed as an outpatient three times a week for 21 months until a suitable cadaver kidney was donated for his transplant. He was notified at home on December 28 and was admitted soon after that to the transplant center. Admission vital signs and laboratory values were:

BP	163/105	Na	137	Ca	8.6
HR	89	K	5.9	PO_4	3.3
Resp	20	Cl	96	BUN	120
Temp	97.7°F	CO_2	15	Hgb	11.1
Weight	97.8 kg	Gluc	131	Hct	35.7
		Creat	19.8	WBC	9.4

Preoperatively he was given methylprednisolone, ATG, and azathioprine. A left kidney was transplanted on December 29. The surgery was uncomplicated. Estimated blood loss was 200 ml and Mr. Holland received 1200 ml of crystalloid IV solution and 4 units of packed red blood cells. He arrived in the ICU awake and extubated, receiving dopamine at 2 μg/kg/

min for renal perfusion and 40% O_2 via face mask. He had a central line, a Jackson-Pratt drain in his left flank, and a Foley catheter. Relevant clinical data included the following:

Vital Signs		ABGs	
BP	134/87	pH	7.48
HR	93	$PaCO_2$	38
Resp	16	PaO_2	147
Temp	98.6°F	SaO_2	98%
		HCO_3	28
CVP	5		

Laboratory Values			
Na	131	PO_4	3.3
K	4.1	BUN	110
Cl	91	Hgb	10.9
CO_2	29	Hct	34.7
Creat	16.5	WBC	13.2
Ca	8.8	Plat	237,000

Relevant values on postoperative day 1 were as follows:

BP	140/84	Na	135	PO_4	3.2
HR	76	K	4.4	BUN	100
Resp	20	Cl	95	Hgb	10.6
Temp	98.6°F	CO_2	22	Hct	33.0
CVP	6	Creat	14.5	WBC	13.7
Weight	98 kg	Ca	8.9	Plat	296,000

Intake	9050 ml
Output	Urine, 7510 ml
Jackson-Pratt drainage	165 ml

Mr. Holland's BUN and creatinine continued to drop over the next 5 days. His urine output averaged >100 ml/hr and he was hemodynamically stable. A temperature spike to 100.4°F on postoperative day 4 was attributed to cellulitis secondary to IM ATG injections. Mr. Holland's BUN was 31 and creatinine 1.6 on day 6. His weight was 97.6 kg. Immunosuppression therapy continued with decreasing doses of methylprednisolone, azathioprine 200 mg q day, and ATG 50 mg q 12 hr. On postoperative day 7, Mr. Holland's temperature was 101.4°F, and his urine output had decreased to an average of 45 ml/hr even with furosomide (Lasix) boluses. He was complaining of slight abdominal tenderness and stated that he did not feel well.

Relevant values on postoperative day 7 were as follows:

BP	195/100	Na	132	Hgb	9.2
HR	85	K	4.2	Hct	27
Resp	28	Cl	109	WBC	25.5
Temp	101.4°F	CO_2	24		
CVP	11	Creat	1.7		
Weight	99.2 kg	BUN	39		

Intake	2280 ml
Output	1080 ml

Renal function continued to deteriorate and on January 9 (postoperative day 11) Mr. Holland's relevant laboratory values were:

Na	132	Hgb	8.4	Intake	1900 ml
K	4.4	Hct	26	Output	2270 ml
Cl	97	WBC	21.8	Weight	101.2 kg
CO_2	22				
Creat	6.9				
BUN	135				

OKT-3 was started on postoperative day 11. A renal biopsy was planned but Mr. Holland's bleeding time was prolonged and his graft site was nontender. By January 13 (postoperative day 15) his creatinine was stabilized and it was decided to continue the OKT-3 and delay the biopsy. Six days later on January 20, 22 days postoperatively, relevant clinical data included:

BP	155/86	Na	138	Hgb	8.9
HR	70	K	4.9	Hct	26
Resp	16	Cl	113	WBC	8.6
Temp	98.6°F	CO_2	20		
Weight	92.4 kg	Creat	2.0		
		Ca	11.1		
Intake	2810 ml	PO_4	2.5		
Output	2935 ml	BUN	31		

He was started on cyclosporin at this time. No further complications occurred and on January 26, 28 days posttransplantation, Mr. Holland was discharged home with the following laboratory values:

BUN	28	Hct	27
Creat	2.0	WBC	3.0
Ca	10.7		
PO_4	4.1		

Discharge medications included:

cyclosporine (Sandimmune), 100 mg/ml, 2½ ml BID
ranitidine, 150 mg at hs

metoclopramide, 10 mg at hs
azathioprine, (Imuran) 150 mg daily or as directed by transplant physician
nystatin, 100,000 units/ml, 5 ml swish and swallow QID
prednisone, 20 mg q day

QUESTIONS AND ANSWERS

1. **What criteria are used to select patients for kidney transplantation?**

Improved transplant results because of changes in immunosuppression have liberalized transplant recipient criteria. In some centers, guidelines for selecting recipients are stated as simply as a person <70 years of age with end-stage renal disease (ESRD) who has the potential for a better quality of life and an estimated life span of >2 years. Other centers look at absolute contraindications as incurable malignancy and refractory noncompliance. Relative contraindications may include chronic pulmonary disease or heart failure, nonfunctioning lower urinary tract, renal disease with high recurrence rate and age >65 or <5 years. Each body system is evaluated and correctable problems such as hypertension, GI ulceration, metabolic bone disease, and severe anemia are treated. Psychiatric evaluation is critical because a successful outcome depends on patient compliance with the general care regimen and immunosuppressive therapy.

2. **Because dialysis is a relatively successful long-term treatment for ESRD, the choice of kidney transplant is different for Mr. Holland than for a heart or liver transplant candidate. What information will assist Mr. Holland in deciding for or against transplantation?**

Mr. Holland needs to be given a clear picture of the risks of surgery and complications associated with transplantation and rejection. He also needs to understand that immunosuppressive therapy must continue for life and the drugs have side effects that can be significant. Because Mr. Holland's ESRD forced early retirement and his hemodialysis three times a week limits his freedom, he may see transplantation as an end to all his problems. In addition, dialysis can only partially regulate electrolytes and fluid volume and cannot stimulate RBC production or control BP as a healthy kidney can. Transplantation can offer the recipient greater independence and an improved life-style if all goes well. As much information as possible should be given to Mr. Holland so that he can make the choice as objectively as possible. He must remember, however, that there are no guarantees.

3. **What are the advantages and disadvantages of a cadaver versus a living donor kidney?**

   Living Donor

Advantages	**Disadvantages**
Greater success rate	Small risk of death for donor: <0.1%
Available graft when no cadaver graft is available	Small risk of complications for donor
Scheduled transplantation	Donor should have annual examination of remaining kidney for life
Less ischemic time with no transport time	Psychological implications with donor and/or recipient

   Cadaver Donor

Advantages	**Disadvantages**
No risk to donor	Shortage of available kidneys
No psychological trauma related to donor if graft fails or is rejected	Undetected disease can be transmitted to recipient
	"On call" transplant; especially after a long wait, recipient may not be prepared physically or psychologically

4. **How are cadaver kidneys preserved until they are transplanted?**

   Adequate fluid volume for renal perfusion is vital until the kidneys are removed. The aorta and vena cava are cannulated from below and ligated above the renal arteries and veins. A cold flush solution of Ringer's lactate with 10,000 units of heparin/liter is used to cool and flush the kidneys while they are being removed. This decreases the "warm ischemic" time, which should be as brief as possible and always <60 min. Once the kidneys are removed from the donor, they can be maintained in two ways. (a) Preservation by perfusion maintains low flow, low pressure perfusion of a cold (6–10°C) solution that provides the kidneys with nutrients and oxygen and removes end products of metabolism. This preservation method can maintain viability up to 72 hr. (b) Kidney preservation using cold storage decreases metabolic needs and therefore increases the tolerance for ischemia. An electrolyte flush and storage solution resembling intracellular composition (high potassium, low sodium) is needed to prevent cell damage. Because the solution closely resembles the electrolyte balance inside the kidney cells, it decreases active transport of sodium out of the cell, decreases lactic acid production and maintains a normal pH, controls cellular swelling, and avoids adverse effects produced by changes in intracellular ion content. Storing the flushed kidneys at <6°C in sterile plastic bags filled with intracellular type solution will maintain viability up to 30 hr.

5. **Describe the surgical procedure briefly relating graft placement and anastomoses to possible postoperative complications.**

   The donor kidney is placed in the recipient's iliac fossa on the same side from which it was removed. Vascular and ureteral anastomoses can be done in a variety of ways. Most commonly the renal artery is attached to the hypogastric or iliac artery and the renal vein is anastomosed to the iliac vein. Clamps are then released and the kidney is reperfused. The ureter may be implanted into the dome of the bladder after creating a submucosal tunnel to prevent reflux. Another option is a uretero-uretero anastomosis. This procedure has a higher incidence of ureteral leak, however. Some type of closed system suction drain, usually a Jackson-Pratt, is placed to evacuate drainage. Although not frequently seen, arterial bleeding can occur from the anastomosis, resulting in hemorrhagic shock. Renal artery thrombosis can result in loss of the graft if not recognized and treated immediately. Some centers recommend that any patient who suddenly becomes anuric in the first 2 days postoperatively should be explored in the Operating Room immediately. Warm ischemic time >90 min leads to kidney death. Renal vein thrombosis causes massive hematuria and enlargement of the kidney, which can be seen on abdominal examination. Renal artery stenosis can occur at the anastomosis suture line or between the suture line and the kidney hilum. This is seen clinically as hypertension that is difficult or impossible to decrease with medication. Dilatation of the stenotic area by angioplasty is now being done in some centers with good results. This procedure has a high risk and patients need to be observed for rupture of vessels postangioplasty. Collection of lymph in the iliac fossa can occur when the lymph vessels are not ligated and can result in obstruction of the renal vein, artery, and/or ureter. Clinically this can be seen as swelling at the site, decreased or absent drainage from the closed system drain, and signs of vascular or ureteral obstruction. Surgical opening of the lymphocele into the peritoneum is the usual treatment because an external lymph fistula requires months to heal. The other complications that must be kept in mind are postrenal. Indications of urinary leakage include significant labial, scrotal, or ipsilateral thigh swelling, decreased urine output, abdominal pain, swelling around the wound, or urine drainage from the incision or Jackson-Pratt drain. Ureteral obstruction can occur from a blood clot or because of a kink or compression of the ureter. Since this usually occurs in the early postoperative period and oliguria is not uncommon in the cadaver kidney, early diagnosis is essential. A sonogram will show presence of hydronephrosis in the calyces. The Foley catheter should be irrigated initially to assess for clots.

6. **Assess Mr. Holland's status upon his return from the Operating Room. Has anything changed on postoperative day 1?**

    Mr. Holland's pulmonary status was satisfactory. Hemodynamically he may have been slightly volume depleted with a CVP of 4, BP of 134/87, and heart rate of 93. He was slightly hyponatremic and hypochloremic and his BUN and creatinine were still quite elevated. By the first postoperative day his BUN and creatinine were slightly decreased, his hemodynamic status appeared normal, his electrolytes were normalizing, and his overall status looked good.

7. **Mr. Holland continued to have a brisk diuresis. What assessments and interventions are important in this phase of recovery?**

    Maintaining hemodynamic stability in order to preserve graft perfusion is very important in the kidney transplant patient. Intravenous fluid volume is monitored carefully to keep the CVP >4.0. BP should be maintained somewhere between 110/60 and 150/90. The goal is to ensure renal perfusion and pressure for an adequate glomerulofiltration rate, but avoid hypertension-induced bleeding from the arterial anastomosis. Fluids were given according to the previous hour's urine output plus 50 ml to maintain a slightly hypervolemic state. Urine output fell below 100–200 ml/hr. Frequent assessment of urinary drainage can identify catheter obstruction or other problems. Bladder rupture may occur if a Foley catheter obstruction is not identified early. Monitoring of electrolytes is important because the donor kidney may be unable to regulate adequately at first and there is electrolyte loss with diuretics. Daily weights are vital to assess for third spacing of fluid.

8. **On postoperative day 7, Mr. Holland's urine output decreased. What other changes are important? What are the possible causes?**

    Mr. Holland's BUN and creatinine had increased slightly, and he was hypertensive and febrile. His weight was up slightly and his CVP was 11. His general feeling of malaise and the tenderness in his abdomen all point to possible acute rejection. A renal blood flow study was consistent with rejection and Mr. Holland received methylprednisolone, 1 gm IV, for 4 days. Methylprednisolone is used in large doses for acute rejection because it impairs recognition of antigens, macrophage response, antibody synthesis, and T-cell proliferation.

9. **Renal function deteriorated further in the next 4 days. To what can this be attributed? What therapy is indicated?**

Obstruction of arterial, venous, or ureter anastomoses were ruled out with blood flow studies and sonograms. It was decided that Mr. Holland had renal insufficiency resulting from his acute rejection episode, which had not responded to steroid therapy. He was started on OKT-3 in addition to his other immunosuppressives. Hemodialysis was used for several days to support his renal function.

10. **What is OKT-3 and how does it work? Explain side effects and precautions needed with this drug's administration.**

OKT-3 (Orthoclone) is a monoclonal anti-T-cell antibody that reacts with most peripheral T-cells. It is directed to a glycoprotein in the human T-cell surface that is essential for T-cell function. OKT-3 reacts with and blocks the function of all T-cells, thereby reversing acute allograft rejection. This drug is given IV bolus in <1 min and never as an infusion or with another drug. OKT-3 must always be administered the first time in an area where resuscitation equipment is available, and most often it is given by a physician the first time or two. Dosage is 5 mg/day for 10–14 days. Side effects include acute pulmonary edema, fever, chills, and respiratory complications such as wheezing and dyspnea. The manufacturer recommends premedication with methylprednisolone and acetaminophen to decrease febrile response. Diphenhydramine IV is recommended prior to the first dose and hydrocortisone IV ½ hr after the first dose of OKT-3. Frequent vital sign checks and fever control should continue as long as the patient is symptomatic.

11. **Cyclosporine is the newest and most specific immunosuppressive drug available. Why was Mr. Holland treated with another regimen?**

Cyclosporine often causes vasoconstriction and nephrotoxicity. Graft rejection is very difficult to distinguish from cyclosporine-induced nephrotoxicity. Clinical symptoms of rejection may be the only way to differentiate between the two and these symptoms are very subtle. Because of Mr. Holland's impaired renal function, he was not a candidate for cyclosporine at this time. Many transplant centers do not administer cyclosporine until the patient's creatinine is 2.5 or less.

12. **On January 24, Mr. Holland's BUN was 31 and creatinine 2.0, so cyclosporine was started. How is this drug given? How is the dose regulated?**

Cyclosporine can be given IV or PO. Mr. Holland was started on 6 mg/kg PO given in divided doses every 12 hr. Cyclosporine is usually mixed with chocolate milk or orange juice but may be diluted in various liquids. The drug should be taken in a consistent diluent 1 hr before or 2 hr after meals at the same time each day to maintain consistent absorption. Sandoz Pharmaceuticals, Inc. recommends storage at room temperature, mixing in a glass container, administering as soon as mixed with the diluent, rinsing the container with more of the same diluent and administering that to the patient as well to make sure the entire dose is given. The pipette used to measure the drug should be wiped clean but not washed with water. Doses for Mr. Holland were based on daily trough levels drawn before the morning dose was given. Using the radioimmunoassay method of measurement, levels were maintained at 250–350 mg/ml. Dosage is usually decreased to 4–5 mg/kg 6–8 weeks after transplantation.

13. **What psychological stresses must Mr. Holland, as a transplant recipient, learn to deal with on an ongoing basis?**

After transplantation, the hope for a cure for ESRD must be balanced against many psychological stresses. Constant threat of rejection, dependency on immunosuppression drugs, assertion of new independence after months of illness and dependency on hemodialysis, powerlessness over graft function, and fear of infection all must be faced honestly.

14. **Patient teaching is a vital part of Mr. Holland's nursing care. What does he need to learn prior to discharge from the hospital?**

In order to improve self-care and compliance, it is very important for Mr. Holland to understand each of his medication's actions, side effects, toxic effects, and method of monitoring. He must be taught symptoms of rejection, and how to monitor and record his weight, urine volume, edema, temperature, and blood pressure. He must know when to call his transplant physician about abnormalities or concerns.

15. **What nursing diagnoses apply to Mr. Holland's renal transplantation?**

Potential for infection related to immunosuppression
Potential for altered pattern of urinary elimination related to obstruction or urine leak
Potential for fluid volume excess related to renal failure
Potential for fluid volume deficit related to diuresis
Knowledge deficit related to kidney transplantation and self-care
Fear related to rejection episode
Powerlessness related to end-stage renal disease, hospitalization, and graft function

SUGGESTED READINGS

Braun E. Kidney transplant recipients your responsibility: surveillance and trouble-shooting. Consultant 1984;24(10):135–142.

Collins G. Kidney preservation by cold storage. In: Cerilli GJ, ed. Organ transplantation and replacement. Philadelphia: JB Lippincott, 1988:296–311.

Keown PA, Stiller CR. Kidney transplantation. Surg Clin North Am 1986;66(3):517–539.

Living with kidney transplantation. East Hanover: NJ, Sandoz Pharmaceuticals, 1988.

MacLeod AM, Catto GRD. Medical aspects of renal transplantation. In: Catto ERD, ed. Clinical transplantation. Boston: MTP Press, 1987:1–29.

Rao KV. Status of renal transplantation: a clinical perspective. Med Clin North Am 1984;68(2):427–453.

Southard JH, Belzer FO. Kidney preservation by perfusion. In: Cerilli GJ, ed. Organ transplantation and replacement. Philadelphia: JB Lippincott, 1988:312–321.

CHAPTER 36

Rhabdomyolysis

Kathleen H. Toto, R	, MSN, CCRN

Bill Ellis, a 20-year-old man, was celebrating his new job with friends by smoking "crack" (cocaine) and running races in an alley. The ambient temperature was 96°F and the relative humidity was high. Upon being discovered by the police, the young men scattered. While attempting to escape, Bill collapsed. The distance he ran was unknown. He stated that his legs became so weak that he fell. He was brought to the Emergency Department by the paramedics, with a chief complaint of weakness and severe pain in his legs.

Physical examination revealed an alert and oriented but extremely anxious young man with a blood pressure of 160/70 mm Hg, heart rate of 120/min, and respirations of 30/min. Cardiac auscultation demonstrated an S_4, S_1, S_2, and a systolic ejection murmur. He complained of shortness of breath and had fine rales in the lower lung fields bilaterally. His abdomen was diffusely tender and bowel sounds were absent. Examination of his extremities revealed mild swelling in his arms, thighs, and calves. Both legs were flaccid and deep tendon reflexes were absent. He was anuric.

Shortly after the examination, Bill had a tonic-clonic seizure. His systolic blood pressure fell to 50 mm Hg and he lost consciousness. Large volumes of intravenous saline were administered to maintain his blood pressure. Initial laboratory data revealed the following:

Serum Electrolytes		ABGs		Serum Enzymes	
Na	141	pH	7.11	CK	4,780
K	6.7	$PaCO_2$	27	LDH	812
Cl	104	PaO_2	97		
CO_2	7	SaO_2	98%	**Clotting Profile**	
Creat	4.5	HCO_3	7	PT	28
Ca	5.0			PTT	>180
Mg	2.0	**Hematology Values**		Platelets	80,000
PO_4	11.2	Hct	30		
BUN	20	WBC	18,400		

The patient was assessed to have a sensory level at T-10. X-rays of the thoracolumbar spine were normal. A 12-lead ECG showed sinus tachycardia with first degree AV block and tall, peaked T waves and a PR interval of 0.22 sec. Bill was given intravenous sodium bicarbonate, dextrose, and insulin. He experienced progressive respiratory distress and hypoventilation. He was intubated, connected to a ventilator, and transferred to the ICU.

A Foley catheter was placed and 15 ml of urine were obtained. A peritoneal lavage was also performed with negative results. A urine sample was sent to the laboratory and the following data were revealed:

Urinalysis

Color	Brownish red, cloudy
Specific gravity	1.008
pH	5.0

Sediment

RBC	0–1/HPF
WBC	4–5/HPF
Epithelial cells	30–40/HPF
Casts	Granular and epithelial

Dipstick		**Urine Chemistries**	
Ketones	1+	Urine Na^+	42 mEq/liter
Protein	2+	Urine osmolality	280 mOsm/kg
Blood	4+		

A subclavian vein access was placed and emergent hemodialysis using a bicarbonate and zero potassium bath was initiated. During dialysis, it was noted that the patient's lower extremities were becoming massively edematous and the pedal pulses were absent.

After 6 hr of hemodialysis, Bill became hemodynamically unstable necessitating the discontinuation of dialysis. Despite aggressive fluid resuscitation and intensive hemodialysis, laboratory data post-dialysis revealed the following:

Serum Electrolytes		**ABGs**		**Serum Enzymes**	
Na	130	pH	7.10	CK	170,000
K	7.5	$PaCO_2$	20	LDH	15,000
Cl	92	PaO_2	80		
CO_2	6	SaO_2	90%		
Creat	7.2	HCO_3	6		
BUN	26				

No further urine output was observed. An emergency surgical consultation was obtained because of the loss of pedal pulses. Fasciotomies of the lower extremities were carried out at the bedside in an attempt to reestablish blood flow to Bill's legs.

Fifteen hours after admission, Bill had received 16 liters of IV fluid but remained hypotensive with a systolic blood pressure of 90 mm Hg and a CVP of 4 mm Hg. Progressive abdominal swelling developed and a bowel infarction due to hypotension was suspected. The patient suddenly developed refractory ventricular tachycardia and was unable to be resuscitated. Bill was pronouned dead 16 hr after admission.

A section of muscle removed at autopsy showed gross rhabdomyolysis.

QUESTIONS AND ANSWERS

1. Define rhabdomyolysis and discuss its etiology.

Rhabdomyolysis can be defined as skeletal muscle injury, reversible or irreversible, that alters the integrity of the cell membrane and allows the escape of intracellular contents into the plasma.

These cell contents include CK, LDH, myoglobin, uric acid, potassium, phosphorus, organic acids, and creatinine. Many of these substances including myoglobin, potassium, organic acids, and/or phosphorus are toxic or potentially lethal at high plasma levels.

Rhabdomyolysis is a relatively common and important clinical condition with a multitude of causes. Few patients have the admitting diagnosis of "rhabdomyolysis" but there may be reference to "myoglobinuria" in the chart. Myoglobin is a protein found in skeletal and smooth muscle cells. It is normally detected in the plasma in small quantities. Myoglobinuria (myoglobin in the urine) occurs when plasma myoglobin concentrations exceed 1.5 mg/dl. High levels of myoglobin in the urine will cause the urine to turn an unusual "tea" color. Myoglobin is nephrotoxic and responsible for the development of acute renal failure in a large percentage of patients with rhabdomyolysis.

There are well over 150 causes of rhabdomyolysis. The causative factors associated with rhabdomyolysis have been compiled from a variety of references and abbreviated as shown in Table 36.1. In each of the categories identified, there is a relationship between deranged energy metabolism and cellular injury.

Discussion of Table 36.1

I. Primary Muscle Injury. Trauma, crush injuries, and burns cause necrosis of muscle cells. The muscle cell membranes become "leaky" and release their intracellular contents into the plasma.

II. Increased Energy Consumption. Muscle cell injury is induced by unmeetable energy demands.

III. Ischemia. A major reduction in cellular oxygen delivery or frank elimination of blood flow causes muscle cell injury.

IV. Decreased Energy Production. Muscle cell injury is caused by a derangement of energy metabolism due to a biochemical disturbance.

V. Drugs. Amphetamines and cocaine (in toxic doses) cause muscle damage secondary to hyperactivity and intense vasoconstriction. Overdoses of heroin, barbiturates, and diazepam may cause coma,

Table 36.1   Causes of Rhabdomyolysis

I. Primary Muscle Injury	**IV. Decreased Energy Production**
Trauma	Severe potassium depletion
Crush injury	Myxedema
Burns	Phosphate depletion
II. Increased Energy Consumption	Hypothermia
Seizures (status epilepticus)	Diabetic ketoacidosis
Fever	**V. Drugs**
Delirium tremens	Cocaine
Thyroid storm	Heroin
Strenuous exercise	Barbiturates
III. Ischemia	Amphetamines
Arterial occlusion	Diazepam
Prolonged immobility	Lovastatin
Prolonged cardiac surgery	Alcohol
Arterial embolism	Phencyclidine (PCP)
Shock	**VI. Infections**
Carbon monoxide poisoning	Septic shock
	Infectious hepatitis
	Viral influenza
	Reye's syndrome
	Toxic shock syndrome
	Tetanus
	Legionnaires' disease

resulting in prolonged immobility and compression of a limb. If perfusion is compromised and ischemia occurs, cellular injury and rhabdomyolysis may result. It is hypothesized that all of the drugs listed above may also be myotoxic to some degree. Alcohol is thought to be a direct muscle toxin, producing changes in muscle cell structure. It is not clear how lovastatin, used to lower serum cholesterol, causes rhabdomyolysis but it has occurred primarily in patients receiving lovastatin concurrently with high doses of cyclosporin, primarily in transplant patients. Rhabdomyolysis has also been seen in patients taking lovastatin and erythromycin concurrently. Phencyclidine-induced rhabdomyolysis is secondary to seizures. Hyperactivity in patients who are fighting restraints may also cause rhabdomyolysis.

VI. Infections.   Infections can cause myositis (muscle inflammation) and may result in muscle cell necrosis. Septic shock can cause rhabdomyolysis due to myositis as well as ischemia from decreased oxygen delivery to the muscle cells.

Several factors contributed to the development of rhabdomyolysis in Bill's case. The primary cause was cocaine intoxication. Rhabdomyolysis associated with cocaine use is usually rapid in onset, as was the case with Bill. The exact mechanism of cocaine-induced rhabdomyolysis is unclear, but it is thought to be related to the following pathophysiologic changes:

Intense vasoconstriction resulting in microinfarctions with skeletal muscle necrosis
Direct toxic effect on muscle metabolism
Malignant hyperthermia
Sleep deprivation with hyperactivity (strenuous exercise)
Fluid losses with inadequate fluid replacement

In addition to his cocaine use, the level of Bill's physical activity (running races and running from the police) also contributed to the development of rhabdomyolysis. The energy requirements of his skeletal muscles could not be met, resulting in cellular damage. When rhabdomyolysis occurs as the result of an individual pushing him- or herself to the point of collapse, causing skeletal muscle injury, it is termed exertional or "self-induced" rhabdomyolysis. The intense skeletal muscle activity that occurred during Bill's seizure in the Emergency Department may also have contributed to the development of rhabdomyolysis.

2. **What are the signs and symptoms of rhabdomyolysis and which laboratory tests are used to diagnose it?**
A patient with rhabdomyolysis may present with or without symptoms. If present, symptoms often include musculoskeletal pain and tenderness, weakness, or muscular swelling. Although these findings provide supportive information, the diagnosis of rhabdomyolysis is based primarily on laboratory data. Laboratory manifestations of rhabdomyolysis include the following:

Elevated serum CK
Orthotolidine (Hematest) positive urine
Few or no RBCs on urinalysis

CK is an enzyme present in abundance in myocardium, skeletal muscle, and brain. Injury to these organs causes release of the enzyme into the blood stream and elevates serum CK. A CK as high as 2.5 million U/liter has been recorded in a patient with massive rhabdomyolysis.
The orthotolidine test, or the dipstick Hematest, is performed to detect hemoglobin in the urine. However, this test cannot differentiate hemoglobin from myoglobin and will test positive if either of these substances is present in the urine. In rhabdomyolysis, the urine will usually test dipstick positive but contain few or no RBCs, indicating the presence of myoglobin rather than hemoglobin. However, a negative dipstick does not rule out the diagnosis of rhabdomyolysis.
Other laboratory manifestations may include:

Visible myoglobinuria (tea-colored urine)
Hyperkalemia

Serum creatinine levels elevated out of proportion to BUN levels
Hypocalcemia
Hyperphosphatemia

The last four criteria are more typically associated with patients who develop acute renal failure in the setting of rhabdomyolysis.

Bill manifested all of the criteria listed above as well as symptoms consistent with rhabdomyolysis. He complained of weakness, diffuse muscle aches, and muscular swelling. He had an elevated serum CK (4780 U/liter), dipstick positive urine with 0–1 RBCs/HPF on urinalysis, and brownish red urine (visible myoglobinuria). He had an elevated serum potassium (6.7 mEq/liter) and phosphorus (11.2 mg/dl) and a low serum calcium (5.0 mg/dl). His serum creatinine was 4.5 mg/dl (normal 0.6–1.2) and his BUN was 20 mg/dl (normal 7–18), with a BUN to creatinine ratio of approximately 5:1. The normal ratio is 10:1. Both BUN and creatinine are produced as a result of protein breakdown. BUN is produced in the liver and creatinine in the muscles and both are eliminated via the kidney. Serum creatinine levels are elevated in the presence of renal failure and muscle injury. Because creatinine is formed in muscle cells, their intracellular creatinine levels are high. In rhabdomyolysis, there is muscle injury, and intracellular creatinine is rapidly released into the plasma, causing significant elevations in the serum creatinine. The BUN was normal on admission, as Bill had not been in renal failure long enough for it to be elevated.

3. **What factors contribute to the development of acute renal failure in rhabdomyolysis?**

    Approximately 16–33% of patients with rhabdomyolysis develop acute renal failure. The two primary factors that promote acute renal failure in the setting of rhabdomyolysis include hypovolemia and acidic urine (urine pH <5.6).

    At a urine pH <5.6, myoglobin dissociates into its toxic component, ferrihemate. The nephrotoxity is, in part, related to the amount of ferrihemate present in the renal tubules. The second and most important factor contributing to the development of acute renal failure is hypovolemia. Many patients with rhabdomyolysis present with intravascular volume depletion. If the patient is volume depleted at the time of injury, or becomes volume depleted as a result of the injury (i.e., blood loss), prerenal failure may result. (See Chapter 34, "Prerenal Azotemia.") Furthermore, myoglobin is more toxic to the renal tubules in volume-depleted patients. Bill was volume depleted at the time of injury, as a result of his increased activity level in a high heat index (elevated temperature and humidity) and failure to replace insensible losses. A final factor that may have contributed to the development of ARF was cocaine's vasoconstrictive effect on the renal vasculature.

4. **Identify the metabolic and systemic complications of rhabdomyolysis.**

    Profound electrolyte disturbances
    Metabolic acidosis
    Hypovolemic shock
    Disseminated intravascular coagulation

The electrolyte disturbances that occur with rhabdomyolysis can be quite impressive. Elevations in serum potassium levels can be seen as early as 12–36 hr after injury. The rapid increase in serum potassium is due to rupture or injury of muscle cell membranes and the release of large amounts of intracellular potassium. The intracellular compartment contains 98% of total body potassium, which is approximately 4000 mEq of potassium in a 70-kg person. Therefore, any injury or event that causes massive cellular destruction could release a fatal dose of potassium into the extracellular space. If the patient with rhabdomyolysis develops ARF, hyperkalemia is even more pronounced. Hyperkalemia was the most likely cause of death in Bill's case, as in many patients with massive rhabdomyolysis.

Profound hypocalcemia may also be seen in rhabdomyolysis. It is attributed to the deposit of calcium salts in injured or necrotic muscle and again is more commonly seen in the rhabdomyolysis patient who develops ARF. It is most prominent in the first 24 hr. Levels as low as 3.5 mg/dl have been observed. The calcium salts deposited in the muscle tissue may mobilize later (during the diuretic phase of ATN) and may cause severe and sometimes fatal hypercalcemia.

Hyperphosphatemia is also common. Muscle cells contain large amounts of phosphorus. In rhabdomyolysis, phosphorus leaks out of the injured muscle cells. The elevated serum phosphorus levels facilitate the deposition of calcium phosphate salts in tissues, thus contributing to an already low serum calcium level. If ARF develops, hyperphosphatemia is potentiated.

A metabolic acidosis, specifically a lactic acidosis, occurs in rhabdomyolysis due to the release of organic acids from damaged muscle cells. The anion gap can be significantly elevated. An arterial pH of <7.20 is a poor prognostic sign. Bill's admission arterial pH was 7.11.

Although hypovolemia is an important precipitating factor in the development of acute renal failure associated with rhabdomyolysis, it may also occur as a complication of rhabdomyolysis. Massive fluid shifts occur early, as damaged muscle cells lose their ability to maintain normal intracellular volume status and cellular swelling occurs.

This is what happened in Bill's case. Aside from being volume depleted at the time of admission, Bill continued to have an intravascular volume deficit despite aggressive fluid resuscitation. He received 16 liters of intravenous crystalloid solution but his maximum CVP was 4 mm Hg. As fluid was administered, it was sequestered inside his damaged skeletal muscle cells. This caused such profound edema that fasciotomies were required to relieve vascular compression.

In massive rhabdomyolysis, disseminated intravascular coagulation (DIC) may be present at the time of admission to the hospital. Rhabdomyolysis can initiate intravascular coagulation by the release of tissue thromboplastin and other activators of the coagulation cascade. DIC is associated with severe forms of rhabdomyolysis and suggests a grave prognosis.

5. Discuss the medical and nursing management of rhabdomyolysis.

Early recognition of rhabdomyolysis is key in preventing the devastating complication of acute renal failure as well as heading off potentially fatal electrolyte imbalances.

Treatment includes:

    a. Volume replacement
    b. Mannitol
    c. Sodium bicarbonate
    d. Normalization of electrolyte imbalances

a. Volume Replacement. Massive rhabdomyolysis associated with hypovolemic shock requires large quantities of volume replacement. Up to 15 liters, or more, may be required during the first 24 hr to adequately maintain circulation. Intravenous normal saline is the fluid of choice. Strict intake and output, as well as daily weights, should be followed. If the patient becomes oliguric and the CVP is within normal limits, the infusion rate should be decreased until the urine output can be reestablished.

b. Mannitol. Mannitol, an osmotic diuretic, should be administered when oliguria persists despite adequate volume replacement. Mannitol, 100 ml of a 25% solution, should be given intravenously over 15 min. The rationale for giving mannitol is to improve renal function by: (*a*) increasing renal perfusion by expanding volume: (*b*) dilatation of renal vasculature: and (*c*) inducing an osmotic diuresis, thereby overcoming tubular obstruction by a "washing out" of tubular debris including toxic substances such as myoglobin. Intravenous Lasix can be given in conjunction with mannitol to induce a diuresis.

c. Sodium Bicarbonate. The rationale for sodium bicarbonate infusion is to cause alkalinization of the urine in order to decrease the nephrotoxicity of myoglobin. At a urine pH <5.6, myoglobin dissociates into ferrihemate, which is toxic to the renal tubules. Sodium bicarbonate (4 ampules) in D_5W, 1000 ml, infused at a rate of 100–200 ml/hr may be given to alkalinize the urine and prevent the dissociation of myoglobin into ferrihemate.

This treatment is controversial, as there are side effects that may outweigh the benefits. In order to alkalinize the urine, large quantities of sodium bicarbonate would need to be administered, resulting in a metabolic alkalosis. This could potentially aggravate the hypocalcemia often present in these patients. In patients with oxygen transport problems, the leftward shift of the oxyhemoglobin dissociation curve induced by the alkalosis could further impair tissue oxygenation.

d. Electrolyte Imbalances. Even severe hypocalcemia is not usually treated in rhabdomyolysis unless tetany occurs, which is rare in these patients. Administration of calcium will only temporarily elevate the serum calcium level. The calcium will eventually deposit in injured tissues, and then tends to mobilize later as the muscles heal and the patient undergoes a diuresis, causing severe or even fatal hypercalcemia. Hyperphosphatemia should be treated with phosphate binding agents such as Basaljel or antacids (Amphojel). Maintenance of adequate urine output is usually sufficient to prevent severe hyperphosphatemia. If the patient is oliguric, dialysis may be needed to help control serum phosphorus levels.

6. **Identify the signs and symptoms of hyperkalemia and discuss its treatment.**

Potassium plays a significant role in nerve conduction and muscle contraction. In hyperkalemia, the resting potential of cells is lowered, causing neuromuscular irritability in both cardiac and smooth muscle cells. The manifestations of hyperkalemia correlate with the degree of serum potassium elevation as well as the rate of development of the hyperkalemia.

The most important complication of hyperkalemia is cardiotoxicity. Levels of potassium above 7 mEq/liter may be lethal. Therefore, hyperkalemia is a medical emergency and its treatment should be instituted immediately.

Signs and symptoms of hyperkalemia include the following:

Cardiac: ECG Changes

Mild elevations
  Tall peaked T waves
  Shortened QT interval
Moderate elevations
  Lengthening PR interval
  Disappearing P waves
  Complete heart block

Severe elevations
   Widening QRS
   Ventricular tachycardia
   Asystole

Neuromuscular

Moderate elevations
   Hyperactive DTRs
   Muscle cramps
   Twitching
   Weakness
Severe elevations
   Paresthesias
   Paralysis
   Respiratory arrest (paralysis of diaphragm)

Gastrointestinal

Mild to moderate elevations
   Abdominal cramps
   Diarrhea
Severe elevations
   Ileus

Bill manifested several signs and symptoms of hyperkalemia at the time of admission. Cardiac manifestations included tall, peaked T waves and a prolonged PR interval of 0.22 sec. Neuromuscular manifestations included weakness and progressive hypoventilation requiring intubation and mechanical ventilation.

He also presented with absent bowel sounds, which suggested an ileus. This was most likely due to hyperkalemia and bowel infarction, which was secondary to intense vasoconstriction caused by cocaine.

Bill's partial paralysis was thought to be due to profound ischemia of the spinal cord, resulting from arterial occlusion or spasm (possibly cocaine induced).

The treatment of hyperkalemia is largely dependent upon the degree of hyperkalemia present and/or the severity of symptoms. As a general rule, a serum potassium >6 mEq/liter (with or without symptoms) requires treatment. Treatment may be divided into two stages: (*a*) restoration of the intracellular to extracellular potassium ratio and (*b*) removal of excess potassium from the body.

Emergency Treatment of Hyperkalemia

Administration of Sodium Bicarbonate (NaHCO$_3$). Sodium bicarbonate raises the blood pH and causes H$^+$ to move out of the cell in an attempt to lower the pH. As H$^+$ moves out, K$^+$ moves into the cell, lowering plasma K$^+$ levels. The onset of action is about 15 min, with effects lasting for several hours. Eventually, the serum pH falls, H$^+$ moves back into the cells, and K^+ leaks back out of the cells. Side effects of $NaHCO_3$ administration include volume overload, hypernatremia and "overshoot" alkalosis.

Administration of Insulin and Glucose. In less emergent situations or as a follow-up to $NaHCO_3$, IV insulin and glucose may also be given to shift K^+ into the cells. The usual regimen is regular insulin, 10–20 units IV push followed by 1–2 ampules $D_{50}W$. The onset of action is immediate, with a duration of 1–2 hr.

Administration of Calcium. The toxic effect of hyperkalemia on the heart can be temporarily counteracted by the IV administration of calcium gluconate (1 gm) or calcium chloride (500 mg). Calcium helps to stabilize cell membranes and increase myocardial contractility. Onset of action is 1–5 min but is relatively transient. It must be administered cautiously to patients receiving digitalis. It is important to remember that calcium does not alter serum potassium levels, it merely counteracts the toxic effects of hyperkalemia on the heart. Therefore, it is only indicated for those patients demonstrating cardiotoxic effects of hyperkalemia.

Removal of Excess K^+ from the Body

Administration of Sodium Polystyrene Sulfonate (Kayexalate). This is an ion exchange resin that will bind approximately 1 mEq/liter of total body potassium for each 1 gm of resin administered. Sodium is liberated in the exchange for potassium, which is bound and then excreted. The usual dosage is 25–50 gm with 100–200 ml of a 20% sorbitol solution. Kayexalate may be administered orally or rectally. When given with sorbitol, mild diarrhea occurs, which facilitates the excretion of potassium.

Dialysis (Peritoneal or Hemodialysis). Dialysis removes potassium from the plasma, using the principle of diffusion. Peritoneal dialysis may be used for patients who are hemodynamically unstable. Acute hemodialysis can be performed immediately in a patient without a permanent vascular access by placing a large bore catheter in the subclavian or femoral vein. Hemodialysis will lower the serum K^+ much more rapidly than peritoneal dialysis.

Bill received almost all of the treatments mentioned above for his hyperkalemia. He was given intravenous sodium bicarbonate, dextrose, and insulin initially to promote the shifting of potassium into the intracellular compartment. Emergent hemodialysis was then initiated to remove plasma potassium. Normally, the dialysate used in hemodialysis contains a potassium level of approximately 2.0–3.0 mEq/liter. Bill was dialyzed against a zero potassium bath, as it was anticipated that his serum potassium levels would continue to rapidly elevate due to the massive cell destruction that was occurring. This was demonstrated by the marked rise in his CK from 4,780 to 170,000 U/liter. He was not given Kayexalate, as this would have been ineffective because he had an ischemic bowel.

Despite this aggressive treatment, his potassium was 7.5 mEq/liter at the conclusion of 6 hr of dialysis against a zero potassium bath. The cause of his death was refractory ventricular tachycardia, which was most likely due to hyperkalemia.

7. What nursing diagnoses apply in this case?

Altered peripheral tissue perfusion related to vasoconstriction

Fluid volume deficit related to insensible losses and intracellular shifting of fluid

Altered renal perfusion related to vasoconstriction and volume depletion

Electrolyte disturbances (hyperkalemia, hypocalcemia, and hyperphosphatemia) related to cell injury and renal dysfunction

Potential for bleeding related to disruption of clotting cascade

Impaired physical mobility related to muscle weakness and partial paralysis

Hyperthermia related to increased activity and cocaine intoxication

Potential for altered family processes related to sudden loss of family member

SUGGESTED READINGS

East C, Alivizatos PA, Grundy SM, Jones PH. Rhabdomyolysis in patients receiving lovastatin after cardiac transplantation. N Engl J Med 1988;318(7):47–48.

Gabow PA, Kaehny WD, Kelleher SP. The spectrum of rhabdomyolysis. Medicine 1982;61(3):141–152.

Grossman RA, Hamilton RW, Morse BM, Penn AS, Goldberg M. Nontraumatic rhabdomyolysis and acute renal failure. N Engl J Med 1974;291(16):807–811.

Kiely MA. Rhabdomyolysis. J Emerg Nurs 1986;12(3):1534–1536.

Knochel JP. Rhabdomyolysis and myoglobinuria. Medical Grand Rounds 1977; May 26. Dallas: Southwestern Medical School.

Knochel JP. Self-induced rhabdomyolysis. Medical Grand Rounds 1987; July 23. Dallas: Southwestern Medical School.

Knochel JP, Barcenas C, Cotton JR, Fuller TJ, Haller R, Carter NW. Hypophosphatemia and rhabdomyolysis. J Clin Invest 1978;62:1240–1246.

Puschett JB, ed. Disorders of fluid and electrolyte balance. New York: Churchill Livingstone, 1985.

Roth D, Alarcón FJ, Fernandez JA, Preston RA, Bourgoignie JJ. Acute rhabdomyolysis associated with cocaine intoxication. N Engl J Med 1988;319(11):673–677.

Thomas MA, Ibels LS. Rhabdomyolysis and acute renal failure. J Med 1985;15:623–628.

Ward MM. Factors predictive of acute renal failure in rhabdomyolysis. Arch Intern Med 1988;148:1553–1557.

Part V

Endocrine System

CHAPTER 37

Adrenal Crisis

Linda Weld, RN, MSN, CCRN

Adam Walker, a 40-year-old man, was admitted to the hospital for a cholecystectomy. Two days after the surgery, he developed hypotension and electrolyte imbalances. Blood was obtained for CBC, electrolytes, and a plasma cortisol level, and IV fluids were started. He was transferred to the ICU, where the following data were obtained:

Vital Signs		Laboratory Data	
BP	80/48	Na	123
HR	126	K	6.6
Resp	18	Cl	88
Temp	100.8°F	CO$_2$	19
		Gluc	60
		Creat	1.0
		BUN	30
		Hgb	15

Upon physical assessment, he was lethargic but oriented ×3, moved all extremities to command, but was unable to lift his legs off the bed against resistance. He denied incisional pain, but complained of acute abdominal pain and nausea. His cardiac monitor showed sinus tachycardia without ectopy but with tall T waves. No murmurs, rubs, or gallops were auscultated. Peripheral pulses were present but diminished. Bilateral breath sounds were audible and clear. His urine output was 15 to 20 ml/hr and was dark yellow without visible sediment. His skin was pale and cool, with hyperpigmented areas on his inner arms and genitalia and bluish black spots visible on his lips.

His plasma cortisol level returned as 3 μg/dl. Intravenous fluids of D$_5$NS were started and a pulmonary artery catheter was inserted. Twenty-five units of synthetic adrenocorticotropic hormone (ACTH) were given intravenously and an ACTH stimulation test was ordered.

Hemodynamic Data

CVP	5
PAP	18/9
PAWP	6
CO	4.8
CI	2.2

QUESTIONS AND ANSWERS

1. What hormones are normally released by the adrenal cortex?

> Aldosterone (mineralocorticoid)
> Androgens
> Cortisol and corticosterone (glucocorticoids)

2. Describe the normal mechanisms that control the secretion of glucocorticoids and mineralocorticoids.

Secretion of cortisol is controlled by ACTH, which is released from the anterior pituitary. The release of ACTH is regulated by corticotropin-releasing factor (CRF) from the hypothalamus. Three factors affect the release of CRF and in turn ACTH: plasma cortisol levels, wake-sleep patterns, and psychological and physical stress. When plasma cortisol levels drop, the hypothalamus releases CRF, which stimulates ACTH. The ACTH causes the adrenal cortex to make more cortisol. When the cortisol level rises, the hypothalamus stops releasing CRF. In people with regular sleep patterns, the maximum ACTH release is in the early morning.

Aldosterone release is stimulated by increases in serum potassium, activation of the renin-angiotensin system, and ACTH in a minor way. The renin-angiotensin system (and thus aldosterone release) is stimulated by hypovolemia, hyperkalemia, and β-adrenergic sympathetic stimulation. Aldosterone release is inhibited by decreases in serum potassium, angiotension II, and ACTH.

3. What are the physiological effects of cortisol and aldosterone?

> Cortisol
> > Enhances gluconeogenesis
> > Decreases glucose utilization in tissues (insulin antagonist)
> > Elevates blood sugar
> > Accelerates protein catabolism
> > Promotes lipolysis
> > Suppresses T-cells and inflammatory response
> > Promotes appetite
> > Increases tissue responsiveness to other hormones such as catecholamines

Aldosterone
Promotes sodium conservation and potassium loss in the distal renal tubule, GI tract, and epithelial cells of the sweat glands.

4. What hormones are normally released by the adrenal medulla?
Epinephrine and norepinephrine (catecholamines)

5. What hormones are deficient in adrenal crisis?
Adrenal crisis involves insufficient levels of glucocorticoids (cortisol and corticosterone) and mineralocorticoids (aldosterone).

6. What are the causes of adrenal crisis?
The causes of adrenal crisis are divided into primary (those affecting the adrenal glands) and secondary (those affecting the pituitary or hypothalamus).

Primary Causes
Idiopathic atrophy, probably due to an autoimmune response
Infection
Hemorrhage
Metastatic disease
Secondary Causes
Hypopituitarism
Suppression of hypothalamic-pituitary axis by exogenous steroids

High steroid levels in the blood from exogenous steroid administration suppress the pituitary's release of ACTH and over time the adrenal cortex will begin to atrophy. This is generally seen with prolonged steroid therapy. Dexamethasone is the synthetic steroid that has the greatest ability to suppress adrenal function.

There are other conditions that may lead to adrenal failure. Patients with an overwhelming bacterial sepsis may show signs of hypoadrenal function. Fulminant meningococcal meningitis may cause a bilateral adrenal hemorrhage known as Waterhouse-Friderichsen syndrome.

7. What are the possible causes of Mr. Walker's adrenal crisis?
Mr. Walker had primary adrenal insufficiency, and the stress of surgery triggered the adrenal crisis. The hyperpigmentation on his arms is due to melanocyte stimulation by an increased level of ACTH. If the ACTH level is increased, the pituitary must be functioning, so the adrenal glands themselves must be at fault (primary cause).

8. **How long after receiving steroids should a patient be presumed to have some adrenal suppression?**

   Any patient who has received steroid replacement for >1 week during the last year is presumed to have some pituitary-adrenal suppression. If a patient has received chronic steroid therapy, it takes up to 9 months for the pituitary/adrenal glands to recover.

   When determining if a patient has received previous steroid therapy, remember that it is not only the oral or parenteral agents that can cause suppression. Steroid agents may be given topically for skin conditions, as well as by inhalation treatments. These agents can also affect the pituitary and adrenal glands' ability to function, particularly if the patient is stressed.

9. **What are the clinical indicators of acute adrenal crisis?**

   Abdominal pain
   Nausea and vomiting
   Diarrhea
   Hypovolemia
   Hyponatremia
   Hypotension
   Hyperkalemia
   Hypoglycemia
   Weakness
   Hyperpigmentation (primary causes)
   Total eosinophil count > 300 cells
   Mild metabolic acidosis

10. **Why does hypotension occur in adrenal crisis?**

    The vascular response to catecholamines is decreased, as is the vascular tone in the periphery. Vasodilatation is the result. In primary causes, aldosterone secretion is decreased, causing severe sodium and water loss from the kidneys. Hypovolemia is the result.

11. **List factors that predispose a patient to an acute adrenal crisis.**

    Infection
    Trauma
    Surgery
    Pregnancy
    Physical stress

12. **Mr. Walker's sodium was 123 mEq/liter. What are the clinical indicators of hyponatremia?**

> Nausea and vomiting
> Anorexia
> Abdominal cramps
> Fatigue, weakness
> Lethargy
> Confusion
> Convulsions
> Coma

13. **What is an ACTH stimulation test?**
    This test is used to differentiate primary from secondary causes of adrenal crisis. That is, is the pituitary at fault, or are the adrenal glands? Intravenous ACTH is given, and serum cortisol levels are checked. If the level increases, a diagnosis of secondary adrenal disease is made, meaning that the adrenal glands are functioning and the problem lies with the pituitary. If no increase in serum cortisol is seen, the problem is primary adrenal disease.

14. **What other diagnostic tests might be done?**

Laboratory Test	Normal Value
Random serum cortisol levels	>20 μg/dl in stressed patient
Plasma cortisol levels at 8:00 AM and 4:00 PM	7–18 μg/dl in AM, 2–10 μg/dl in PM
Urine 17-hydroxycorticoids	2–10 mg/24 hr
Urine 17-ketosteroids	7–25 mg/24 hr (males)
	7-15 mg/24 hr (females)
Plasma aldosterone levels	2–9 ng/dl in supine patient
Plasma ACTH levels	<80 pg/ml at 8 AM

15. **What is the usual medical treatment for adrenal crisis?**
    The first step is rapid fluid replacement with a solution such as D_5NS to raise the serum sodium and glucose as well as to replace the volume deficit. Initially, fluids are given very rapidly, up to 500 ml/hr. The other cornerstone of treatment is steroid replacement, with 100 mg of hydrocortisone succinate given intravenously every 6 hr. If the patient has a metabolic acidosis, sodium bicarbonate may be given if the pH is <7.20. Two hours after resuscitation is started, laboratory values should be rechecked.

16. **What is Addison's disease?**
    Addison's disease is the chronic form of adrenal cortical insufficiency. Adrenal crisis is also referred to as Addisonian crisis.

17. Describe the treatment of Addison's disease.

Patients with Addison's disease receive chronic replacement of mineralocorticoids as well as corticosteroids. Because of the normal variation of cortisol levels during the day, the corticosteroids are given orally in divided doses with a larger dosage in the morning. An example would be 20 mg of hydrocortisone in the morning and 10 mg in the evening. Cortisone acetate and prednisone may also be used. Fludrocortisone acetate is the usual agent given to replace the mineralocorticoids or aldosterone.

18. What information should the nurse give Mr. Walker and his family about his disease?

During illness or any type of infection, the dosages of his drugs will need to be adjusted and physicians or dentists should be informed of his condition prior to any procedure. The family should be instructed on how to give dexamethasone (a synthetic glucocorticoid) parenterally in case of an emergency.

19. What nursing diagnoses apply in this case?

Fluid volume deficit related to hormonal imbalances
Sleep pattern disturbances related to environmental stimuli
Diarrhea related to increased intestinal motility
Potential for cardiac dysrhythmias related to abnormal electrolyte levels
Impaired physical mobility related to muscle fatigue and weakness
Pain related to a surgical incision and hormonal imbalances
Altered role performance related to acute unexpected illness

SUGGESTED READINGS

Bullas JB, Pfister S. Adrenal insufficiency. Crit Care Nurse 1985;5(1):8–11.

Chernow B, Wiley CS, Zaloga GP. Critical care endocrinology. In: Shoemaker CW, Ayres S, Grenvik A, Holbrook PR, Thompson WC, eds. Textbook of critical care. 2nd ed. Philadelphia: WB Saunders, 1989.

Geelhoed GW, Chernow B, eds. Endocrine aspects of acute illness. New York: Churchill Livingstone, 1985.

Larson CA. The critical path of adrenocortical insufficiency. Nursing 1984;14(10): 66–69.

Miller PH. Primary aldosteronism: a challenging case. Dimens Crit Care Nurs 1984;3(2):84–90.

Sanford SJ. Endocrine anatomy and physiology. In: Kinney MR, Packa DR, Dunbar SB, eds. AACN's clinical reference for critical care nursing. 2nd ed. New York: McGraw-Hill, 1988.

CHAPTER 38

Diabetes Insipidus

Rochelle Logston Boggs, RN, MSN, CCRN, CEN

Steven Williams is a 20-year-old college student who was injured in a single car automobile accident. The vehicle he was driving apparently missed a curve and plunged down an embankment. On admission to the Emergency Department, Steven was in mild distress. He was combative and restless and had fresh blood coming from his left ear. There was crusted blood in both nares and marked bilateral ecchymosis and edema. He was easy to arouse, used loud and abusive language, and although oriented, he seemed to have little recall of circumstances surrounding the accident.

Steven's vital signs were as follows: BP 100/64, heart rate 120, and respiratory rate 20/min. His CBC and serum electrolytes were within normal limits. His skull x-rays demonstrated pneumocephalus, with air outlining the pituitary stalk and inferior hypothalamus, and a linear skull fracture in the left temporal region. The remainder of the physical examination was unremarkable. Following initial assessment and stabilization in the Emergency Department, Steven was admitted to the Neurosurgical ICU for further care and observation.

Steven's urine output during the first 5 hr in the Neurosurgical ICU was as follows:

9:00 AM	100 ml
10:00 AM	110 ml
11:00 AM	180 ml
12:00 PM	260 ml
1:00 PM	560 ml

At 1:30 PM the urine osmolality was measured and found to be 180 mOsm/kg, and the specific gravity was 1.006. Aqueous vasopressin (Pitressin), 10 units, was given SC at 3:00 PM. Steven's urine osmolality and volume measured q 15 min over the next 2 hr was as follows:

3:15	150 ml	185 mOsm/kg
3:30	130 ml	240 mOsm/kg
3:45	90 ml	290 mOsm/kg
4:00	60 ml	330 mOsm/kg
4:15	55 ml	360 mOsm/kg
4:30	40 ml	390 mOsm/kg
4:45	30 ml	420 mOsm/kg
5:00	25 ml	530 mOsm/kg
5:15	20 ml	605 mOsm/kg

The diagnosis of neurogenic DI was made, and aqueous vasopressin, 10 units SC was continued q 6 hr for the next 5 days. After 5 days, his urine output averaged 60 ml/hr and his urine osmolality was 350 mOsm/kg.

On the eighth day of hospitalization, Steven complained of a severe occipital headache. He also demonstrated nuchal rigidity and a fever of 101.2°F. A lumbar puncture was performed and showed an opening pressure of 110 cm H_2O. The cerebrospinal fluid was cloudy and contained a Gram-negative rod later identified as *Escherichia coli*. Steven was diagnosed with meningitis, and intravenous chloramphenicol, gentamicin, and ampicillin were started.

Two days later, Steven complained of severe thirst and demonstrated polydipsia and polyuria. His urine osmolality was 160 mOsm/kg. He was administered exogenous antidiuretic hormone (ADH) (aqueous vasopressin) and once again he responded promptly with a decrease in urine output and an increase in urine osmolality. Subsequently, nasal 1-desamino-8-D-arginine vasopressin (DDAVP) was given and urinary output and thirst decreased. Throughout his ICU stay Steven was managed with intranasal DDAVP 0.05 ml q day.

QUESTIONS AND ANSWERS

1. Define DI.

DI is a condition in which excessive urination of dilute urine and excessive thirst occur and persist. In most instances it results from an inability to concentrate urine, caused by a deficiency in the synthesis or release of ADH from the posterior pituitary gland (neurogenic) or a decrease in kidney responsiveness to ADH (nephrogenic). In both types, water reabsorption by the renal tubules is decreased, resulting in a profound diuresis of a dilute urine.

2. What factors contributed to the development of Steven's DI?

Severe head trauma with documented disruption of the pituitary stalk and hypothalamus
Acute bacterial meningitis

The etiology of diabetes insipidus (Table 38.1) can be addressed under two major categories, including neurogenic causes and nephrogenic causes. Neurogenic causes are related to decreased secretion of ADH from the posterior pituitary, while nephrogenic causes are due to decreased renal responsiveness to ADH. In addition to the two major categories, DI may result from psychogenic or pharmacologic causes.

Table 38.1. Etiology of DI

Neurogenic	Nephrogenic	Pharmacologic Induced	Psychogenic
Brain trauma Neurosurgery (especially in hypothalamic- pituitary area) Tumors involving th'hypothalamic- pituitary area Meningitis Encephalitis Cerebral aneurysms Familial, idiopathic Radiotherapeutic ablation of the pituitary	Inability of kidney to respond to ADH	Drugs affecting secretion of ADH from the posterior pituitary: phenytoin Drugs affecting renal responsiveness to ADH: lithium, demeclocycline	Compulsive water drinking

3. **What are the typical clinical symptoms of DI?**

   DI typically manifests as polydipsia, polyuria (5–40 liters/day), and severe thirst. If left untreated, DI can lead to hypovolemia, resulting in hypotension and decreased cerebral perfusion. The serum osmolality and serum sodium will increase, producing neurologic symptoms such as confusion, irritability, and seizures.

4. **What laboratory tests can be used to diagnosis DI in a critically ill patient? What are the results consistent with a diagnosis of DI?**

   > Urine osmolality <200 mOsm/kg
   > Urine specific gravity <1.007
   > Serum osmolality >300 mOsm/kg
   > Serum sodium >147 mEq/liter
   > Decreased plasma ADH

5. **What is a vasopressin test? How can aqueous vasopressin be used to differentiate neurogenic from nephrogenic DI?**

   A vasopressin test involves administration of aqueous vasopressin SC followed by measurements of urine osmolality and volume q 15 min for 2 hr.

   Administration of aqueous vasopressin will cause a decrease in urine output and increase in urine osmolality in the case of neurogenic DI. This is because the exogenous ADH (Pitressin) acts on the kidney to effect water conservation.

Administration of exogenous vasopressin will not decrease urine output or increase urine osmolality in the case of nephrogenic DI. The kidney is not responsive to ADH, so administration of exogenous ADH will have no effect. The urine osmolality will remain <200 mOsm/kg in nephrogenic DI. In Steven's case, the initial dose of aqueous Pitressin increased his urine osmolality to 605 mOsm/kg. This confirmed the neurogenic etiology of Steven's DI.

6. What is a water deprivation test?

A water deprivation test involves preliminary measurements of weight, serum and urine osmolality, and urine specific gravity. Water deprivation is generally carried out for a 16-hr period during which fluid intake is prohibited. The above parameters are measured and recorded. Next, 5 units of vasopressin are administered SC and a final urine collection is obtained 1–2 hr later.

A negative water deprivation test (ruling out DI) would be evidenced by:

Urine specific gravity >1.020
Urine osmolality >800 mOsm/kg

A positive water deprivation test would be evidenced by:

Loss of 3–5% body weight
Urine specific gravity not increasing for 3 hr after water deprivation is completed

The water deprivation test is not usually done on critically ill patients, as it may result in hypernatremia, severe dehydration, and hypovolemic shock. It is appropriately used in the stable patient outside of the ICU in whom DI is suspected.

7. What does the medical management of DI usually involve?

Rehydration with hypotonic IV fluids to replace free water lost in the dilute urine. Fluid replacement is rapid until normovolemia is restored, and then it is based on the urine output.
Exogenous vasopressin (Pitressin) administration (Table 38.2)
Chlorpropamide stimulates ADH release and kidney responsiveness to ADH in nephrogenic DI.
Thiazide diuretics combined with sodium restriction enhance water reabsorption in nephrogenic DI.

8. What are the potential side effects of exogenous vasopressin (Pitressin)?

Potential side effects of vasopressin include angina, MI, abdominal or uterine cramping, increased peristalsis, and water intoxication.

Table 38.2. Exogenous vasopressin preparations for treatment of DI

Agent	Dose	Route	Duration	Indications/Usage
			hr	
Aqueous vasopressin	5–10 units	SC, IM	3–6	Severe DI in unconscious or conscious patients Diagnostic testing Acute management post-trauma or surgery
Vasopressin tannate in oil	2.5–5 units	IM	24–72	Long-term management Failure to respond is due to faulty mixing or injection techniques Side effects include smooth muscle contraction, angina, abdominal cramps
Lypressin	5–10 units	Nasal spray	3–8	Severe transient or permanent DI Short acting Generally nonirritating
Desmopressin (DDAVP) acetate	5–20 μg	Nasal spray, SC, IV	12–24	Severe transient or permanent DI

The physician should be notified promptly if the patient experiences chest pain. Nitroglycerin may be ordered.

The serum sodium should be monitored so that water intoxication will be detected early. Symptoms of water intoxication may include altered level of consciousness, headache, nausea, and seizures.

9. **It is not uncommon for patients sustaining head injury to have concomitant facial trauma. How would DDAVP be administered to patients having injuries to the nose that would prevent intranasal administration?**

   DDAVP can be administered subcutaneously or intravenously; however, the duration of action differs with each route.

10. **Which is more common, permanent or transient DI?**

    Transient DI is more common. It generally occurs during the first few days following surgery and is usually a result of edema to the hypothalamus and/or neurohypophysis. The duration of transient DI varies from several days to weeks. Permanent (chronic) DI occurs when the supraoptic nuclei in the hypothalamus and the proximal end of the pituitary stalk are destroyed.

11. An important nursing diagnosis in Steven's case was actual or potential fluid volume deficit due to excessive urinary water loss. What nursing actions are important in relation to this diagnosis?

> Record accurate I & O.
>
> Maintain adequate hydration. In unconscious or intubated patients, it is customary to administer 1 ml of hypotonic IV fluid/ml of urine output.
>
> Weigh patient daily.
>
> Monitor for signs of dehydration, including poor skin turgor, dry mucous membranes, tachycardia, and BP, CVP, or PAWP below baseline.
>
> Monitor laboratory studies including serum sodium, serum and urine osmolality, and urine specific gravity. Report abnormalities to physician.

12. What other nursing diagnoses are relevant to Steven's DI problems?

> Knowledge deficit related to diabetes insipidus
>
> Sleep pattern disturbance related to polyuria and nocturia
>
> Altered patterns of urinary elimination, increased, related to insufficient ADH
>
> Diarrhea related to the inward flux of body water into the gastrointestinal tract

SUGGESTED READINGS

Colbassani H Jr, Barrow D. Fluid and electrolyte disorders. Contemp Neurosurg 1987;9,10:1–4.

Gotch P. The endocrine system. In: Alspach JG, Williams SM. Core curriculum for critical care nurses. 3rd ed. Philadelphia: WB Saunders, 1985:468–476.

McGinnis G. Central nervous system I: head injuries. In: Cardona V, Hurn P, Mason P, Scanlon-Schilpp A, Veise-Berry S. Trauma nursing from resuscitation through rehabilitation. Philadelphia: WB Saunders, 1988:407–408.

Ricci M, ed. Core curriculum for neuroscience nursing. Park Ridge, IL: American Association of Neuroscience Nurses. 1984:446–448.

Sanford S. Endocrine patient-care problems. In: Kinney MR, Packa DR, Dunbar SB. AACN's clinical reference for critical care nursing. New York: McGraw-Hill, 1988:1089–1092.

Swearingen PL, Sommers MS, Miller K. Manual of critical care applying nursing diagnoses to adult critical illness. St. Louis: CV Mosby, 1988.

CHAPTER 39

Diabetic Ketoacidosis

Terry L. Jones, RN, BSN, CCRN

Roberto Enrico is a 37-year-old known insulin-dependent diabetic who was found stuporous but responsive to vigorous shaking in his home by a neighbor. He was immediately transported to the Emergency Department of the nearest hospital. The initial assessment revealed warm, dry, flushed skin, poor skin turgor, rapid, deep respirations, and a fruity odor to his breath. A diabetic alert bracelet was present, prompting the nurse to perform a bedside serum glucose determination. The reading exceeded the upper limits of the dextrometer. The nurse notified the physician immediately and started a peripheral IV of NS to run at a wide open bolus rate. Further assessment and laboratory data revealed the following:

ABGs (Room Air)		Electrolyte Panel		CBC	
pH	7.0	Na	124	Hgb	12
$PaCO_2$	17	K	6.2	Hct	36
PaO_2	90	Cl	92	WBC	24
SaO_2	94%	CO_2	6	Plat	358
HCO_3	4	Gluc	704		
		Creat	1.9		

Vital Signs		Other
BP	80/40	+ Serum ketones to 1 : 16 dilution
HR	118	+ Urine ketones
Resp	24	Anion gap 26
Temp	37°C	Lungs clear to auscultation

A diagnosis of diabetic ketoacidosis (DKA) was made. Two sets of blood cultures were obtained, as were urine and sputum cultures. The IV of NS continued to infuse at a wide open rate. Serum glucose determinations and electrolyte panels were ordered every hour, with ABGs q 2 hr. The laboratory results are given in Table 39.1.

QUESTIONS AND ANSWERS

1. **Which type of diabetes is most frequently the cause of DKA?**
    Type I insulin dependent.

Table 39.1. Flow sheet—diabetic coma

Date and Hour	Blood Chemistries								Acetone						Urine			Insulin	Parenteral Intake		
	Bun	Creat.	Na	K	CO$_2$	Cl	Gluc.	D-Stix	Undil	1:1	1:2	1:4	1:8	1:16	Vol.	Sugar	Acet.	Type/Amount/Time	Type/Amount		
																			NS	D$_5$½NS	KCl
9/1/88 3:15 PM		1.9	124	6.2	6	92	704	1+	++	++	+	+	+	Tr[a]	500	+++	Lg[b]	Regular 50 units IV push	1000		
4:15		2.0	127	4.5	8	87	625	1+							500			Regular 50 units IV push	1000		40 mEq KCl
5:15		2.0	129	3.7	7	92	538	1+							250			Regular 50 units IV push	200		40 mEq KPO$_4$
6:15		1.9	131	3.2	9	93	387	371							205			Regular 50 units IV push	200		40 mEq KPO$_4$
7:15		1.8	131	2.9	9	95	300	294							205			Regular 50 units IV push		200	40 mEq KCl
8:15		1.8	135	2.8	17	100	284	270							190			Regular 25 units IV push		200	40 mEq KPO$_4$
9:15		1.6	131	3.1	19	97	235	227							110			Regular 12 units SC		200	40 mEq KCl

[a] Tr, trace.
[b] Lg, large.

353

2. **DKA develops as a result of the combined effects of a relative or absolute insulin deficiency and a relative or absolute increase in glucagon concentration. Through what mechanism does insulin deficiency contribute to the clinical presentation of the patient with DKA?**

   Insulin plays a vital role in the metabolism of the three basic nutritional substrates, including carbohydrate, protein, and fat. Whenever there is a lack of insulin, whether absolute, as in the case of untreated Type I diabetes, or relative, as in situations of increased insulin demand such as infection, the normal pathways for metabolism of these substrates are disrupted. Without adequate insulin, glucose cannot be transported across the cell membrane for use in normal metabolic processes. Consequently, serum glucose levels rise and a state of hyperglycemia develops.

   When the serum glucose level exceeds the renal threshold, glucose is lost via the tubules into the urine. This creates an increase in osmolarity in the renal tubules and an osmotic diuresis ensues. As a result, water and electrolyte depletion develops.

   Even though serum glucose levels are elevated, the inability of the cells to use glucose results in cellular starvation. This stimulates the body's homeostatic mechanisms to increase gluconeogenesis, which is the production of glucose from other sources. Consequently, the protein in muscle tissue is catabolized and amino acids are liberated. Amino acids are transformed into glucose, causing the serum glucose to rise even further. In addition, adipose tissue is catabolized, freeing the gluconeogenic precursor glycerol. This further compounds the hyperglycemia. It is not uncommon for patients in DKA to present with serum glucose levels of 300–800 mg/dl (Table 39.2).

3. **Through what mechanism does the concentration of glucagon contribute to the clinical presentation of a patient with DKA?**

   When cells are deprived of glucose, homeostatic mechanisms cause an increase in glucagon release from the pancreas. Catecholamines released during the stress response cause a similar increase in glucagon release. Glucagon facilitates gluconeogenesis, thus contributing to the hyperglycemia. Osmotic diuresis, volume and electrolyte depletion, and dehydration follow.

   An additional effect of glucagon involves activation of the ketogenic process, which is responsible for the metabolic acidosis characteristic of DKA. When adipose tissue is broken down into glycerol and free fatty acids, glucagon causes oxidation of the fatty acids and ketone formation. The ketones bind with available buffers, deplete the body's buffer systems, and produce a metabolic acidosis.

Table 39.2. Pathophysiologic alterations responsible for the clinical presentation of DKA

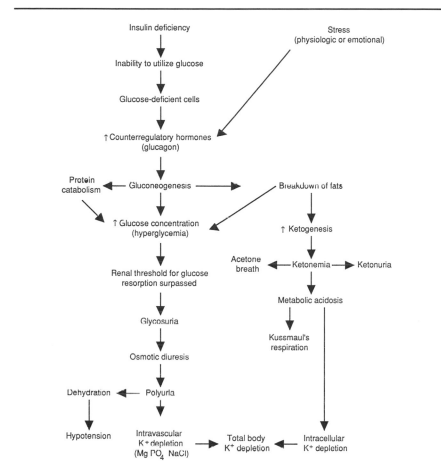

4. **What classic signs of DKA were evident in Mr. Enrico's presentation?**

Hyperglycemia
Ketonemia
Ketonuria
Kussmaul's respirations
Acetone breath
Dehydration
Metabolic acidosis

5. **In addition to Kussmaul's respirations, the nurse documented a fruity odor to Mr. Enrico's breath. Why does this occur in DKA?**

    Exhalation of the acetone formed during the ketogenic process causes a characteristic sweet or fruity odor.

6. **How does the body attempt to compensate for the metabolic acidosis?**

    In response to a fall in serum pH below about 7.2, the respiratory center in the brain is stimulated. The result is an increase in depth and rate of respiration for the purpose of eliminating CO_2 (an acid) and thus raising the pH. This characteristic rapid, deep respiratory pattern is termed Kussmaul's respirations.

7. **Upon identification of a metabolic acidosis, the nurse calculated an anion gap and found it to be 26. How is an anion gap calculated? What is the significance of the anion gap in DKA?**

    Normally, there are approximately the same number of measured anions (negative ions) as cations (positive ions) circulating in the blood. The primary anions are Cl and CO_2, whereas the primary cation is Na. If the Cl and CO_2 are added together and subtracted from Na, the difference should be a number no higher than 15. The slight difference in measured cations and anions is due to the presence of small quantities of such normal unmeasured anions as albumin, phosphate, and sulfate.

    For example:

    Na   138
    Cl   100
    CO_2 25
    138 − (100 + 25) = 13 (normal anion gap)

    On the other hand, if a number higher than 15 is obtained when the sum of Cl and CO_2 is subtracted from Na, an abnormal anion gap exists. This indicates that the number of measured circulating anions is less than the number of measured circulating cations. An anion gap indicates a metabolic acidosis.

    In DKA, the number of unmeasured anions (ketones) increases, while the number of measured anions (CO_2 and Cl) decreases. Therefore, because there is a decrease in measured anions, the difference between measured cations and anions will be greater than 15, and an increased anion gap exists.

For example:

Na   130
Cl   94
CO_2 8
$130 - (94 + 8) = 28$ (abnormal anion gap)

The anion gap is a useful parameter in monitoring insulin therapy in DKA. As glucose metabolism is restored toward normal and ketogenesis is reversed, the number of unmeasured anions (ketones) will decrease. The number of measured anions (CO_2 and Cl) will increase, the difference between measured cations and anions will decrease, and the gap will close.

8. **Despite having a pH of 7.0, Mr. Enrico was not treated with sodium bicarbonate. Why not?**

Recall the effect of 2,3-DPG and pH on the oxyhemoglobin dissociaton curve. As a result of the alternate metabolic pathways occurring in DKA, there is a decrease in 2,3-DPG. A decrease in 2,3-DPG usually causes the oxyhemoglobin dissociaton curve to shift to the left, thus increasing the affinity of hemoglobin for oxygen and potentially impairing the dissociation of oxygen from hemoglobin at the tissue level. However, the drop in pH that occurs during DKA shifts the curve to the right, thus decreasing the affinity of hemoglobin for oxygen. Shifts in opposite directions in effect counteract each other, thus preventing a significant shift in either direction. If sodium bicarbonate is administered, the pH will suddenly increase, causing the curve to shift to the left, potentially impairing oxygen release at the tissue level. Administration of sodium bicarbonate should be reserved for those instances when the pH is <6.9–7.0.

9. **What are the three main components of therapy in DKA?**

> Insulin
> Electrolyte replacement
> Fluid replacement

10. **Insulin therapy is considered the cornerstone of treatment for DKA. What is the preferred route and type of insulin for treatment of DKA in its initial stages?**

In the initial stages of DKA, it is imperative that a rapid-acting insulin be used so that reversal of the ketogenic process may begin as soon as possible. Regular insulin is therefore the insulin of choice and the recommended route is intravenous. Regular insulin is the only type of insulin that can be given intravenously. However, the potency of regular insulin may be reduced by 20–80% when administered through plastic IV tubing. Consequently, when giving it IV push, it should be given in the injection port as close to the IV insertion site as possible. Onset of action is immediate, with its peak effect occurring in 30–60 min. This allows for a relatively controlled manipulation of the blood glucose level. In fact, when this route is used, the glucose level will fall at a predictable rate of 75–100 mg/dl/ hr. When given via the subcutaneous route, its onset of action is much slower and its absorption may be delayed because of volume depletion and poor tissue perfusion. The subcutaneous route is therefore undesirable for the initial treatment of DKA.

11. **Mr. Enrico's blood glucose on admission was 704 mg/dl. He was immediately given 50 units of regular insulin IV push. Is this unusual?**

    There are two opinions regarding dosage and frequency of insulin administration in DKA. While some clinicians advocate a loading dose of 10–30 units IV push followed by a continuous low dose infusion of 2–12 units/hr, others support the high dose IV push approach. If the continuous infusion is to be used, care must be taken to minimize alterations in potency resulting from administration techniques. Insulin drips should be mixed in glass bottles and delivered via special IV tubing such as that used for IV nitroglycerin. If such tubing is not available, some of the drug will be absorbed by the tubing, necessitating increasing the infusion rate and careful blood glucose monitoring until the desired effect is obtained.

    The high dose approach, which was used for Mr. Enrico, involves administering 25–50 units of regular insulin IV push q 1–2 hr until the anion gap is closed. Clinicians who advocate this approach believe that some patients present with a degree of insulin resistance. For these patients, high dose insulin has the advantage of ensuring saturation of the insulin receptors despite the presence of competing antibodies.

    Regardless of the approach used, frequent close blood glucose monitoring is essential to prevent hypoglycemia. It is recommended that electrolyte panels and bedside serum glucose determinations be checked q 1–2 hr until the anion gap is closed. Placement of a heparin lock is suggested to prevent the unnecessary discomfort of frequent venipuncture.

12. **Through what mechanism does insulin affect the anion gap?**

    Insulin acts to facilitate transport of glucose across the cell membrane into the cell, where it can be used in various metabolic processes. Once this occurs, the body is no longer stimulated to produce glucose from other sources and thus gluconeogenesis decreases. As fat metabolism ceases and ketones are no longer produced, the number of unmeasured anions drops, closing the gap between measured cations and measured anions.

Mr. Enrico required 50 units of regular insulin every hour for 5 hr based on his response to therapy. After 2 hr of treatment, KCl, 40 mEq, was added to each liter of IV fluid. Refer to Table 39.1 for his response to these therapeutic interventions.

13. Notice that although Mr. Enrico's serum potassium was initially 6.2 mEq/liter, it dropped rapidly after treatment was started. What is the physiologic basis for the rapidly decreasing potassium?

Metabolic acidosis causes potassium ions to move from the cells into the serum. Although the serum K^+ level may appear normal, intracellular potassium depletion exists. When the osmotic diuresis occurs, potassium is lost in the urine. Then, with the administration of insulin, K^+ is transported into the cells along with glucose. This further decreases the serum K^+ level. It is not uncommon to see a drop in the serum K^+ during the first few hours of treatment for DKA. For this reason, it is important to monitor the serum K^+ closely (every 1–2 hr until the gap is closed and subcutaneous insulin is used). Potassium replacement should begin as soon as the K^+ level approaches the normal value.

14. How should K^+ be replaced in the patient with DKA?

Because of the total body K^+ depletion described above, it is not uncommon to give as much as 200–300 mEq of K^+ within the first 12 hr of therapy for DKA. As soon as the serum K^+ is <5 mEq/liter, 20–40 mEq of K^+ should be added to each liter of IV fluid. This can be in the form of KCl or KPO_4, depending on the patient's serum phosphorus level. As the IV infusion rate is decreased, it may be necessary to cautiously administer supplemental IV piggyback doses of KCl.

15. What causes phosphorus depletion in DKA?

Phosphorus is lost in the urine as a result of the osmotic diuresis. In addition, phosphorus is required for the chemical reaction completing glucose metabolism. Therefore, as insulin is given and glucose metabolism is restored, the serum phosphorus will drop even further.

Phosphorus is required for the production of 2,3-DPG; a low serum phosphorus will decrease the amount of available 2,3-DPG, thus shifting the oxyhemoglobin dissociation curve to the left. If the hypophosphatemia is not corrected, once the acidosis is corrected and the curve moves back in a leftward direction, oxyhemoglobin dissociation may be impaired and cellular oxygen deprivation may result.

The normal serum phosphorus is 2.7–4.5 mg/dl. Serum phosphorus levels must be monitored and replacement therapy instituted as necessary.

16. **Mr. Enrico presented with dry, flushed skin, poor skin turgor, tachycardia, and hypotension. These signs indicated volume depletion, which resulted from the osmotic diuresis. What is the IV fluid of choice for fluid resuscitation of a patient with DKA?**

    Patients in DKA typically present with a fluid loss of 3–5 liters. However, it is not uncommon to administer 10 liters of IV fluids within the first 12 hr of therapy. Since Na and Cl are also depleted as a result of the osmotic diuresis, the initial fluid of choice is NS. A wide open or bolus rate is indicated in most instances for the first 1–2 hr, after which the rate is titrated to maintain adequate blood pressure and urine output.

17. **Despite being hypotensive, Mr. Enrico was not started on vasopressors. Why not?**

    The hypotension associated with DKA is usually the result of severe volume depletion. Vasopressors should be reserved for those few patients who do not respond to fluid resuscitation.

18. **At 7:15 PM, Mr. Enrico's blood glucose was still 300 mg/dl, yet he was started on D$_5$½NS. Why?**

    At this point, Mr. Enrico still had an anion gap of 27 (131 − (9 + 95) = 27). This indicated that ketones were still being produced, and additional insulin was needed to restore normal glucose metabolism. Because the glucose was approaching the normal range, the risk of precipitating hypoglycemia and subsequent cerebral edema existed. Therefore, when the serum glucose reaches 250–300 mg/dl, dextrose should be added to the IV fluid (D$_5$W, D$_5$NS, D$_5$½NS, or D$_{10}$W). Additional insulin should be given until the anion gap is closed.

19. **Although urine and serum were assessed for ketones to make the diagnosis of DKA, they were not monitored as frequently as other parameters in the assessment of response to treatment. Why?**

    While measuring plasma ketones using the nitroprusside test is helpful in confirming the diagnosis of DKA, most clinicians suggest that frequent measurement thereafter is not clinically helpful. Although this particular test usually yields strongly positive results in undiluted plasma, it may not represent the full extent of the ketosis because it measures only one of the two ketones elevated in DKA. A better idea of the severity of ketosis can be obtained by measuring ketones at various dilutions of the plasma until they disappear.

However, the key parameters for assessing ketosis in DKA from a purely clinical standpoint are serum pH and the anion gap.

20. When Mr. Enrico presented to the Emergency Department, his temperature was 37°C. Even so, blood, urine, and sputum cultures were sent. Why?

Infection is second only to omission of the prescribed dose of insulin by the insulin-dependent diabetic in terms of frequency as a precipitating factor in DKA. It is therefore essential to search for infection and identify causative organisms so the appropriate treatment can be instituted.

21. The IV insulin was discontinued at 9:15 PM, and Mr. Enrico was started on subcutaneous regular insulin per sliding scale. Why was this change made?

When the anion gap is closed and the serum glucose falls below 300 mg/dl, the IV route is changed to SC. When the patient begins taking PO feedings, an intermediate insulin such as NPH may be started in an attempt to reestablish the patient's previous maintenance regimen.

22. What are some possible nursing diagnoses that apply to Mr. Enrico?

Potential for injury related to self-care deficit secondary to altered mental status

Noncompliance related to irrational belief regarding consequences of uncontrolled diabetes

Knowledge deficit related to lack of teaching regarding signs and symptoms of hyperglycemia

Altered nutrition: less than body requirements related to insufficient insulin

Fluid volume deficit related to hyperglycemia and osmotic diuresis

Potential for infection related to altered host defense mechanisms and ICU environment

SUGGESTED READINGS

Alspach J, Williams S, eds. Core curriculum for critical care nursing. 3rd ed. Philadelphia: WB Saunders, 1985.

Braunwald E, Isselbacher KJ, Petersdorf RG, Wilson JD, Martin JB, Fauci AS, eds. Harrison's principles of internal medicine. 11th ed. New York: McGraw-Hill, 1987.

Davidson M. Diabetes mellitus diagnosis and treatment. 2nd ed. New York: John Wiley & Sons, 1986.

Gahart B. Intravenous medications. 5th ed. St. Louis: CV Mosby, 1989.

Kenner C, Guzzetta C, Dossey B. Critical care nursing body mind spirit. 2nd ed. Boston: Little, Brown, 1985.

McCarthy J. The continuum of diabetic coma. AJN 1985;85(8):879–883.

Sabo CE, Michael SR. Diabetic ketoacidosis: pathophysiology nursing diagnosis and nursing interventions. Focus Crit Care 1989;16(1):21–28.

Shoemaker W, Ayres S, Grenvik A, Holbrook P, Thompson W. Textbook of critical care. 2nd ed. Philadelphia: WB Saunders, 1989.

CHAPTER 40

SIADH

Rochelle Logston Boggs, RN, MSN, CCRN, CEN

John Evans, a 28-year-old construction worker, was injured when his motorcycle slid under a pickup truck. He sustained an open skull fracture which was depressed, compound, and comminuted with extrusion of brain matter in the right frontal area. Multiple facial lacerations were present.

Following initial assessment in the Emergency Department, Mr. Evans was sent to the Operating Room where a partial right frontal lobectomy with exenteration of both frontal sinuses and a pericranial patch graft for a dural tear were performed. Right supraorbital rim and nasal antral frontal fractures were reconstructed using calvarium bone grafts. Facial and intra-oral lacerations were repaired at this time. He had multiple fractures of his right hand, which was edematous but had an intact radial pulse. Due to the extent of his neurological problems, he was admitted to the Neurosurgical ICU postoperatively.

Upon physical assessment, he was intubated and being hyperventilated. Pupils were round, equal and reacted sluggishly to light. He responded to deep pain with decerebrate posturing on the left side. His Glasgow Coma Scale score was 4: eye opening 1, verbal response 1, motor response 2. A partial listing of laboratory data follows:

Na	136
K	3.3
Cl	101
Creat	0.9
Hgb	12.2
Hct	37.4
BUN	9
Serum osmolality	282

Via two peripheral antecubital IV lines, 0.45% normal saline was infusing at a rate of 100 ml/hr. Urinary output was >50 ml/hr. During the first 3 days of Mr. Evans' postoperative course, vital signs, clinical data, and neurological status remained relatively stable. However, by the 4th post-operative day, the serum sodium level had dropped from a 2-day previous level of 135 to 124 mEq/liter. The remaining laboratory data were as follows:

K	3.0	Urine	30–40 ml/hr
Cl	88	output	
Creat	0.4	Urine	1100
Hgb	13.4	osmolality	mOsm/kg

Hct	39.6	Urine specific	1.030
BUN	6	gravity	
Serum osmolality	268		

Mr. Evans' Glasgow Coma Scale score remained unchanged.

QUESTIONS AND ANSWERS

1. What is ADH?

ADH is antidiuretic hormone, also referred to as vasopressin. ADH is secreted by the posterior pituitary. It increases water reabsorption in the distal renal tubules and collecting ducts, thereby controlling the osmolality of the extracellular fluid. In pharmacologic amounts, it causes arteriolar constriction.

2. What factor normally inhibits ADH release?

Decrease in plasma osmolality.

3. What is SIADH?

SIADH occurs when there is continuous secretion of ADH in spite of abnormally low serum osmolality or when extracellular fluid volume is normal or expanded. Under these conditions, the neurons of the hypothalamus would normally inhibit the synthesis of ADH in the supraoptic nuclei. However, in SIADH, secretion of ADH is excessive, causing inappropriate water retention by the kidney and a resultant hyponatremia in the extracellular fluid.

4. What feedback mechanisms are responsible for communicating abnormal plasma volume or osmolality values to the posterior pituitary?

Osmoreceptors of the hypothalamus sense changes in plasma osmolality. When the plasma is hypoosmolar, the osmoreceptors inhibit the release of ADH. However, when the plasma is hyperosmolar, the osmoreceptors stimulate the release of ADH. Baroreceptors of the carotid and aortic bodies respond to changes in blood pressure. When blood pressure is low, baroreceptors stimulate the secretion of ADH. ADH secretion increases blood volume and constricts peripheral arterioles in order to increase blood pressure. Stretch receptors of the atria and pulmonary arteries respond to changes in blood volume. During a hypovolemic state, ADH is stimulated by the vagal-hypothalamic-hypophyseal pathway. ADH increases the reabsorption of water in the distal tubules and thus increases circulating blood volume. When pain, fear, and major trauma are experienced, the limbic system communicates these stress responses to the hypothalamus, which influences the release of ADH.

5. **Which circumstances surrounding Mr. Evans' case would most likely precipitate SIADH?**

   Cerebral trauma, cranial surgery, general anesthesia, ventilator support, supine positioning.

   A multitude of factors can precipitate SIADH. The most common ones involve central hypersecretion of ADH, which may be induced by: trauma, surgery, vascular lesions, subarachnoid hemorrhage, cerebral infarctions, subdural hematomas, brain tumors, metabolic encephalopathy, and infections such as meningitis, Guillain-Barré syndrome, and encephalitis.

   Pharmacologic agents can precipitate the occurrence of SIADH by increasing the secretion of ADH or potentiating its action. Such agents include:

   > Analgesic agents (morphine, meperidine, acetaminophen)
   > Barbiturates
   > General anesthetics
   > Antineoplastic agents (vincristine, cyclophosphamide)
   > Anticonvulsants (carbamazepine)
   > Psychotropic agents (thorazine)
   > Antilipidemic agents (clofibrate)
   > β-Blocking agents
   > Nicotine
   > Thiazide diuretics
   > Tricyclic antidepressants

   A variety of nonhypothalamic conditions can trigger an excessive production of a chemical substance similar or identical to ADH, resulting in SIADH. These conditions include: carcinomas of the lung, pancreas, gastrointestinal tract, prostate, and lymphoid tissue, and infectious processes due to lung abscesses, pneumonitis, and tuberculosis.

   Recumbant positioning and positive pressure ventilation may also precipitate SIADH.

   With the multiplicity of precipitating factors, it is understandable why patients in the critical care setting are at an increased risk of developing SIADH.

6. **SIADH has often been referred to as cerebral salt wasting. Is cerebral salt wasting a component of SIADH?**

   No. Cerebral salt wasting is a separate syndrome. In 1981, Nelson and coworkers described a population of neurosurgical patients that clinically presented similar symptomatology and laboratory findings as patients diagnosed with SIADH (1). Differentiating findings included decreases in red blood cell mass, plasma volume, and total blood volume along with failure to respond to water restriction. It was concluded that these disorders could have resulted from an unidentified natriuretic influence of the brain, which negatively affected the kidneys' ability to conserve sodium. This picture accurately describes "cerebral salt wasting."

7. **When the critical care nurse assessed Mr. Evans, what signs and symptoms did the patient manifest that would indicate SIADH?**

   Mr. Evans was at risk for the development of SIADH because of the injuries he sustained. However, his only clinical symptoms were coma and sluggish deep tendon reflexes. The signs and symptoms associated with SIADH are directly related to the degree of hyponatremia and the rapidity with which it develops. Nonspecific symptoms include fatigue, headache, restlessness, muscle cramps, abdominal cramps, personality changes, sluggish deep tendon reflexes, lethargy, anorexia, nausea/vomiting, diarrhea, confusion, and irritability. These generally occur with a slow drop in serum sodium. Stupor, coma, seizures, and death are more often associated with a rapid decline in serum sodium, especially with serum levels below 120 mEq/liter.

8. **Which diagnostic studies are useful in diagnosing SIADH?**

   Urine specific gravity, urine osmolality, serum sodium, and serum osmolality. The following chart compares normal laboratory values to those typical of SIADH.

Laboratory Parameters	Normal Value	SIADH
Urine specific gravity	1.002–1.030	>1.010
Urine osmolality	50–1400 mOsm/kg	>900 mOsm/kg
Serum osmolality	275–295 mOsm/kg	<275 mOsm/kg
Serum sodium	136–146 mEq/liter	<130 mEq/liter
K	3.5–5.1 mEq/liter	Normal
BUN	7–18 mg/dl	Normal
Creat	0.6–1.2 mg/dl	Normal

9. **What types of drugs are used in the treatment of SIADH?**

   Demeclocycline in doses of 600–1200 mg/day is used to inhibit the action of ADH at the renal tubular level. Lithium carbonate also inhibits the action of ADH at the renal tubular level. However, it is not widely used due to its renal toxic effects.

10. **Can PAWP be used as an indirect method to accurately measure the expanding fluid volume?**

    No. The increase in extracellular fluid volume occurs in the interstitial as well as the intravascular space. The PAWP reflects only intravascular volume. There is no accurate bedside method presently available to accurately measure the total expanding extracellular fluid volume.

11. **Is water restriction the best possible way to manage hyponatremia?**

    Yes, generally. However, this usually presents a challenge to the nursing staff, as the patient has a strong urge to drink. The persistent water intake together with excessive ADH lead to excessive body water and dilutional hyponatremia.

12. **What nursing interventions are helpful in limiting fluid intake in patients with SIADH?**

    > Meticulous recording of intake and output
    > Keeping water pitchers away from the bedside
    > Placing a sign at the bedside to communicate fluid restriction
    > Communication and education of the patient and family as to the rationale for fluid restriction

13. **Initially Mr. Evans exhibited a dilutional hyponatremia. Should salt replacement occur with this finding?**

    Not generally. The severity of stress or injury as well as the metabolic and hormonal response determine the degree and duration of posttraumatic sodium retention. During this 2–5-day period, serum sodium retention is not necessarily reflected in serum sodium values. Those values may inaccurately reflect a mild dilutional hyponatremia. Therefore, salt replacement is not indicated unless serum sodium levels drop below 125 mEq/liter, particularly if the patient becomes symptomatic. Serial monitoring of the serum sodium level is indicated.

14. **What types of intravenous fluids are likely to be ordered?**

    A 3% saline solution, which includes equal proportions of sodium and chloride, 513 mEq/liter, is indicated for patients presenting the more severe neurological symptoms. Forced diureseis with Lasix, 20–40 mg, is indicated during severe symptoms in order to eliminate free water and correct the hyponatremia. The maintenance fluid of choice is 0.9% saline solution, or in some instances 0.45% saline solution.

The use of hypotonic dextrose type solutions in the presence of cerebral injury can initiate or exacerbate cerebral edema and should not be used.

15. What nursing interventions should be used with caution in patients with SIADH?

Patients with decreased serum osmolality should avoid those therapies that further dilute body fluids, including tap water enemas and irrigation of nasogastric tubes with water.

16. What nursing diagnoses are pertinent to the patient with SIADH?

Fluid volume overload related to water intoxication Anxiety response related to inability to control thirst drive Impaired physical mobility related to depressed level of consciousness

REFERENCE

1. Nelson P, Seif S, Maroon J, Robinson A. Hyponatremia in intracranial disease: perhaps not the syndrome of inappropri- ate secretion of antidiuretic hormone (SIADH). J Neurosurg 1981;55:938.

SUGGESTED READINGS

Gotch P. The endocrine system. In: Alspach J, Williams S, eds. Core curriculum for critical care nursing. 3rd ed. Philadelphia: WB Saunders, 1985:471–474.

Guyton A. Textbook of medical physiology. 7th ed. Philadelphia: WB Saunders, 1986.

Johndrow P, Thornton, S. Syndrome of inappropriate antidiuretic hormone a growing concern. Focus on Crit Care. 1985:12(5): 29–34.

Part VI

Gastrointestinal System

CHAPTER 41

Abdominal Trauma

Kimmith M. Jones, RN, BS, CCRN

Harry Henderson is a 28-year-old man who was driving while intoxicated, fell asleep at the wheel, and was involved in a one-car accident. He was not wearing a seat belt and was thrown forward, forcing the steering wheel into his chest and abdomen.

Upon arrival in the Emergency Department, Mr. Henderson was awake and oriented × 3 but slightly combative. There was a 2-cm scalp laceration over his left frontal area. His pupils were equal and reactive at 5 mm. His BP was 90/56, heart rate 126, and respirations 24 and shallow. He had abrasions over his left lower rib cage and abdomen, and his breath sounds were diminished on the left. There was hyperresonance to percussion on the left side, and Mr. Henderson stated that it hurt to breathe. Sub-cutaneous emphysema was present from the left nipple line to the left upper abdominal quadrant. His abdomen was round and firm, with no audible bowel sounds. He was uncooperative during the abdominal examination, thrashing around on the stretcher. He complained of left shoulder pain while lying flat. Relevant laboratory data included:

ABGs		CBC		Electrolytes		Urinalysis
pH	7.30	Hct	39	Na	138	WNL
$PaCO_2$	50	Hgb	14	K	4.0	
PaO_2	76	WBC	13,000	Cl	100	
SaO_2	92%	RBC	4.4	CO_2	24	
HCO_3	24	Plat	350,000	Creat	0.7	

The following treatments were performed:

1. A left chest tube was placed. Upon insertion, a large gush of air was heard. Breath sounds following insertion were audible bilaterally with equal chest excursion.
2. 40% O_2 was administered via face mask.
3. A 16-gauge intravenous catheter was inserted in the right antecubital area, and an infusion of 1000 ml of Ringer's lactate (RL) was begun.
4. An orogastric tube was inserted. The contents tested negative for blood. An orogastric tube is the route of choice when a basal skull

fracture or cribriform plate fracture may be present. This route decreases the chance of an intracranial intubation and the development of sinusitis.
5. A Foley catheter was inserted. The urine was negative for blood.
6. A peritoneal lavage was performed, and the following results were obtained from the peritoneal fluid:

RBC	114,000 cells/mm^3
WBC	524 cells/mm^3
Amylase	30 U/liter
Bacteria	Absent
Bile	Absent
Feces	Absent

A chest x-ray revealed fractures of ribs 5–10 on the left and a well-inflated left lung with the chest tube in place.

Mr. Henderson remained hypotensive after rapid infusion of 2 liters of RL, so he was taken to the Operating Room where he was found to have a ruptured spleen. A splenectomy was performed, and he was brought to the Surgical ICU.

Upon admission to the unit, Mr. Henderson's vital signs and ventilator settings were:

BP	92/56	Mode	Assist control
HR	128	Rate	14
Resp	14	FIO$_2$	0.40
Temp	36.2°C	Tidal volume	900 ml

He had a pulmonary artery catheter in place with the following hemodynamic parameters:

CVP	1
PAP	18/3
PAWP	3
CO	3.4
SVR	1576

After 2 units of whole blood and 1000 ml of RL were administered, these parameters stabilized into their normal ranges.

QUESTIONS AND ANSWERS

1. **What are the two mechanisms of injury involved in abdominal trauma?**

    Blunt Trauma. Blunt trauma most often causes injuries to solid organs. The mechanisms surrounding blunt trauma include crushing, shearing, and burst forces. Death occurs most frequently with blunt trauma because of delays in diagnosis. Severe blunt injuries can be

masked by less severe but more obvious injuries or wounds. Injuries
from blunt trauma usually involve more than one body system. For
example, along with a GI problem, a patient who has sustained blunt
trauma may have a neurological injury, cardiac contusion, pneumothorax, or fractures.

Penetrating Trauma. Injuries resulting from penetrating trauma
usually do not have multisystem involvement and are most often
caused by stabbings, gunshot wounds, or impalement.

2. **Which organs sustain injury most often during blunt abdominal
   trauma?**

   Spleen
   Liver
   Small intestine
   Kidneys
   Bladder

3. **Which organs are most often injured with penetrating trauma?**

   Small intestine
   Liver

4. **What diagnostic procedure is commonly used to determine intraperitoneal trauma?**
   Peritoneal lavage is a commonly used, highly accurate procedure
   for detecting intraabdominal trauma. This diagnostic tool is mainly
   used during the resuscitative phase of patient care. It is routinely
   used when physical examination findings are questionable or when a
   patient is unable to participate in the examination. Peritoneal lavage
   is not organ specific and is not accurate in diagnosing retroperitoneal
   injuries.

5. **How is peritoneal lavage performed?**
   Before this procedure is begun, a Foley catheter and a gastric tube
   must be in place. This decreases the chance of accidental perforation
   of the stomach or bladder.
   Xylocaine with epinephrine is used to anesthetize the area and
   decrease the bleeding from surrounding vessels. With the open technique a midline incision is made one-third of the distance from the
   umbilicus to the symphysis pubis after the skin is prepped and
   draped. Then the linea alba is identified and incised, allowing the
   peritoneal cavity to be entered under direct vision. A peritoneal
   lavage catheter is then inserted and directed toward the pelvis. A
   syringe is then placed on the end of the catheter, and an attempt is

made to aspirate peritoneal fluid. If any nonclotting blood is retrieved, a hemoperitoneum is confirmed, and an exploratory laparotomy is required. If no blood is retrieved, 1000 ml of an isotonic solution is infused into the peritoneal cavity. For children and small adults, 10–15 ml of solution/kg of body weight is infused. The patient should then be gently rotated from side to side to distribute the fluid. He or she should be flat during this procedure to allow the fluid to reach the diaphragm. The fluid is then removed by gravity and sent to the laboratory for analysis. The catheter is removed, and the incision is sutured closed.

6. What constitutes a positive peritoneal lavage?

Although some variability exists among different institutions, the most widely accepted criteria include:

Aspiration of any nonclotting blood
Lavage fluid appears bloody
RBC count $> 100,000$ cells/mm^3
WBC count > 500 cells/mm^3
Presence of bacteria, bile, or fecal material
Amylase level $>$ serum level

7. What signs and symptoms eliminate the need for a peritoneal lavage, with the patient being transported directly to the Operating Room?

Evidence of hollow organ rupture on x-ray
Obvious abdominal wall defects
Rapidly increasing abdominal distention
Hypotension unresponsive to fluid boluses
Unquestionable positive abdominal examination on the cooperative and appropriate patient

8. What other diagnostic tests may be used when intraabdominal trauma is suspected?

Paracentesis

Paracentesis may be performed when the patient is hypotensive or unconscious, as it can be accomplished quickly and easily. Any nonclotting blood is considered a positive tap and indicates the need for an exploratory laparotomy. A negative tap is not definitive, and other procedures are needed to rule out abdominal injury.

Computed Tomography (CT Scan)

CT is a sensitive, noninvasive procedure that is currently being evaluated for its effectiveness in identifying abdominal trauma. It is most useful in diagnosing trauma to the liver, spleen, kidney, and pancreas. If it is used alone, continual reevaluation by repeat CT scan must be performed. The accuracy of CT is significantly improved with the use of IV or oral contrast media.

Radiographic Films

AP and left lateral decubitus films of the abdomen are taken and used to detect the presence of intraabdominal fluid or air and alterations in visceral contour. Evidence of enlarged or distorted organs on x-ray may indicate subcapsular hematomas or bleeding confined to an area.

An upright chest film is also taken to look for free air under the diaphragm, which signifies rupture of a hollow organ. The chest x-ray will also help identify the presence of associated chest injuries.

Damage to skeletal structures evident on x-ray should increase one's suspicion of abdominal injuries under those structures (e.g., rib fractures over the liver or spleen alert the practitioner that there may be underlying injuries to these organs).

Negative x-rays do not rule out the presence of intraabdominal injury. The amount of blood that has accumulated may not be enough to be detected by x-rays.

Serum Amylase

Serum amylase should be obtained. Elevations should raise an index of suspicion for intestinal or pancreatic injury. However, the most recent literature questions its reliability in predicting patients with or without injury.

Hemoglobin and Hematocrit

These tell little about acute blood loss. It takes 6–8 hr after the acute injury for these values to accurately reflect blood loss. Hgb and Hct are generally not used as the only guide to volume replacement because of the fluid shifts that occur following trauma.

Other Diagnostic Tests

Other laboratory tests that are obtained on abdominal trauma patients include:

Type and cross-match	PT, PTT, fibrinogen
ABG	Electrolytes
Urinalysis	Calcium
Toxicology screen	BUN, creatinine
Serial Hct and WBC	

9. **What are the signs and symptoms of peritoneal irritation?**

The symptoms of peritoneal irritation are:

Abdominal wall rigidity
Guarding
Generalized pain or tenderness
Abdominal distention and loss of bowel sounds
Rebound tenderness
Pain on movement or cough
Splinting of abdominal muscles and thoracic breathing
Unexplained shock

All of these symptoms are a result of the peritoneal membranes being irritated by bowel contents, enzymes, blood, urine, or bile.

Patients who have peritoneal irritation are most comfortable with their legs bent to decrease tension on the psoas muscle.

Signs of peritoneal irritation are:

Cullen's Sign. A bluish discoloration around the umbilicus may indicate peritoneal bleeding.

Grey Turner's Sign. Ecchymosis over the flank area is a sign of retroperitoneal bleeding.

Coopernail's Sign. Ecchymosis of the scrotum or labia indicates a pelvic fracture with hemorrhage into the perineal area.

10. What are Kehr's sign and Ballance's sign?

Kehr's Sign. When this is present, the patient complains of pain at the top of the left shoulder. The patient must be lying flat or in the Trendelenburg position to elicit this type of pain. It is caused by the irritation of the inferior surface of the diaphragm from intraperitoneal blood.

Ballance's Sign. On physical examination a fixed dullness is percussed over the left flank area with dullness in the right flank area that disappears when the patient's position is changed. This finding indicates the presence of a large quantity of clots in the perisplenic area with free blood in the remainder of the abdomen.

11. What is the medical management for injury to the spleen?

Surgery. The severity of the injury will determine the extent of the surgery. With minor splenic injuries a splenorrhaphy may be appropriate. Splenorrhaphy may consist of the application of hemostatic agents to the spleen to stop bleeding, or the débridement of necrotic tissue and suture repair, or partial splenic resection. With more severe injuries a total splenectomy may be necessary.

Splenectomy with autotransplantation is another alternative. This involves removal of the spleen followed by transplantation of a portion of the splenic tissue into a pouch made in the greater omentum. The goal is for this transplanted tissue to develop a blood supply and be effective in filtering bacteria from the blood to prevent lifelong problems with immunity. Recent research has questioned the effectiveness of this procedure. Nonoperative management of splenic injuries is advocated by many authors, especially in children.

12. What are the possible complications of abdominal trauma?

Ileus	Stress ulcers
Peritonitis	Cholycystitis
Sepsis	Abscess formation
Body image changes	Fistula formation
Hypovolemia	Pain

The potential for development of complications emphasizes the importance of continual nursing assessment for these patients.

13. Following splenectomy, what is the most life-threatening complication that may develop?

Overwhelming postsplenectomy sepsis (OPSI)—Animal studies have shown that following removal of the spleen immunological defects are present. These defects include:

Impaired ability to clear blood-borne particles
Decreased activity of alveolar macrophages against pneumococci
Decreased response of antibodies to specific antigens
An alteration in the levels of immunoglobulins
Decreased T-cell function
Decreased ability to phagocytize bacteria in conjunction with an absence of circulating tuftsin. Tuftsin stimulates the motility and phagocytic activity of polymorphonuclear leukocytes by direct action.
Decreased antibody response to intravenous immunization.

The incidence of OPSI is 0.58–0.86% in healthy patients who have had splenectomies. This is compared with an incidence of 0.01% of severe sepsis in healthy patients who still have their spleens. Eighty percent of OPSI occurs within the first 2 years after surgery but may occur up to 30 years after splenectomy.

Currently, the way to prevent this complication is with the polyvalent pneumococcal vaccine (Pneumovax 23). This vaccine, which was released in 1983, encourages immunity for 23 of the most prevalent pneumococcal bacteria. It should be given to all asplenic patients during their hospitalization. Usually this is given on the general surgical floor, due to the immunosuppressed state of patients in the intensive care units.

Asplenic patients need to be educated about their lifelong increased risk of infection and the need to inform health professionals of their splenectomy.

14. List the appropriate nursing diagnoses and nursing interventions that would pertain to Mr. Henderson.

Nursing Diagnosis.   Potential for infection related to invasive monitoring lines and presence of drainage devices

Monitor WBC and CBC differential
Monitor temperature every 2–4 hr and notify MD of increasing temperature
Assist with changing invasive lines per hospital policy
Change line dressings with sterile technique every day
Assess line insertion sites for redness, swelling, or drainage every day and notify MD of abnormal findings
Monitor and document amount and character of drainage from drainage devices every shift
Administer antibiotics as ordered
Monitor therapeutic drug levels for the antibiotics administered

Nursing Diagnosis.   Impaired gas exchange related to pneumothorax

Assess and document breath sounds every 2 hr
Monitor arterial blood gases and notify MD of abnormal results
Suction patient as indicated by nursing assessment
Hyperoxygenate prior to and following suctioning
Assess proper functioning of chest tube every 2 hr and notify MD of abnormal findings
Assess pulmonary secretions for color, consistency, and odor and notify MD of changes
Assess mechanical ventilator every 2–4 hr
Monitor peak inspiratory pressures (PIP) and notify MD of sudden rise in PIP
Assess daily chest x-ray for changes in infiltrates and reexpansion of affected lung
Perform chest physiotherapy and postural drainage every 4 hr as indicated by nursing assessment
Turn patient every 2 hr
Monitor arterial oxygen saturation via pulse oximeter and notify MD of sudden drop in saturation

Nursing Diagnosis.   Fluid volume deficit related to ruptured spleen and blood loss

Monitor vital signs every hour
Monitor intake and output every hour
Assess for signs of shock—increasing heart rate, decreasing blood pressure, decreasing skin temperature, decreasing urinary output, and change in level of conciousness
Assess abdominal girth every 4 hr and notify MD of increasing girth and firmness
Infuse IV fluids as ordered
Monitor hemoglobin and hematocrit and notify MD of decreasing trends

Monitor pulmonary artery pressures every 1–2 hr and notify MD of abnormal findings

Nursing Diagnosis. Knowledge deficit related to lifelong impact of splenectomy

Assess patient's level of understanding of splenectomy
Provide reading material for patient and family that is related to decreased immunity due to splenectomy
Encourage questions from patient and family
Arrange family conference with MD, nurse, patient, and family to answer questions and concerns

Nursing Diagnosis. Impaired verbal communication related to oral endotracheal tube

Assess patient for communication barriers such as impaired hearing, impaired sight, and foreign language
Use interpreters, picture cards, letter boards, or sign language as alternate means of communication
Explain purpose and importance of endotracheal tube to patient and family

Nursing Diagnosis. Impaired social interaction related to hospitalization

Allow visitors at scheduled visiting times
Encourage family to touch and talk to patient about events outside of hospital
Read mail to patient and allow family to read to patient
Interact with patient on an adult to adult level and encourage the same of the family
Encourage family to bring in one or two personal belongings or pictures to provide stimulation other than ICU environment

Nursing Diagnosis. Sleep pattern disturbance related to ICU environment

Assess normal sleeping pattern of patient and attempt to keep it regular
Keep lights low during sleep and "on" during wake periods
Cluster care to avoid disturbing sleep
Keep noise to a minimum during sleep
Provide privacy during sleeping periods
Attempt to maintain normal day-night schedule

SUGGESTED READINGS

Bastnagel-Mason PJ. Abdominal trauma. In: Cardona VD, Hurn PD, Mason PJ, Scanlon-Schilpp AM, Veise-Berry SW, eds. Trauma nursing from resuscitation through rehabilitation. Philadelphia: WB Saunders, 1988:491–524.

Green JB, Shackford SR, Sise MH, Fridlaund P. Late septic complications in adults following splenectomy for trauma: A prospective analysis in 144 patients. J Trauma 1986; 26(11):999–1003.

Kenner CV, Guzzetta CE, Dossey BM. Critical care nursing, Body, Mind, Spirit. 2nd ed. Boston: Little, Brown & Co, 1985.

Llende M, Santiago-Delpin EA, Lavergne J. Immunobiological consequences of splenectomy: A review. J Surg Res 1986; 40:84–85.

Moore FA, Moore EE, Moore GE, Millikan JS. Risk of splenic salvage after trauma. Analysis of 200 adults. Am J Surg 1984;148:800–805.

Schwartz SI, Shires GT, Spencer FC, Principles of surgery. 5th ed. New York: McGraw-Hill, 1989.

CHAPTER 42

Fulminant Hepatic Failure

Virginia Byrn Huddleston, RN, MSN, CCRN

Karen Holder, a 28-year-old woman, is admitted to the Emergency Department in an incoherent state. She has a 10-year history of intravenous drug abuse and was diagnosed with acute hepatitis B in the hospital clinic 2 weeks prior to this admission. Upon neurological examination, asterixis and hyperactive reflexes are noted. Ms. Holder's speech is unintelligible, and she has a generalized seizure 45 min after admission.

Cardiopulmonary assessment reveals sinus tachycardia with occasional PVCs, S_1S_2, minimal peripheral edema, and clear breath sounds bilaterally. Her respirations are rapid and shallow. Severe fetor hepaticus (foul-smelling breath) is noted at this time. Jaundice and mucosal bleeding are also present. Examination of the abdomen reveals hepatomegaly and tenderness to deep palpation. Bowel sounds are absent. A Foley catheter is placed and drains 100 ml of dark amber urine. A diagnosis of stage III acute hepatic encephalopathy in association with fulminant hepatic failure (FHF) is made, and Ms. Holder is admitted to the ICU. Blood samples are drawn with the following results:

Laboratory Values		ABGs	
Na	126	pH	7.51
K	3.1	$PaCO_2$	30
Gluc	55	PaO_2	85
Creat	2.3	SaO_2	95%
Mg	1.0	HCO_3	30
Alk Phos	150		
AST	2500		
SGPT	2200		

QUESTIONS AND ANSWERS

1. **The liver is a complex, dynamic organ. Describe its major physiological functions.**

    The functions of the liver can be divided into three categories: metabolic, circulatory/immune, and secretory/excretory.

    Metabolic

    Carbohydrate
    Glycogen storage
    Conversion of galactose and fructose to glucose
    Gluconeogenesis

Blood glucose homeostasis
Formation of other chemical compounds from intermediates of
carbohydrate metabolism
Protein
Deamination of amino acids for energy or conversion to carbohydrate
or lipid
Ureagenesis (to remove NH_3)
Plasma protein synthesis
Amino acid interconversions
Lipid
β-Oxidation of fatty acids $\rightarrow$ ATP
Formation of ketones
Formation of most lipoproteins
Cholesterol synthesis (bile salts)
Phospholipid synthesis (cell membrane)
Conversion of carbohydrate/protein $\rightarrow$ lipid
Miscellaneous
Vitamin storage
Synthesis of coagulation factors
Iron storage
Detoxification, modification, or excretion of drugs, hormones, toxins

Circulatory/Immune

Storage and filtration of blood
Half of total body lymph formation
Kupffer cell—phagocytizes 99% of intestinal bacteria translocated into
the portal circulation

Secretory/Excretory

Bile production
Bilirubin metabolism

2. **Due to the diverse functions of the liver, hepatic failure can have
devastating consequences. What are precipitating factors commonly
associated with both acute and chronic hepatic failure?**

Acute

Viral hepatitis
Hepatoxic chemicals—acetaminophen, halothane, methotrexate, tetra-
cycline
Acute fatty liver of pregnancy
Circulatory failure
Hepatic vascular occlusion
Yellow fever
Septic shock
Reye's syndrome

The three most common causes of acute hepatic failure are viral hepatitis, acute overdose, and halothane.

Chronic

Cirrhosis
Alcoholic liver disease
Viral hepatitis
Parasitic disease—schistosomiasis, malaria
Intestinal bypass procedures
Chronic biliary infection
Extrahepatic obstruction
α_1-Antitrypsin deficiency
Wilson's disease
Chronic CHF
Congenital syphilis
Galactosemia
Glycogen storage disease
Sarcoidosis
Cystic fibrosis
Hepatic malignancies

3. **Describe the pathophysiology of hepatic injury occurring in Ms. Holder's case.**

The terminal event in FHF is hepatocyte injury with concomitant impairment of hepatocellular function. Although the etiology of this event is often identifiable, the exact pathogenesis of hepatocellular necrosis remains elusive. As in many other disease processes, such as pancreatitis and multisystem organ failure, current research focuses on the activation and liberation of numerous chemical and immunological mediators. (See Appendix F.) The hepatocyte plasma membrane may play an integral role in hepatic failure, contingent upon its response to the various etiological factors, including viral invasion and hepatoxic drugs.

Calcium ions have also been implicated in sustaining the destructive process, because they are able to cross the damaged membrane and potentiate necrosis. The amount of viral antigen present, the magnitude of the cellular immune response, and the number of hepatocytes invaded may all play a role in the progression of acute viral hepatitis to FHF.

As the hepatocytes lose their ability to function, derangements occur in the hepatic homeostatic mechanisms. Alterations in carbohydrate, protein, and lipid metabolism, as well as coagulation and detoxification functions, occur. These incite a variety of complications that lead to further physiological perturbations and, in many cases, death.

4. What complications are seen in FHF?

Due to the complex nature of hepatic function, numerous complications are seen in FHF. They include:

Hepatic encephalopathy secondary to circulating toxins

Cerebral edema secondary to alterations in vasogenic, cytotoxic, or interstitial cerebral homeostatic mechanisms, which represents the most frequent cause of death in FHF

Coagulopathies secondary to decreases in circulating platelets and clotting factors

Hypotension secondary to hemorrhage, bacterial invasion, cardiopulmonary abnormalities, and central vasomotor depression (↓ cardiac output, ↓ SVR, ↓ heart rate)

Inadequate ventilation secondary to intrapulmonary shunting, dilatation of vascular bed, and central depression

Pulmonary edema secondary to pulmonary vasodilatation and cerebral edema

Electrolyte imbalances secondary to vomiting, increased aldosterone, failure of sodium/potassium pump, and altered renal handling of fluid and electrolytes

Acid-base disturbances secondary to lactic acid accumulation, hyperventilation, and electrolyte abnormalities

Renal dysfunction secondary to hepatorenal syndrome and hypovolemia

Hypoglycemia secondary to increases in circulating insulin not metabolized by the liver, impaired hepatic glucose release, and decreases in glycogen stores

Cardiac abnormalities secondary to dysrhythmias and central vasomotor depression

Infection secondary to inadequate portal clearance of intestinal bacteria, inhibition of PMN function, low serum complement levels, immobility, and decreased LOC

Portal hypertension secondary to intrahepatic block due to massive necrosis of hepatocytes

Upper GI hemorrhage secondary to mucosal ulceration and portal hypertension if the process continues

5. On day 2, Ms. Holder becomes severely obtunded. Over the course of the next 24 hr, she becomes comatose and shows an abnormal EEG. A diagnosis of stage IV hepatic encephalopathy is made. Explain the development and progression of this process. How does it differ from that seen in chronic hepatic failure?

Hepatic encephalopathy (HE) is the most common complication of FHF, and its presentation is actually required as part of the differential diagnosis of the disease process. The etiology and pathogenesis of its development remain speculative, but current thought does differentiate it from the hepatic encephalopathy occurring in chronic liver disease and failure. The portal systemic shunting of blood to collaterals, important in the hepatic encephalopathy of chronic disease, is not present in FHF.

Inadequately metabolized vasoactive substances and humoral toxins generated by the dysfunctional liver could induce hepatic encephalopathy through several mechanisms, including inhibition of enzymes necessary for cellular oxidation, suppression of neurotransmission, or accumulation of false neurotransmitters. Alterations in the blood-brain barrier, osmotic regulation, and hypoxic changes in the cerebral tissue may make the brain more susceptible to even normal circulating levels of certain mediators. Hypotension, hypoglycemia, and cerebral edema also contribute to the pathophysiological and functional changes seen in the hepatic encephalopathy of FHF.

Treatment for hepatic encephalopathy is limited to supportive care and elimination of the secondary causes. Charcoal hemoperfusion, administration of dopamine agonists, and alterations of the plasma amino acid profile have been attempted, but results remain inconclusive.

6. **On day 4, Ms. Holder's urine output begins to drop. Serial laboratory studies over the succeeding 48 hr show an increasing BUN and creatinine and decreasing urine sodium. Clinical tests also reveal a decrease in glomerular filtration rate (GFR). What is a possible explanation for this clinical picture?**

Acute renal failure in the presence of liver disease is not uncommon and may be related to a variety of etiological factors. The diagnosis of hepatorenal syndrome (HRS) is primarily one of exclusion and can be made only after examination of clinical, laboratory, and anatomic findings rule out ATN, hypotensive prerenal azotemia, or other known causes of renal failure.

Despite extensive research of the HRS, the pathogenesis of the process has not been elucidated. Although alterations in renal function may be progressive and severe, most data indicate a functional renal failure in a previously healthy kidney. Minimal pathological abnormalitites are noted in relation to the syndrome. The currently described pathophysiological mechanism focuses on alterations in renal hemodynamics, leading to selective renal hypoperfusion with cortical ischemia, decreases in GFR, and increases in intrarenal vascular resistance. If the alterations are due to ineffective circulating plasma volume, HRS is ruled out.

Due to the complicated factors associated with severe liver dysfunction and its treatment (GI bleeding, abnormal renal handling of sodium and water, sodium restriction, diuresis, ascites, peripheral edema, decreased cardiac output, decreased SVR, increased circulating levels of renin, angiotensin, and catecholamines), it is often difficult to determine effective circulating volume and causes for acute renal failure. Several explanations for HRS have been advanced. These include:

Alterations in kallikrein-kinin system
Increased sympathetic nervous system activity
Metabolites of arachidonic acid—prostaglandins, thromboxanes, and leukotrienes
Endotoxins—shown to cause potent vasoconstriction
Atrial natriuretic factor—involved in fluid balance
Alterations in the renin-angiotensin axis
Decreased deactivation of circulating hormones
Hepatic encephalopathy—false neurotransmitters may lead to alterations in vascular adrenergic tone

7. What treatment modalities are employed in the HRS?

Since the mechanisms involved in the HRS remain undefined, treatment for the syndrome also remains symptom based and supportive. Effective circulating plasma volume must be maintained. While the plasma volume may appear adequate, as demonstrated by normal hemodynamic parameters, the volume may be maldistributed and ineffective in maintaining adequate perfusion to specific organs.

For this reason, sodium and fluid restriction, diuresis, and dialysis may be instituted. A LeVeen shunt may also be placed to prevent progressive ascitic buildup. Nutritional support to maintain adequate energy stores and decrease peripheral edema by repletion of serum albumin levels is also added to the overall regimen. Calcium antagonists have been shown to decrease renal vascular resistance and increase GFR and may play an integral role in the future of HRS management. At present, treatment of the underlying liver failure remains the focus of HRS intervention.

8. Ms. Holder's sodium is 126 mEq/liter. Why does this occur when the kidney is actually retaining sodium?

Although there is abnormal renal retention of sodium in FHF, serum sodium levels are often below normal limits in FHF because of the kidney's marked inability to excrete adequate amounts of free water. Cell membrane sodium pump failure has also been cited as a cause of decreased serum sodium.

Because sodium is such an integral electrolyte in total body fluid homeostasis, alterations in its serum levels may represent several different fluid states of the circulating volume. Hyponatremia may exist in normovolemic or hypervolemic states. Hypervolemic hyponatremia may exist due to an increased retention of fluid. Excess total body sodium may be present but masked by increased fluid accumulation.

9. What is the normal serum sodium level? What are the signs and symptoms of hyponatremia and hypernatremia?

The normal serum sodium level is 136–146 mEq/liter. The severity of signs and symptoms seen with abnormal levels is dependent on the degree and rate of development of the condition. Many of the indicators are neurological and secondary to changes in the cellular hydration of the tissues of the CNS.

Hyponatremia	**Hypernatremia**
Nausea/vomiting	Lethargy
Muscle irritability	Muscle weakness
Malaise	Twitching
Headache	Generalized seizures
Lethargy	Pulmonary edema
Generalized seizures	Coma
Coma	

10. Why does Ms. Holder have an increased susceptibility to infection?

As with any ICU patient, susceptibility to infection is increased for a multiplicity of reasons. Immobility, decreased LOC, and inadequate ventilation increase the risk of pneumonia. The use of numerous invasive lines and procedures also provides additional avenues of infection. In addition to the above factors, inadequate clearance of intestinal bacteria from the portal circulation by injured Kupffer cells (liver macrophages), inhibition of PMN function by humoral toxins, and low serum complement levels place Ms. Holder at further disposition to bacterial invasion. Overzealous use of antibiotics and improper technique and handwashing not only increase the risk of infection but also favor the colonization of nosocomial infections more resistant to standard therapy.

Standard monitoring of these patients is not enough to prevent and identify infectious processes. Fever, leukocytosis, and other clinical signs and symptoms of sepsis are often absent in FHF, so the critical care nurse must constantly be aware of ways to prevent and identify infection in this patient population. Strict adherence to aseptic technique by the nurse and other staff must be followed. Daily cultures of blood, urine, and sputum may be indicated. Adherence to institutional policy concerning site care and line changes is important.

Meticulous skin care, pulmonary toilet, and mobility are all necessary to decrease the risk of infection.

Femoral sites should be avoided for laboratory phlebotomy and line placement. Subtle changes in LOC, cardiovascular status, and fluid and electrolyte balance should be monitored, but changes may be difficult to assess in a patient already exhibiting alterations in these areas. Critical care nurses at the bedside 24 hr a day are in a key role to identify and initiate intervention in these changing systems.

11. What nursing diagnoses apply in this case?

Fluid volume excess related to hepatorenal syndrome and CNS dysfunction

Alteration in tissue perfusion: cerebral related to hypotension, alteration in blood-brain barrier, and circulating mediators

Impaired gas exchange related to decreased LOC, immobility, and intrapulmonary shunting

Alteration in nutrition: less than body requirements related to abnormal hepatic metabolism, circulating hormone levels, and inadequate intake

Potential for infection related to numerous lines, decreased liver function, immobility, LOC, and pulmonary abnormalities

Anxiety related to patient condition, ICU environment, and confusion secondary to hepatorenal syndrome

SUGGESTED READINGS

Adinaro D. Liver failure and pancreatitis: fluid and electrolyte concerns. Nurs Clin North Am 1987;22(4):843–852.

Epstein M. Hepatorenal syndrome. In: Epstein M, ed. The kidney in liver disease. 3rd ed. Baltimore: Williams & Wilkins, 1988:89–118.

Guyton AC. Textbok of medical physiology. 7th ed. Philadelphia: WB Saunders, 1986.

Jones EA, Schafer DF. Fulminant hepatic failure. In: Zakim D, Boyer TD, eds. Hepatology. A textbook of liver disease. Philadelphia: WB Saunders, 1982:415–445.

Kokko JP, Tannen RL, eds. Fluids and electrolytes. Philadelphia: WB Saunders, 1986.

Levy M. Pathophysiology of the hepatorenal syndrome and potential for therapy. Am J Cardiol 1987;60:661–72I.

Zieve L. Hepatic encephalopathy. In: Schiff L, Schiff ER, eds. Diseases of the liver. 6th ed. Philadelphia: JB Lippincott, 1987:925–948.

CHAPTER 43

Liver Transplantation

Connie Glass, RN, MSN, CCRN

Jane Arnold is a 45-year-old divorced secretary who lives alone. She has no children, and her parents live in another state. In 1981, after a partial gastrectomy for a gastric ulcer, she was transfused with several units of blood. Shortly thereafter Ms. Arnold was diagnosed with non-A, non-B hepatitis. She subsequently developed chronic liver failure, which resulted in portal hypertension, ascites, and bleeding esophageal varices. She was admitted to the hospital on November 10, 1988 for transplant evaluation. Her physical examination revealed a nonicteric, cachetic woman, alert and conversant, with no asterixis, splenomegaly, or bright red GI bleeding. She had moderate ascites with a liver 12 cm below the left costal margin and melanotic stool. She was 5 feet, 5 inches tall and weighed 43 kg.

Vital Signs		Laboratory Values			
BP	110/60	Na	125	PT	3/11
HR	84	K	5.8	PTT	27/25
Resp	28	Cl	101	Fibrinogen	276
Temp	97.5°F	CO_2	13	AST	92
		Gluc	3	ALT	70
ABGs (room air)		BUN	51	Alk Phos	94
pH	7.38	Creat	3.2	T. Bili	0.9
$PaCO_2$	25	WBC	17.1	TP	5.2
PaO_2	111	RBC	2.1	Albumin	2.7
SaO_2	95%	Hgb	6.3	Plat	31,000
HCO_3	15	Hct	18.2		

After an extensive workup, Ms. Arnold was listed on the organ procurement computer. On February 7, 1989, she received a liver transplant with the surgery lasting 14 hr. She received 56 units of packed red blood cells, 52 units of fresh frozen plasma, and 52 units of platelets during surgery. When she arrived in the ICU, her ventilator settings and blood gases were as follows:

Mode	SIMV	pH	7.60
Rate	8	$PaCO_2$	37
FIO_2	0.50	PaO_2	223
Tidal volume	500	SaO_2	98%
		HCO_3	36

Her weight was 45.1 kg. Other parameters and laboratory values were:

Hemodynamic Parameters		Laboratory Values			
BP	120/70	Na	154	Albumin	3.2
HR	90	K	2.8	Alk Phos	42
CVP	5	Cl	108	ALT	288
PAP	16	CO_2	37	AST	474
PAWP	8	Gluc	254	BUN	17
CO	5	Creat	1.1	Fibrinogen	268
SVR	1312	Ca	8.0	PT	13/12
		Hgb	9.7	PTT	29/26
		Hct	28.2	T. Bili	2.0
		WBC	23.5	TP	4.9
		Plat	28,000		

Ms. Arnold was given 100 ml albumin and started on 10% dextran at 25 ml/hr. Fluids were given to increase her PAWP to 12–15 mm Hg. After 12 hr in the ICU, her fluid balance was 3670 ml intake and 3125 ml output. Bile drainage from the T-tube for the first 24 hr was 150 ml. Total parenteral nutrition was started at 2 liters/24 hr on the second postoperative day because of her drop in albumin to 2.9.

On the third postoperative day, Ms. Arnold's clinical data showed a normal coagulation profile and 230 ml bile drainage from the T-tube for 24 hr. Her weight was 42.7 kg, and her ventilator settings remained unchanged from ICU admission.

Laboratory Values		ABGs		Vital Signs	
Albumin	2.9	pH	7.54	BP	140/86
Alk Phos	71	$PaCO_2$	39	HR	83
ALT	858	PaO_2	71	Resp	8
AST	1062	SaO_2	93%	CVP	15
T. Bili	2.6	HCO_3	34	PAP	29/22
				PAWP	20

Her ABGs gradually deteriorated over the next 12 hr, even with an increase in FIO_2 and the addition of PEEP. She also received furosemide (Lasix) as 40 mg bolus twice. At 7:00 PM on postoperative day 5 on an FIO_2 of 1.0, tidal volume 500 ml, SIMV 8, PEEP + 15 cm H_2O, the following values were recorded.

ABGs		Hemodynamic Parameters	
pH	7.44	BP	140/86
$PaCO_2$	50	HR	90
PaO_2	75	RAP	15
SaO_2	93%	PAP	29/22
HCO_3	32	PAWP	21

A continuous Lasix infusion was started at 70 mg/hr, and Ms. Arnold's condition gradually improved. After 8 hr on an FIO_2 of 0.50 and PEEP + 12 cm H_2O, her ABGs were:

pH	7.51
$PaCO_2$	45
PaO_2	187
SaO_2	98%
HCO_3	34

On postoperative day 6, Ms. Arnold was extubated. Her Lasix infusion was discontinued. She had active bowel sounds and was begun on clear liquids with the plan to decrease the hyperalimentation as her caloric intake increased. Her caloric needs were assessed at 2000 kcal for maintenance and 2500 kcal for repletion.

Laboratory Values

Albumin	3.8
Chol	122
TP	5.9
Transferrin	219

On postoperative day 10, Ms. Arnold was transferred to the transplant floor with her condition stable and her transplanted liver functioning properly.

QUESTIONS AND ANSWERS

1. **Although the first human orthotopic liver transplant was performed in 1963, the procedure had a 1-year survival rate of only 30% until the late 1970s. What changes have increased the 1-year survival in adults and children to over 80%?**

   Increases in survival of liver transplant recipients can be attributed to:

   Development of more effective operative techniques

   Increased procurement and access of donor organs by better maintenance of harvested livers. By cold flushing and storage in an intracellular electrolyte solution closely resembling the electrolyte balance inside the liver cells, the donor liver can remain functional up to 10 hr. This high-potassium–low-sodium solution controls cell swelling and avoids adverse effects produced by changes in intracellular ion content.

   New immunosuppressive therapy with more specific action on the T-lymphocyte. This has decreased the need for total immune system suppression, therefore reducing the risk of infection while decreasing the incidence of rejection.

2. **What are some indications for liver transplant? What in Ms. Arnold's history and clinical profile indicates the need for transplant?**

   Irreversible end-stage liver disease that has proven refractory to medical and/or surgical therapy is the criteria for liver transplantation common to all centers. Specific indications include chronic hepatitis with cirrhosis, sclerosing cholangitis, primary biliary cirrhosis, and metabolic diseases of the liver. Ms. Arnold's liver failure with ascites, malnutrition, and recurrent variceal bleeds indicated her need for a donor organ.

3. **Hepatorenal syndrome is a major sequela to end-stage liver disease. Is this a relative contraindication for transplantation? Will Ms. Arnold's renal insufficiency create problems for her after transplantation?**

   Hepatorenal syndrome, although a major complication of hepatic failure, is not a contraindication for transplantation. No anatomical or histological changes occur in the kidneys, which makes this a functional disorder. In animal studies, kidneys in failure because of hepatorenal syndrome have been transplanted into other animals and have functioned adequately. It is theorized that hepatorenal syndrome is caused by endotoxins released by the failing liver or circulating vasoconstrictor substances that decrease renal perfusion. (See Chapter 42, "Fulminant Hepatic Failure.") Ms. Arnold's kidney function should improve after transplantation.

4. **Transplantation is divided into three phases. Name and briefly describe each. What is the most difficult phase of the operation and why?**

   Transplantation of the liver is a very complex operation requiring 8–24 hr. The three phases of this surgical procedure are:

   Donor Hepatectomy

   The donor liver is removed and is carefully inspected for abnormalities. Attention is given to color and texture to exclude ischemic injury. Cautious dissection is done to preserve the vascular structures leading into and out of the liver as well as the common bile duct. The liver is infused with 4°C Ringer's lactate to a temperature of 30°C, then flushed with an intracellular electrolyte solution and immersed in this cold solution in a sterile plastic bag. The donor organ is transported in an iced cooler but protected from direct contact with the ice to prevent burns. Adequate postoperative function is enhanced if the vascular anastomoses can be completed within 5–6 hr.

   Recipient Hepatectomy and Anhepatic Phase

   During the removal of the donor liver, the recipient liver is being excised. Because of scarring of the cirrhotic liver, portal hypertension, and possible previous surgeries or coagulopathy, this portion of the transplantation is the most difficult. A venovenous bypass is used to shunt blood from the inferior vena cava and splanchnic circulation back to the right heart via the axillary, subclavian, or jugular vein. This increases the right heart preload and decreases venous hypertension and bleeding.

Transplantation (Figure 43.1)

Vascular anastomoses of the suprahepatic vena cava and portal vein are followed by flushing of the donor liver with Ringer's lactate solution to remove the high-potassium intracellular solution and any air bubbles. Anastomoses of the inferior vena cava, hepatic artery, and biliary tree are then completed.

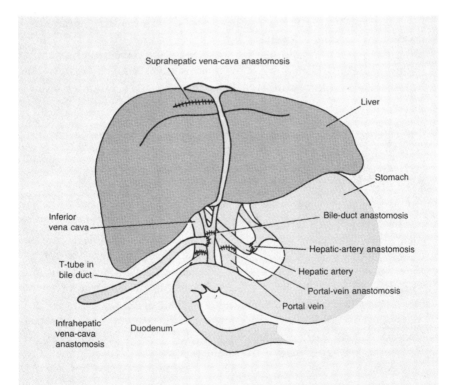

Figure 43.1. End-to-end anastomosis between donor and recipient common bile ducts. (From Miller HD. Liver transplantation: postoperative ICU care. Crit Care Nurse 1988;8(6):25.)

5. **What is the leading cause of death in both adults and children following liver transplantation? What were Ms. Arnold's specific risk factors for developing this complication?**

   Infection is the leading cause of death in both adults and children following liver transplantation. Ms. Arnold was at risk for infection because of her malnourished pretransplant state and the 14-hr surgery. Intraoperative and postoperative venous, arterial, and urinary catheters, mechanical ventilation, and abdominal and biliary T-tube drains provided ports of entry for bacteria and viruses. Postoperative recovery is often complicated by systemic fungal infections and Gram-negative enteric organisms, as well as nosocomial pulmonary and opportunistic infections such as herpes and cytomegalovirus. Immune system depression by antirejection drugs makes infection a greater risk in transplant patients than in other surgical patients.

6. **Electrolyte imbalances can be a problem in the immediate posttransplantation phase. Ms. Arnold's sodium was 154, potassium 2.8, carbon dioxide 37, calcium 8.0, and pH 7.60. Explain these abnormalities.**

   Metabolic alkalosis results from increased sodium retention and bicarbonate reabsorption by the kidneys and hypokalemia as a result of both renal potassium loss and donor liver potassium uptake. This metabolic alkalosis is also a result of the metabolism of the blood preservative sodium citrate into bicarbonate as the new liver begins to function. Acetazolamide (Diamox) was given to Ms. Arnold to treat the metabolic alkalosis. This drug causes chloride sparing and bicarbonate excretion. Potassium chloride infusions were given to increase her serum potassium. Abnormally low calcium is a result of the citrate in the banked blood binding with ionized calcium. Intraoperative washing of RBC prior to administration can decrease the amount of citrate the patient receives. Replacement is based on ionized calcium levels, since serum calcium is minimally affected by this binding process.

7. **On postoperative day 3, Ms. Arnold's AST increased to 1062 and her ALT to 858, yet her total bilirubin was 0.6. She had 230 ml of bile from the T-tube over the past 24 hr. When does acute rejection occur? Would rejection be suspected in Ms. Arnold? What physical signs would be present? How is rejection diagnosed and treated?**

   Although compatibility of ABO blood group between donor and recipient is considered a necessity for transplantation, matching human lymphocyte antigens (HLA) is not always done. Acute graft rejection usually occurs between postoperative days 6 and 21, although it can occur at any time. The patient may experience upper abdominal pain, depression, loss of appetite, fever, and tachycardia. Although Ms. Arnold had an increase in AST and ALT, the total bilirubin was normal. Her coagulation profile was normal and her bile output was good. Hepatic ischemia from occlusion of the portal vein or hepatic artery, biliary obstruction, perihepatic infections, sepsis, and drug toxicity can all produce clinical and laboratory findings compatible with rejection and must be ruled out. Rejection is defined differently in various centers, with some relying on clinical criteria and others requiring biopsy and histological diagnosis. Because Ms. Arnold did not have clinical signs and her liver function test results began to decrease the following day, she was not biopsied, nor was she treated for acute rejection. Ischemia was ruled out and obstruction was considered unlikely, since her bile output was increased. Acute rejection is treated with large doses of methylprednisolone. This drug impairs antigen recognition and macrophage response so that lymphocytes are not attracted to the graft and those already there redistribute away from the donor organ.

8. **How does chronic rejection differ from acute rejection, and how is it identified?**

   Chronic rejection has clinical features that are less obvious than those of acute rejection. Histological changes include progressive loss of bile ducts, portal inflammation and infiltrates, and narrowing in the hepatic artery lumen. Chronic rejection may not respond to steroid therapy and in some centers is an indication for retransplantation.

9. **What immunosuppressive regimen is usually used for liver transplant patients?**

   Immunosuppressive therapy is variable according to patient response and center protocol. Combined drugs allow for more adequate graft acceptance with fewer side effects because lower doses can be given. Large doses of methylprednisolone are given initially in most centers along with antithymocyte globulin (ATG), azathioprine (Imuran), and cyclosporine (Sandimmune). (See Chapter 2, "Cardiac Transplantation," for more information on these drugs.)

10. **To what would you attribute Ms. Arnold's change in pulmonary status on postoperative day 3?**

    After abdominal surgery, patients often experience third spacing of fluid, especially if they have a low intravascular colloidal osmotic pressure. At first glance, one might suspect ARDS, because of Ms.

Arnold's inability to oxygenate adequately despite increasing FIO_2 and the addition of PEEP. However, her hemodynamic profile indicates volume overload with elevation of filling pressures and no hypotension. Since her weight is unchanged, reabsorption of third-space fluid rather than additional intake increased her intravascular volume. Because of decreased renal function, Ms. Arnold could not excrete this fluid rapidly enough and developed pulmonary edema. Her pulmonary status improved with diuresis.

11. **A flexible T-tube is placed intraoperatively in the common bile duct and brought out through the skin. How does the amount of bile draining from Ms. Arnold's T-tube indicate liver function?**

    The normal liver makes 600–1000 ml of bile every 24 hr. The ability to assess and measure the bile draining from the liver helps evaluate liver function. In the first 24 hr after transplantation, Ms. Arnold's new liver made 150 ml of bile. An early output of 50–100 ml of bile every 8 hr indicates good liver function. Ms. Arnold's bile drainage was monitored every 8 hr, and her output continued to increase. Golden brown bile is considered normal, and any change of color, consistency, or chalk-like sediment is a warning sign. T-tubes are left open to drain for approximately 2–3 weeks after surgery. They are then clamped but left in place to function as a stent to the anastomosis for 6–9 months.

12. **Evaluate Ms. Arnold's nutritional status on postoperative day 6. Why is nutrition of importance in the liver transplant patient?**

    Some of the normal functions of the liver include synthesis of amino acids and albumin; storage of fat soluble vitamins; and formation of lipoproteins, cholesterol, and phospholipids. When liver failure occurs, these vital nutritional functions are impaired. In addition, albumin is also lost in ascites. To heal and maintain WBC function, nutritional needs must be met, especially in immunosuppressed patients. Ms. Arnold was started on 2 liters of total parenteral nutrition and IV lipids on her second postoperative day. By day 6, her nutritional indicators had all moved into the low normal range. Adequate nutrition can usually be achieved with 1–1½ gm of protein per kilogram of body weight plus carbohydrates and fats daily.

13. **Ms. Arnold will soon be moving from the ICU to the transplant floor. What psychological concerns might the nurse expect to deal with at this point?**

    Having experienced 8 years of chronic illness from liver failure and a 2-month wait for a donor liver, Ms. Arnold has now experienced 9 days of intensive nursing care during which she has successfully moved through the critical phase of her transplantation. Her nurses could expect her to have a variety of responses to this period in her recovery. Ms. Arnold may have fears related to transfer from the ICU or to possible rejection of her new liver. Mood swings related to steroid therapy may occur, including indecisiveness, withdrawal, pessimism, and depression. Ms. Arnold may have expected to feel much better by this time. She may worry about complications such as drug side effects or infection. Feelings of powerlessness from long-term illness and hospitalization may increase her dependency on the nursing staff. Talking with her about these psychological concerns before transfer fom the ICU may assist her in adjusting to the next phase of her recovery. Ms. Arnold may need time to just talk about her feelings, her hopes and fears, and her expectations for the next days and weeks. Her adjustment to her transplanted liver may be improved if she is able to ventilate her feelings.

Another response not uncommon in the transplanted patient is a feeling of euphoria. Survival through the ICU phase may make Ms. Arnold feel she has beaten the odds and will have a rapid and uncomplicated recovery with this hurdle overcome. Helping her maintain perspective and set realistic goals is an important nursing intervention. This may avoid depression if complications develop.

14. **What nursing diagnoses would apply to Ms. Arnold's intensive care hospital course?**

> Altered nutrition—less than body requirements
> Potential for infection related to surgery, invasive lines, and immuno-
> suppression
> Fluid volume excess
> Potential fluid volume deficit
> Impaired gas exchange related to fluid volume overload
> Potential for impaired skin integrity related to nutritional status and
> immobility
> Impaired verbal communication related to intubation
> Pain
> Body image disturbance related to surgical incision
> Powerlessness related to hospitalization
> Sleep pattern disturbance related to environment
> Fear related to organ rejection and infection

15. Ms. Arnold recovered and was discharged home. Six months later she is admitted to a community hospital with chest pain. What are some important nursing considerations related to her earlier liver transplantation?

Ms. Arnold must be on lifelong immunosuppressive therapy. Nurses caring for her may not be familiar with drugs, dosages, side effects, methods of administration, and methods of monitoring drug levels. This information must be made available to the staff.

Subtle signs of liver rejection may be difficult to identify. Abdominal pain, excessive fatigue, loss of appetite, low-grade fever, or decreased pigment in the stool should signal the nurse to suspect rejection. Liver function tests should be followed closely. Infection is an ever-present risk of immunosuppression, and special care should be taken to avoid putting Ms. Arnold at increased risk. The first sign of infection should be seen as a red flag, and cultures should be done and treatment begun immediately. Ms. Arnold can assist the staff in learning about the care of the recovered transplant patient. It is important for nurses to be willing to listen to the patient and learn from her in order to be able to care for her.

SUGGESTED READINGS

Harwood CH, Cook CV. Cyclosporine in transplantation. Heart Lung 1985;14(6): 529–540.

Jenkins RL, Benotti PN, Bothe AA, Rossi RL. Liver transplantation. Surg Clin North Am 1985;65(1):103–122.

Maddrey WC, ed. Transplantation of the liver. New York: Elsevier, 1988.

McMaster P, Kirby RM, Gunson BK. Liver transplantation. In: Catto GRD, ed. Clinical transplantation. Boston: MTP Press, 1987.

Miller D. Liver transplantation: postoperative ICU care. Crit Care Nurse 1988; 8(6):19–31.

Smith SL. Liver transplantation: implications for critical care. Heart Lung 1985; 14(6):617–628.

CHAPTER 44

Lower GI Bleed

Lisa Morra Martin, RN, BSN, CCRN

Doris Jasper is a 65-year-old woman who presents to the Emergency Department complaining of rectal bleeding since last night. She has had four or five episodes with bright red blood filling the commode. She had no previous history of similar episodes, no change in bowel habits, and no change in her appetite or weight. She does complain of chronic constipation, yet denies abdominal pain, nausea, or vomiting. She has no other medical problems, except one previous admission 3 years ago for diverticulitis, and denies any history of bleeding abnormalities. Her vital signs upon presentation are:

Lying		Sitting
BP	130/70	110/50
HR	110	130
Resp	18	20
Temp	98.5°F	

Physical examination reveals a mildly obese woman in no distress who is alert and cooperative. Her skin is pale, dry, and cool. Her heart sounds are clearly audible, and no murmurs or gallops are present. She has bilateral clear breath sounds, and her respirations are unlabored. Her abdomen is soft and nontender, bowel sounds are hyperactive, and rectal examination reveals bright red blood and no masses.

A 16-gauge intravenous catheter is inserted in Ms. Jasper's left arm, and Ringer's lactate solution is started. Blood is drawn for type and cross-match and laboratory analysis. An ECG is done, which upon evaluation is found to be unremarkable. A nasogastric tube is inserted, and 90 ml of green aspirate is obtained. This aspirate tests negative for the presence of blood. Laboratory analysis reveals electrolytes, arterial blood gases, and coagulation studies to be within normal limits. Ms. Jasper's hematocrit is noted to be 27% and her hemoglobin 9.

A Foley catheter is inserted and a subclavian central line is placed, which following a chest x-ray is found to be in good position. Her CVP is 1. Fluid resuscitation is continued with infusion of Ringer's lactate. Ms. Jasper is then prepared for proctoscopic examination.

After 2 hr and approximately 3 liters of fluid, Ms. Jasper's repeat hematocrit is 21%. She has had two further episodes of bleeding. Proctoscopic examination reveals no masses or hemorrhoids and bright red blood coming from above 25 cm. Blood transfusion therapy is initiated, and she is taken to nuclear medicine for a tagged red blood cell study.

The nuclear medicine study identifies active bleeding in the ascending colon. Selective arteriography of the superior mesenteric artery identifies bleeding from a branch of the iliocolic artery, and an intraarterial infusion of vasopressin is started. Ms. Jasper was then admitted to the ICU for further care.

QUESTIONS AND ANSWERS

1. What are the most common causes of severe lower GI blceding?

In Children and Young Adults
Meckel's diverticulum
Juvenile polyps
Inflammatory bowel disease

In Adults
Diverticular disease
Inflammatory bowel disease
Polyps
Cancer
Arteriovenous malformation

In Adults over 60 Years of Age
Angiodysplasia
Diverticular disease
Polyps
Cancer
Ischemic colitis

Rare
Infections
Rare tumors
Coagulopathies
Drug-induced ulceration
Vascular abnormalities
Varices

Although other causes are possible, considering her age of 65 and her history of diverticulitis, diverticular disease is the most likely cause of Ms. Jasper's bleeding. This diagnosis was confirmed by the arteriogram.

Diverticular disease is extremely common in Western nations. The incidence increases with age and occurs in at least 10% of patients over the age of 40. It is also estimated that at least one-half of the population may expect to develop diverticula of the colon in their lifetime.

Diverticula represent a herniation of the mucosa through the wall of the colon at a point of entry of a blood vessel. The blood vessel can become stretched over the dome of the diverticula and may degenerate and spontaneously rupture, causing brisk bleeding. The etiology of the development of diverticular disease is not completely understood; however, diet appears to be the most important factor. Although diverticula are most commonly located on the left colon, bleeding occurs most often from the right colon as in Ms. Jasper's case.

2. **What are the most important initial steps in the management of Ms. Jasper?**

Initial efforts should be focused on fluid resuscitation, general determination of volume of blood loss, and localization of the source of bleeding.

3. **What parameters should be followed to determine adequacy of resuscitation?**

Ms. Jasper was noted to have orthostatic changes in BP and heart rate, indicating a relatively severe volume deficit. A CVP line and a Foley catheter are excellent means to monitor fluid replacement. Urine output of 0.5–1 ml/kg/hr usually indicates sufficient volume replacement. Monitoring central venous pressures is especially helpful in elderly patients who may have compromised cardiac function.

4. **Why did Ms. Jasper require a nasogastric tube?**

Although the bright red rectal bleeding indicated a probable lower GI source, bright red rectal bleeding can occasionally result from rapid upper GI bleeding. Moreover, a negative aspirate for blood from the nasogastric tube does not completely exclude an upper GI source. If what appears to be bile-stained fluid is aspirated, as in the green fluid aspirated in Ms. Jasper's case, an upper GI source is very unlikely. If any question exists during evaluation, endoscopy should be performed to rule out an upper gastrointestinal source of bleeding.

5. **What are the indications for blood transfusion?**

Indications for blood transfusion are variable, depending on the age of the patient, associated medical problems, and cardiovascular stability. In diseases of surgical concern, the most common indication for blood transfusion is the restoration of circulating blood volume. Blood volume may be determined by various techniques, yet once again a number of factors may affect values for "normal blood volume." As a result, volume alone is not an absolute indication for transfusion.

Rapid determination of a low hematocrit in a patient who is hypotensive is helpful in judging the need for early transfusion. This assessment may be misleading in situations of acute blood loss, as the hematocrit may be normal despite a markedly diminished blood volume. It is also important to obtain a history regarding bleeding abnormalities and to evaluate results from coagulation studies, as transfusion of clotting factors may be necessary.

6. **What are the signs and symptoms of a blood transfusion reaction?**
    Hemolytic reactions, those reactions due to incompatibility of A, B, O, and Rh groups as well as other independent systems, are characterized by intravascular destruction of red blood cells and resultant hemoglobinemia and hemoglobinuria. Clinical manifestations of such a reaction may vary, yet if the patient is awake, the most common symptoms are the sensations of pain and heat along the vein used for infusion, flushing of the face, lumbar pain, and constricting chest pain. The patient may also experience fever, chills, respiratory distress, tachycardia, and hypotension.
    Abnormal bleeding and persistent hypotension despite adequate volume replacement may be indicative of a transfusion reaction in the anesthetized patient undergoing surgical intervention. Morbidity and mortality from hemolytic reactions are high if a patient receives an entire unit of incompatible blood.
    Finally, allergic reactions result from the transfusion of antibodies from hypersensitive donors or the transfusion of antigens to which the patient is hypersensitive. Reactions are usually mild and are evidenced by urticaria and fever. On rare occasions, reactions are severe enough to cause anaphylactic shock.

7. **Why were a nuclear imaging study and arteriography performed?**
    There are numerous techniques available for the diagnosis and treatment of acute lower gastrointestinal bleeding. Approximately 80% of cases may be treated conservatively, yet 10–20% will require emergency surgery. The source of bleeding is often difficult to identify intraoperatively. Therefore, in individuals suspected to be actively bleeding, every effort should be made to identify the site of bleeding through the use of nuclear imaging, arteriography, and colonoscopy.
    Following exclusion of an upper gastrointestinal source and rectal pathology, technetium scanning was chosen for Ms. Jasper because it is the most sensitive method by which active bleeding can be determined. This study may detect bleeding at rates as low as 0.05–0.1 ml/min. Arteriography, although successful in many cases, has

limitations. Bleeding rates of 0.5–1 ml/min are necessary to enable detection, which results in a high rate of false-negative examinations. To reduce the number of false-negative arteriograms, the more sensitive nuclear imaging may be performed to improve diagnostic yield.

8. What other treatment options are available for Ms. Jasper?
    The exact therapy instituted is dependent on multiple factors, including cause of bleeding, age, associated medical problems, history of colonic bleeding, previous complications of diverticular disease, and the experience of the treating physician. Additional proposed therapy may include embolization of the bleeding vessel with autologous clot or a number of other agents. This procedure carries the risk of bowel infarction, and patients must be observed closely for this serious complication. In addition, emergency surgical resection is advocated by many authors as the treatment of choice. Careful patient selection is important, as emergent surgery in this setting can be associated with high morbidity and mortality.

9. What are the complications of vasopressin infusion therapy?
    See Chapter 47, "Portal Hypertension with Upper GI Bleeding."

10. What nursing diagnoses apply in Ms. Jasper's case?

> Fluid volume deficit related to active bleeding
> Alteration in comfort related to presence of NG tube
> Alteration in nutrition: less than body requirements related to NPO status
> Anxiety related to unfamiliar environment
> Potential for injury related to blood transfusion reaction

SUGGESTED READINGS

Cameron JL. Current surgical therapy-3. Toronto: BC Decker, 1989.

Hunt RH. Acute colonic hemorrhage. In: Bouchier I, Allan RN, Hodgsdon H, Keighley M, eds. Textbook of gastroenterology. London: WB Saunders, 1984:308–317.

Peterson WL. Gastrointestinal bleeding. In: Wickland E, ed. Gastrointestinal disease. 4th ed. Philadelphia: WB Saunders, 1989: 411–417.

Sabiston DC Jr, ed. Textbook of surgery, the biological basis of modern surgical practice. 13th ed. Philadelphia: WB Saunders, 1986.

Schwartz SI. Hemostasis, surgical bleeding and transfusion. In: Principles of Surgery. 5th ed. New York: McGraw-Hill, 1989: 105–133.

Treat MR, Forde KA. Colonoscopy, technetium scanning, and angiography in acute rectal bleeding—an algorithm for their combined use. Surg Gastroenterol 1983; 2:135–138.

CHAPTER 45

Pancreatitis

Virginia Byrn Huddleston, RN, MSN, CCRN

Sam Petty is a 43-year-old man employed by a local factory. He has a history of alcohol abuse with previous admissions for GI bleeding and acute pancreatitis. He is brought to the Emergency Department by ambulance with complaints of severe epigastric pain and intractable nausea and vomiting following a weekend of heavy drinking. On arrival, he is hypotensive, and fluid resuscitation is begun. After initial stabilization in the Emergency Department, he is transferred to the ICU. A pulmonary artery catheter and radial arterial line are inserted. Ultrasonography reveals an enlarged and edematous pancreas, and a diagnosis of acute pancreatitis is made.

Upon admission to the unit, Mr. Petty is oriented to person and place, anxious, and uncooperative. His temperature is 101.5°F. He is tachycardiac, diaphoretic, and tachypneic. Auscultation of the chest reveals clear breath sounds bilaterally. His abdomen is distended without bowel sounds, and guarding is noted on palpation. He continues to complain of severe epigastric pain despite receiving meperidine in the Emergency Department. A Foley catheter is placed, and the measured output is 50 ml of dark, amber urine. Other clinical data include:

Hemodynamic Parameters		Laboratory Values	
PAP	15/8	K	3.5
CVP	1	Gluc	180
PAWP	2	Ca	7.4
CO	3.8	Mg	1.3
BP	85/50	Hct	48
HR	130	WBC	20,000
		Albumin	1.5
		Amylase	650
		Lipase	30
		PT	18
		PTT	28

Vigorous fluid resuscitation is continued with both colloid and crystalloid solutions. A nasogastric tube is inserted, and 100 mg meperidine is given IM. Forty percent face mask and serial laboratory studies are also ordered.

QUESTIONS AND ANSWERS

1. What are the two most common precipitating factors associated with acute pancreatitis?

> Biliary tract disease
> Alcohol abuse

Other precipitating factors include:

> Pancreatic duct obstruction
> Duodenal disorders
> Trauma
> Immunological processes
> Pregnancy
> Vascular disorders
> Hypothermia
> End-stage renal disease
> Drugs (diuretics, estrogens, azathioprine, sulfonamides, methyldopa, tetracycline, mercaptopurine, corticosteroids)
> Hyperlipemia
> Surgery
> Tumors
> Infection
> Carcinoma
> Hypercalcemia
> Scorpion venom
> Hypoperfusion

Although many factors have been associated with the onset of acute pancreatitis, over 90% of the cases are attributed to biliary tract disease, alcohol abuse, or idiopathic factors.

2. Describe the pathophysiological cascade mechanism currently thought to occur in acute pancreatitis at the local level.

> Original insult (from obstruction, reflux, etc.)
> Release of prematurely activated proteolytic and lipolytic enzymes into pancreatic tissue
> Increased microvascular permeability
> Interstitial edema and retroperitoneal fluid accumulation
> Pancreatic tissue and peripancreatic fat necrosis
> Release of arachidonic acid metabolites from damaged cell membranes, causing coagulation and vascular abnormalities
> Progressive acinar cell damage and continued release of destructive enzymes (autodigestion)

3. **Despite aggressive fluid resuscitation, Mr. Petty remains hemodynamically labile. What is a possible explanation of this pathophysiology at the systemic level?**

   As autodigestion occurs in the pancreas, numerous bioactive substances are released into the systemic circulation. Trypsin can activate several zymogen and conversion pathways, including kininogen to kinin/bradykinin, prothrombin to thrombin, and proelastase to elastase. Bradykinin in concert with other vasoactive substances can lead to increased leukocyte chemotaxis, capillary permeability, vasodilatation, hypotension, and shock. Alterations in the coagulation pathways may lead to local or systemic thrombosis, especially in the mesenteric circulation. Elastin in blood vessels is broken down by elastase, leading to further vessel damage, inflammation, edema, and vascular instability. Increased amounts of fluid are then sequestered into the tissues, particularly the pancreatic parenchyma and peripancreatic tissue.

4. **Mr. Petty's total serum calcium is 7.4. Is this a common finding in acute pancreatitis? What is the significance of this calcium level in his case?**

   Hypocalcemia is a common finding in acute pancreatitis; however, the exact etiology remains under investigation. Serum calcium exists in both ionized (47%) and nonionized (53%) forms. The total serum calcium reported on the laboratory results is a sum of both forms. The nonionized form is bound to proteins (primarily albumin) and other molecules, such as phosphate, citrate, and sulfate. Because changes in the pH, circulating levels of albumin, and concentrations of the other molecules can alter the ratio of ionized to nonionized calcium as well as the total serum calcium level, care must be taken not to interpret the calcium level in isolation. It is the calcium circulating in the ionized form that is necessary for the proper functioning of nerve conduction, muscle contraction, coagulation pathways, and other calcium-dependent enzymatic processes. Thus, it is the level of the ionized form that must be kept within therapeutic ranges. Since many laboratories measure total calcium only, a corrected value for total calcium must be calculated that takes into account abnormal albumin levels. Because hypoalbuminemia is also common in acute pancreatitis, Mr. Petty's observed hypocalcemia may be related to a decrease in the protein-bound nonionized form. The ionized level may be within the normal range. Other explanations for a further decrease in circulating calcium include abnormal production or degradation of parathyroid hormone and altered end-organ responsiveness to parathyroid hormone.

5. **Given a calcium level of 7.4 and an albumin level of 1.5, calculate the corrected total serum calcium. Why is it important to make this calculation before treating the patient?**

    $$\text{Corrected calcium} = \text{Total calcium} + 0.8\,(4.0 - \text{albumin})$$
    $$= 7.4 + 0.8\,(4.0 - 1.5)$$
    $$= 7.4 + 0.8\,(2.5)$$
    $$= 7.4 + 2.0$$
    $$\text{Corrected calcium} = 9.4$$

    Since the albumin concentration is low, there is less bound, nonionized calcium; therefore, the total calcium level is low. The ionized calcium level is minimally altered by the hypoalbuminemia and exists in its normal range, indicated by a corrected total serum calcium of 9.4; therefore, treating the patient with calcium supplementation could lead to hypercalcemia and its associated complications. Treatment should occur only if the patient becomes symptomatic or total serum calcium is significantly reduced beyond that accounted for by the decreased albumin.

6. **List the signs and symptoms of hypocalcemia and hypercalcemia.**

Hypocalcemia	Hypercalcemia
Muscle cramps	Anorexia
Paresthesias	Nausea, vomiting
Irritability, anxiety	Muscle weakness
Dysrhythmias (prolonged QT)	Lethargy, apathy
Carpopedal spasms	Confusion, depression
Laryngeal stridor	Dysrhythmias
Tetany	Polyuria, polydipsia
Positive Chvostek, Trousseau signs	

7. **Complications are common in acute pancreatitis. Explain the reason for frequent complications and give the common examples.**
    The pancreas lies almost totally in the retroperitoneum. The lack of encapsulation promotes the free spread of the inflammatory process to many of the adjacent organs, including the duodenum, common bile duct, diaphragm, mesenteric vasculature, small and large bowel, and posterior mediastinum. The liberation of various metabolites and vasoactive substances from the damaged pancreas causes further damage to these organs and systems. Complications of acute pancreatitis include:

Pseudocyst
Hypocalcemia
Fistulas
Pleural effusion
ARDS
Abscess
Peritonitis
Acute renal failure
Septicemia
Mesenteric thrombosis

8. **On day 4, Mr. Petty's PaO$_2$ falls to 50 mm Hg without evidence of parenchymal changes on chest x-ray. Severe progressive hypoxemia develops over the next 48 hr with diffuse pulmonary infiltrates now present on chest x-ray. A diagnosis of ARDS is made. What is the initial cause of the hypoxemia? What is the suspected mechanism for the ensuing development of ARDS?**

The initial hypoxemia is caused by a $\dot{V}/\dot{Q}$ mismatch. The early hypoxemia is related to the presence of microthrombi in the pulmonary circulation, secondary to the circulating toxins and vasoactive substances released from the damaged pancreas. Loss of blood flow to portions of the pulmonary vasculature and overperfusion of the nonembolized areas of the lung precipitates the $\dot{V}/\dot{Q}$ mismatch and hypoxemia. Pleural effusion may also contribute to the development of the hypoxemia.

The development of ARDS becomes more common as the severity of the attack increases. The normal pathophysiology of ARDS is demonstrated, including loss of alveolocapillary integrity, increased microvascular permeability, interstitial and intraalveolar edema, and progressive alveolar collapse. Many of the circulating mediators seen in acute pancreatitis have been implicated in the pathogenesis of ARDS, specifically phospholipase A and high concentrations of free fatty acids. Cellular membranes and pulmonary surfactant, a phospholipid, may both be damaged by these compounds.

9. **On day 10, Mr. Petty's amylase remains elevated, so he undergoes follow-up ultrasonography. A pseudocyst is discovered. What is a pseudocyst? What nursing interventions are important in caring for a patient with this local complication of acute pancreatitis?**

A pseudocyst is a collection of fluid, tissue, and necrotic debris surrounded by a nonepithelial-lined wall. The wall is commonly necrotic granulation tissue, which may eventually become fibrotic or "mature." The pseudocyst may continue to grow, especially if a connection with the pancreatic duct exists. Since a pseudocyst will often resolve spontaneously within 6 weeks, surgical intervention is often postponed unless a complication occurs. Besides awaiting potential spontaneous resolution, drainage is also delayed to allow the pseudocyst wall time to mature. The mature pseudocyst is more easily drained and develops fewer complications postoperatively.

Because actual intervention is often postponed, the nurse at the bedside must continually monitor the patient for signs and symptoms of pseudocyst complications, including rupture, hemorrhage, obstruction, and infection. Clinical indicators of complications include:

Fever
Leukocytosis
Elevated amylase
Sudden epigastric pain
Hemodynamic instability
GI bleeding
Nausea/vomiting
Sudden diarrhea
Respiratory distress
Paralytic ileus
Jaundice
Decrease in LOC

10. What is the normal serum amylase level? What is the significance of the amylase level in acute pancreatitis?

Normal serum amylase is 25–125 U/liter. Amylase, one of the digestive enzymes secreted by the pancreas, becomes elevated if damage to the pancreas occurs. While a patient with acute pancreatitis may show a level 3–5 times above normal, the magnitude of the increase is not directly correlated with the severity of the disease. Other factors, such as length of time since onset and previous pancreatic damage, may affect the values seen on admission.

The return of the amylase to normal levels is also not an accurate guide to the degree of recovery from the attack. Amylase levels may also be elevated in other clinical syndromes; therefore, the use of amylase as a diagnostic criterion must be used in tandem with other components of the clinical picture, such as physical findings, ultrasonography, and computed tomography.

11. What therapeutic modalities are used in the treatment of acute pancreatitis?

While new therapeutic agents such as enzyme inhibitors have come on the scene in recent years, none have proven significantly effective in controlled clinical trials, so supportive management remains the hallmark of the treatment regimen in acute pancreatitis. The focus of care remains on correcting the initiating factors, prompt fluid resuscitation, pain control, and suppression of pancreatic secretion. Administration of fluids, both crystalloid and colloid, hemodynamic monitoring, and frequent assessment of laboratory values are crucial. The patient is made NPO in an attempt to decrease pancreatic activity. A nasogastric tube may be inserted if severe nausea and vomiting, gastric distention, or paralytic ileus are present.

Peritoneal lavage has recently been promoted to aid in removal of necrotic debris and activated enzymes from the peritoneal cavity. The procedure has been shown to decrease the incidence and severity of cardiovascular and pulmonary complications, but not the progression of the pancreatitis itself.

Nursing assessment focuses on hemodynamic monitoring, identification of developing complications, and assessment of the effectiveness of the therapeutic regimen, including pain control and restoration of electrolyte balance. Surgical intervention may be required if the diagnosis is unclear, life-threatening complications occur, or severe necrosis is suspected.

12. Mr. Petty is complaining of severe epigastric pain. What is the drug of choice in treating pain in acute pancreatitis and why?

Meperidine is the usual choice of pain medication in acute pancreatitis because it is thought to cause less spasm of the sphincter of Oddi and smooth muscle of the pancreatic and biliary ducts. The sphincter of Oddi is situated at the terminal end of the common bile duct and controls the emptying of bile and pancreatic juices into the duodenum. Other narcotics are thought to cause an increased incidence of spasm in the sphincter, thus leading to increased reflux of bile and pancreatic fluids into the pancreas, further complications, and increased pain.

13. What nursing diagnoses apply in this case?

Fluid volume deficit related to fluid sequestration in tissues, emesis, NG suction, and diarrhea

Alteration in tissue perfusion related to decreased circulating volume, decreased vascular integrity, and inflammatory processes

Impaired gas exchange related to pleural effusion and ARDS

Pain related to inflammatory processes in the abdomen

Fear related to ICU environment and severity of illness

Alteration in nutrition: less than body requirements related to NPO status, high caloric needs secondary to infectious process, and protein catabolism

SUGGESTED READINGS

Adinaro D. Liver failure and pancreatitis: Fluid and electrolyte concerns. Nurs Clin North Am 1987;22(4):843–852.

Ammann R, Warshaw AL. Acute pancreatitis: Clinical aspects and medical and surgical management. In: Berk JE, ed. Bockus gastroenterology. 4th ed. Philadelphia: WB Saunders, 1985:3993–4019.

Barkin JS, Goldberg H, Bradley EL. Cysts and pseudocysts of the pancreas. In: Berk JE, ed. Bockus gastroenterology. 4th ed. Philadelphia: WB Saunders, 1985:4145–4157.

Creutzfeldt W, Lankisch PG. Acute pancreatitis: etiology and pathogenesis. In: Berk JE, ed. Bockus gastroenterology. 4th ed. Philadelphia: WB Saunders, 1985:3971–3992.

Kaldor PK. Pathophysiology and diagnosis of gastrointestinal problems. In: Kinney MR, Packa DR, Dunbar SB, eds. AACN's clinical reference for critical-care nursing. New York: McGraw-Hill, 1988:1340–1362.

Pak CY. Calcium disorders: Hypercalcemia and hypocalcemia. In: Kokko JP, Tannen RL, eds. Fluids and electrolytes. Philadelphia: WB Saunders, 1986:472–501.

Sabesin S. Countering the dangers of acute pancreatitis. Emerg Med 1987;19:70–96.

Soergel KH. Acute pancreatitis. In: Sleisenger MH, Fordtran JS, eds. Gastrointestinal disease: pathophysiology, diagnosis, management. 4th ed. Philadelphia: WB Saunders, 1988:1814–1842.

CHAPTER 46

Peritonitis

Barbara Hackett, RN, BSN, CCRN

John Wilson is a 45-year-old man who works on an assembly line at a defense plant. He presented to the Emergency Department complaining of severe midepigastric pain of 16 hr duration, which suddenly got much worse immediately prior to admission. He denied nausea and vomiting and stated that the pain got worse when he moved. His medical history included frequent episodes of epigastric pain that were relieved by eating or by drinking milk. He is also a cigarette smoker and has accrued a 60-pack/year history. He has never been hospitalized and has not seen a physician in over 5 years.

Physical assessment revealed a 45-year-old man who was in severe discomfort, lying very still on his back with his knees flexed, appearing hesitant to move. The abdomen was firm and rigid with rebound tenderness, which was worst in the midepigastrium. Bowel sounds were absent, and a rectal examination revealed guaiac-positive stool. Relevant clinical data included:

Vital Signs			Laboratory Values	
BP	118/70 (lying)	90/50 (sitting)	Creat	1.8
HR	118 (lying)	140 (sitting)	BUN	60
Resp	26		WBC	18,000
Temp	38°C		Amylase	130
			LFTs	Within normal limits

A 16-gauge intravenous catheter was inserted, and 1000 ml Ringer's lactate was started at the maximum rate. A Foley catheter was inserted and 150 ml of dark, concentrated urine was obtained. A CVP line was inserted in the right subclavian, with an initial reading of 3 cm H_2O. An NG tube was inserted, yielding dark green aspirate that was guaiac negative. A KUB was done, as was an upright chest x-ray, which showed free air under the diaphragm. There was no pneumothorax, and the central line was in good position.

Three liters of Ringer's lactate were infused over 90 min, with CVP values checked q 15 min along with frequent auscultation of the lungs. The urine output and orthostatic tilt were checked q 30 min.

When Mr. Wilson's urine output increased to 0.5 ml/kg/hr and his tilt was negative, he was given Ancef 2 gm IV piggyback and taken to the

Operating Room for an exploratory laparotomy. A perforated duodenal ulcer was diagnosed and repaired.

After a brief stay in the Recovery Room, Mr. Wilson was admitted to the Surgical ICU with a diagnosis of status post (S/P) perforated duodenal ulcer repair and peritonitis. He was awake and oriented but drowsy, and was receiving 40% oxygen via aerosol mask. Ringer's lactate was being infused at 150 ml/hr, his CVP was 8 cm H_2O, and his vital signs were stable, though he was febrile at 38.5°C. He had an NG tube in his left naris that was attached to low wall suction, and no bowel sounds were audible. A midline dressing was dry and intact. His laboratory results were basically unchanged from admission, except that his BUN had dropped from 60 to 34 mg/dl and his creatinine from 1.8 to 1.3 mg/dl.

QUESTIONS AND ANSWERS

1. **What is the peritoneum? How does the peritoneum help protect the body from infection?**

   The peritoneum is a semipermeable membrane that encloses the abdominal viscera and mesentery like a sac. The peritoneum secretes a small amount of fluid into the peritoneal cavity each day. This fluid reduces friction between the viscera during peristalsis.

   When the peritoneum is contaminated by chemicals or bacteria, it responds with localized vascular dilatation and increased capillary permeability. Polymorphonuclear leukocytes migrate into the peritoneal cavity, where they phagocytize bacteria and foreign material. A fibroplastic exudate is formed and serves to wall off the inflammation, preventing diffuse peritonitis. If the contamination is massive or prolonged, this protective mechanism fails, and diffuse peritonitis results.

2. **Mr. Wilson's postoperative diagnosis was S/P perforated duodenal ulcer and peritonitis. What is peritonitis, and what was the etiology of Mr. Wilson's peritonitis?**

   Peritonitis by definition is an inflammation of the peritoneum. It may be a local or a generalized process in an acute or chronic form. In acute peritonitis, peristalsis decreases or stops, fluid absorption from the distal small bowel and colon is impaired, and the intestinal lumen becomes distended with gas and fluid. Fluid accumulates in the peritoneal cavity due to the increased capillary permeability, causing severe volume depletion which is sometimes followed by cardiac and renal dysfunction. The etiology of the inflammation can be either chemical or bacterial. Chemical peritonitis is often the result of bile or pancreatic juices leaking into the peritoneum. Bacterial peritonitis can occur with the rupture of any abdominal organ or the gastrointestinal tract or following a penetrating abdominal wound.

Mr. Wilson's peritonitis was initially chemical, caused by the digestive juices of the duodenum spilling into the peritoneal cavity. A secondary bacterial peritonitis may develop due to the bacterial overgrowth of the contamination. The peritoneal cavity is very resistant to contamination, and unless overwhelming in quantity or duration, the response will remain localized with a resultant abscess formation. The mortality rate is high for any extensive peritonitis that is not treated aggressively within 72 hr. Other causes of bacterial peritonitis include:

Appendicitis
Perforated diverticulitis
Gangrenous gallbladder
Gangrenous obstruction of small bowel
Incarcerated hernia of small bowel
Perforated carcinoma
Foreign body
Ulcerative colitis

3. What are the clinical features of peritonitis?

Abdominal pain—location depends on cause and extent of inflammation
Abdominal distention
Nausea
Vomiting
Inability to pass flatus or feces
Hypotension
Tachycardia
Thirst
Oliguria
Fever

4. Why is Mr. Wilson's WBC count elevated?

The increased WBC count in peritonitis occurs secondary to mobilization of WBC in response to peritoneal irritation. There will primarily be a rise in polymorphonuclear leukocytes.

5. What is the likely explanation for Mr. Wilson's tachypnea?

Patients with peritonitis typically breathe in a rapid, shallow fashion to avoid pain caused by respiratory excursion.

6. What x-ray findings were significant in Mr. Wilson's case?

The presence of free air as seen best on the upright chest x-ray is of marked clinical significance because its presence indicates the rupture of an intraabdominal viscus. Dilated loops of small or large bowel are nonspecific findings in peritonitis and may indicate an ileus.

7. **What was the rationale for NG tube placement in Mr. Wilson's case?**

    Mr. Wilson had an ileus, as indicated by the absence of bowel sounds and his abdominal x-ray findings. As previously mentioned, gas and fluid accumulate in the GI tract of the patient with peritonitis. Mr. Wilson's NG tube was placed to decompress his stomach and help relieve his pain. It also provided access to his stomach contents so that they could be checked for blood. Mr. Wilson's gastric aspirate was guaiac negative.

8. **In the Emergency Department, Mr. Wilson demonstrated a positive orthostatic tilt test. How is this test done, and what does it mean?**

    This is a simple clinical test that involves checking the BP and heart rate first with the patient lying flat and then with the patient sitting up. If the BP falls by at least 10–20 mm systolic or the heart rate rises by 10–20 beats/min, the tilt test is positive, and it is likely that the patient is volume depleted.

9. **In addition to a positive tilt, what other parameters indicated that Mr. Wilson was volume depleted in the Emergency Department?**

    Mr. Wilson's resting heart rate, CVP, BUN, and scant, concentrated urine output indicated volume depletion. In a young, previously healthy person, the urine output is the best guideline for adequate fluid resuscitation. The surgeon will most likely use the urine output as the indicator of when the patient is adequately fluid resuscitated and ready to go to the Operating Room. Accurately measuring and recording the urine output is an essential nursing responsibility during fluid resuscitation and should be done at least every hour. Generally, 0.5–1.0 ml/kg (average of 30 ml/hr) is considered to be an adequate urine output.

10. **Why was Mr. Wilson's urine output decreased preoperatively?**

    Oliguria is a classical finding in peritonitis and results from intravascular volume depletion. As previously described, the failure of fluid reabsorption in the distal small bowel and colon along with third spacing of fluid in the peritoneal cavity significantly depletes the intravascular fluid volume. This decrease in preload reduces the cardiac output. Since 20% of the cardiac output passes through the renal arteries, there is a significant decrease in renal perfusion, and therefore the patient is predisposed to a prerenal form of renal failure. Mr. Wilson's volume depletion was appropriately treated with rapid administration of crystalloid solutions. Inotropes or vasopressors should not be used to treat hypotension until adequate intravascular volume is assured. Careful monitoring of fluid volume with appropriate replacement therapy continued to be a priority postoperatively.

11. **What was the significance of Mr. Wilson's creatinine of 1.8 and BUN of 60 preoperatively? Why did the BUN drop to 34 postoperatively?**

    Mr. Wilson's volume depletion resulted in a mild form of prerenal azotemia. Inadequate renal perfusion resulted in a mildly elevated creatinine and a significantly elevated BUN. This was most likely due to hypovolemia. In hypovolemic states, the underperfused kidney actively reabsorbs water, sodium, and BUN to restore plasma volume. The creatinine rises slightly due to a fall in glomerular filtration rather than active renal reabsorption of creatinine. The result is mild elevation in the serum creatinine and a larger elevation in the serum BUN. (For a more complete discussion see Chapter 34, "Prerenal Azotemia.") When Mr. Wilson's volume depletion was corrected, his BUN started returning toward normal.

12. **What was the significance of Mr Wilson's amylase of 130?**

    Pancreatitis and peritonitis have many of the same presenting symptoms, and pancreatitis is a cause of peritonitis. Amylase is an enzyme that is secreted primarily by the pancreas. Acute pancreatitis causes an elevated amylase. Since Mr. Wilson's amylase was within the normal range (25–125 U/liter), pancreatitis was ruled out.

13. **Once the free air was visualized on the upright chest x-ray, the decision was made to take Mr. Wilson to surgery as soon as he was adequately fluid resuscitated. Was administration of pain medication appropriate at this point?**

    Once the likely source of pain has been identified and the appropriate operative permit obtained, pain medication can be given. In Mr. Wilson's case, morphine sulfate at a dose of 2 mg was given via IV push and was repeated to a total of 8 mg over 30 min. The BP, heart rate, and respiratory rate were checked before and after each dose. The IM route should not be used in the volume-depleted patient, as the drug will be poorly absorbed. If there is any question as to the source of the pain, medication should be withheld to avoid masking the symptoms. In patients with peritonitis, the supine position with knees flexed may help ease the pain. Abdominal pain may occur as a result of the buildup of gastric contents. Therefore, the patency of the NG tube should be ensured, as should the function of the suction apparatus. In addition, emotional support and reassurance should be offered.

14. What nursing diagnoses apply in this case?

Altered nutrition: less than body requirements related to NPO status
Potential for infection related to altered skin integrity
Potential fluid volume deficit and decreased cardiac output related to hypovolemia, sepsis, or shock
Ineffective breathing pattern related to splinting
Impaired skin integrity related to intravascular lines and drains
Impaired verbal communication related to presence of endotracheal tube
Sleep pattern disturbance related to environment
Pain
Anxiety

SUGGESTED READINGS

Braunwald E, Isselbacher KJ, Petersdorf RG, Wilson JD, Martin JB, Fauci AS, eds. *Harrison's principles of internal medicine*. 11th ed. New York: McGraw-Hill, 1987.
Common causes of peritonitis. *Hospital Medicine*. 1983;19(4):121.
McCormack A, Itkin J, Cloud C. RN master care plan: if your patient develops peritonitis. RN 1987; 50(3):31–32.
Kaldor KK. Medical and Surgical Therapies for Gastrointestinal Problems. In: Kinney MR, Packa DR, Dunbar SB, eds. AACN's clinical reference for critical care nursing, 2nd ed. New York: McGraw-Hill, 1988:1370–1373.
Kaldor KK. Pathophysiology and diagnosis of gastrointestinal problems. In: Kinney MR, Packa DR, Dunbar, SB. AACN's clinical reference for critical care nursing, 2nd ed. New York: McGraw-Hill, 1988:1349–1351.
Swearingen PL, Sommers MS, Miller K. Manual of critical care applying nursing diagnoses to adult critical illness. St Louis: CV Mosby, 1988.

CHAPTER 47

Portal Hypertension with Upper GI Bleed

Virginia Byrn Huddleston, RN, MSN, CCRN

Jorge Garcia is a 48-year-old man who presents to the Emergency Department with a 3-day history of hematemesis. Both bright red blood and coffee-ground emesis are described. On initial assessment, Mr. Garcia is found to be neurologically intact. Auscultation of his chest reveals an audible S_1S_2, without murmur or gallop, and fine bibasilar rales. One-plus pitting edema is palpable in his lower extremities. His skin and sclera are markedly icteric, and spider angiomas are noted over a grossly distended, ascitic abdomen. He complains of "light-headedness" and demonstrates a positive tilt test. A CBC reveals a hematocrit of 10%. He is admitted to the ICU, where he undergoes placement of a central line into the right internal jugular vein and a left radial arterial line without incident. Initial hemodynamic parameters and laboratory values are:

Hemodynamic Parameters		Laboratory Values			
PAP	18/4	Na	136	Albumin	1.8
PAWP	1	K	3.0	Alk Phos	200
CVP	1	Gluc	65	PT	17
CO	6.2	Ca	6.8	PTT	32
SVR	813	Mg	1.0	AST	1100
BP	88/52	Hgb	3.1	SGPT	1000
HR	126	Hct	10	T. Bili	5.0

QUESTIONS AND ANSWERS

1. **List the sources and precipitating factors associated with upper gastrointestinal bleeding (UGIB).**

   Sources
   Peptic ulceration
   Gastric erosion
   Gastritis
   Esophageal varices
   Gastric varices
   Aortoenteric fistula
   Hemobilia
   Gastric malignancies
   Mallory-Weiss tear

415

Precipitating factors
   ↑ gastric acid secretion
   ↑ gastrin release
   ↓ gastric emptying
Inadequate acid buffering in duodenum
Genetic predisposition
Bile acid injury
Abnormal gastric motility
   ↑ ETOH intake
   ↑ aspirin intake
Corticosteroids
Nicotine
Trauma
Surgery
Shock
Frequent vomiting

Although the most frequent cause of UGIB is peptic ulceration of the duodenum, this patient population rarely requires ICU monitoring. Admissions to the ICU are more frequently associated with esophageal varices and the less common Mallory-Weiss tear.

2. Describe the pathophysiological mechanism involved in the development of portal hypertension and esophageal varices in alcoholic liver disease.

Two afferent vessels supply blood to the liver: the oxygen-rich hepatic artery and the portal vein, which drains the venous blood of the GI system (splanchnic organs) and spleen. Both afferent vessels deliver blood through their terminal branches to the liver sinusoids and then on to the hepatic vein, which drains into the inferior vena cava. Obstruction to flow at any site along the above pathway can precipitate portal hypertension. In alcoholic liver disease, resistance occurs in the sinusoids. Excessive alcohol intake and metabolism lead to an increased production of metabolic toxins. Hepatocyte damage and necrosis result, stimulating a fibroblastic response. Vascular anatomy is distorted by fibrosis, nodule formation, and the deposition of a basement membrane-like substance in the sinusoids (space of Disse).

As resistance increases in the sinusoidal vascular bed, portal venous pressure rises, veins proximal to the sinusoids dilate, and blood is shunted through naturally occurring portal systemic anastomoses. These anastomoses include the gastric veins in the lower esophagus, periumbilical veins in the anterior abdominal wall, and retroperitoneal veins draining the spleen, pancreas, and colon. Because the veins in the esophagus are located superficially and are exposed to the mechanical damage of ETOH intake and frequent vomiting, they are more likely to rupture than the other varices.

The development of portal HTN is both beneficial and detrimental to the patient. Portal HTN leads to the severe complications of variceal bleeding, splenomegaly, and ascites; yet maintenance of portal pressures greater than the increased sinusoidal resistance is necessary to sustain portal flow and hepatic function.

3. **Following saline lavage with an Ewald tube, diagnostic endoscopy reveals large esophageal varices 2–4 cm above the gastroesophageal junction. Sclerotherapy is then performed. What is the purpose of this treatment? What nursing interventions are important in caring for a patient undergoing this procedure?**

Endoscopic variceal sclerotherapy (EVS) is now the most common method of treatment in acute variceal hemorrhage. Chronic sclerotherapy may then be instituted to prevent further rebleeding.

The purpose of EVS is to sclerose (scar) the varix, thus halting or preventing further hemorrhage. Various sclerosants, including sodium morrhuate, sodium tetradecyl sulfate (STD), and ethanolamine, are used and may be injected into an intravariceal or paravariceal site.

Nursing interventions during the procedure include providing the patient with information concerning the procedure, positioning the patient, and administering sedation. The nurse also continuously observes the patient for any signs of distress during the procedure. The focus of care following the procedure includes assessing for further bleeding and monitoring for complications. Complications of EVS include:

> Dysphagia
> Aspiration
> Esophageal perforation
> Mediastinitis
> Substernal pain
> Mucosal ulcerations
> Esophageal strictures
> Septicemia

4. **Eight hours after sclerotherapy, Mr. Garcia has an episode of massive hematemesis. He becomes hemodynamically unstable, and his respirations become labored. A four-lumen esophagogastric (Minnesota) tube is inserted, and a continuous infusion of vasopressin (Pitressin) is**

begun at 0.4 units/min. What is the purpose of the esophagogastric tube? What complications is Mr. Garcia at risk for while the tube is in place?

The esophagogastric (Minnesota) tube is used in the treatment of gastric bleeding and bleeding esophageal varices. It has the following four lumens:

Gastric balloon
Esophageal balloon
Gastric aspirate lumen
Esophageal aspirate lumen

When the gastric and esophageal balloons are inflated, they create a tamponade effect. The gastric aspirate lumen is used to drain the stomach and give antacids. The esophageal aspirate lumen lies just above the esophageal balloon and is attached to suction to prevent aspiration of oropharyngeal secretions.

During placement of the esophagogastric tube, Mr. Garcia is most at risk for aspiration, asphyxiation, and esophageal rupture. Endotracheal intubation decreases the risk of aspiration and asphyxiation in the event of improper placement or upward migration of the gastric balloon. A stat chest x-ray should be taken to document proper placement of the tube before the balloon is fully inflated.

Once the tube is in place, Mr. Garcia remains at risk for numerous complications including aspiration, pain, esophageal rupture, and gastroesophageal junction injury. If the tube being used does not have an esophageal aspiration port (such as a Sengstaken-Blakemore tube), a Salem sump should be placed into the esophagus and attached to suction to prevent aspiration of blood from continued bleeding or mucus stimulated by the presence of the esophageal balloon.

Frequent checks are made of the esophageal balloon pressure by using a stopcock-mercury manometer setup. To prevent esophageal erosion or ulceration, pressures should not exceed 35–40 mm Hg. The balloon may also be deflated according to institutional protocol at standard intervals. Daily x-rays are taken to verify proper tube placement and assess for upward migration of the gastric balloon. Stabilization of the tube is of utmost importance to prevent this complication and is usually achieved by anchoring the tube to a helmet face mask or weight system. This system also provides a means of applying upward traction on the tube, thereby ensuring that the gastric balloon is pulled up against the gastroesophageal junction.

5. **Shortly after the vasopressin infusion is begun, Mr. Garcia begins complaining of chest pain. What is the mechanism of action of vasopressin? Why is chest pain a common complication?**

Vasopressin causes extensive vasoconstriction, especially of the splanchnic arteriolar system. It occurs naturally in the body as antidiuretic hormone (ADH), which is produced in minute quantities by the posterior pituitary.

By increasing mesenteric vascular resistance, portal venous blood flow (inflow) is reduced, and a concomitant decrease occurs in portal venous pressure and esophageal variceal pressure. Vasopressin is also thought to interact with other blood pressure–controlling systems (baroreceptors, renin-angiotensin axis, sympathetic nervous system, prostaglandins) to cause a fall in cardiac output secondary to a baroreflex.

Unfortunately, vasopressin has systemic effects that may lead to dangerous side effects. Myocardial ischemia and decreased coronary blood flow are not uncommon, and they are the most likely source of Mr. Garcia's chest pain. NTG is often used simultaneously with a vasopressin infusion to maximize coronary blood flow and perfusion. Nitrates have also been shown to lower portal pressures without compromising hepatic inflow.

6. **What other complications are associated with vasopressin infusion?**

Left ventricular failure secondary to decreased coronary and endocardial blood flow, decreased cardiac output, myocardial ischemia or infarction, and dysrhythmias

Abdominal cramping secondary to splanchnic vasoconstriction and mesenteric ischemia

Hyponatremia secondary to free water retention and antidiuretic action

Bradycardia secondary to reflex responses to hypertension

Hypertension secondary to systemic vasoconstriction

Care must be taken as the patient is weaned from the vasopressin infusion, because rebound effects are common. Hypotension may occur as the patient vasodilates or rebleeding occurs, so NTG is usually weaned at this time. A large diuresis may be noted as the circulating ADH returns to a physiological level. Electrolytes should be monitored closely, especially sodium and potassium.

Somatostatin has recently been acclaimed in the literature for its superiority to vasopressin. It is a peptide hormone with similar action to vasopressin (splanchnic vasoconstriction) but with fewer systemic side effects.

7. **Mr. Garcia is noted to have gross ascites (free fluid in the peritoneal space). Describe the mechanisms currently thought to cause the development of ascites.**

    The etiology and pathogenesis of ascites development are multifactorial and debatable. Because alcoholic cirrhosis often follows a long-term course before ascites eventually develops, alterations in many different processes (hormonal, cellular, nutritional, and hemodynamic) may affect both compartmental fluid sequestration and renal handling of sodium and water.

    As the cirrhotic process continues, extensive scarring and fibrosis induce further increases in hepatic congestion and vascular hydrostatic pressure. Normal Starling forces are overcome, and fluid extravasates into the hepatic interstitium. When the lymphatic drainage can no longer keep pace with the copious production of third-space fluid, ascites collects in the peritoneum.

    Since the hepatic sinusoid is already extremely permeable to plasma proteins, a minimal oncotic gradient exists, so changes in circulating plasma levels of albumin do not greatly affect the initial development of ascites. After the basement membrane material has been deposited in the later stages of the disease, an oncotic gradient is established. At this point, inadequate production of albumin by the failing liver enhances further fluid movement into the peritoneum, in accordance with Starling's law of capillary dynamics.

    The progression of ascites is potentiated by the renal retention of sodium and water as the kidney attempts to replace fluid losses into the peritoneum. Renal homeostatic mechanisms are also affected by circulating humoral substances not fully metabolized by the damaged liver, including aldosterone, catecholamines, angiotensin II, endotoxins, thromboxanes, and prostaglandins.

    Other researchers have also suggested that alterations in renal function may actually precede and initiate ascitic fluid accumulation. This "overflow" hypothesis attributes an expanding splanchnic venous bed and development of portal systemic collateral channels as the very early initiating factors of ascites formation.

8. **What complications are associated with ascites? What interventions are used to control or resolve ascitic fluid accumulation?**

    The presence of gross ascites indicates hepatic decompensation. The actual presence of large amounts of fluid in the peritoneal cavity increases portal pressure and the risk of variceal bleeding. Further alterations in effective circulating volume may initiate or exacerbate the hepatorenal syndrome. Pulmonary atelectasis, pleural effusion, and primary bacterial peritonitis may also result from ascites. The weight of the fluid on the inferior vena cava impedes venous return. Decreased cardiac output, continued activation of hormonal fluid homeostatic mechanisms, and peripheral edema result.

Treatment of ascites remains controversial. Decreased sodium intake and mild diuresis (usually with spironolactone) are the accepted standards at this time. A peritoneovenous (LeVeen) shunt is also recommended in selected cases to move ascitic fluid back into the vascular space. Iatrogenic complications are not uncommon with ascitic treatment. Vigorous diuresis can potentiate azotemia, hypokalemia, hyponatremia, and hepatic encephalopathy. Hypokalemic metabolic alkalosis favors ammonia toxicity. Complications associated with placement of a LeVeen shunt include coagulopathies, pulmonary edema, air embolism, sepsis, peritonitis, and occlusion. Clinical indicators of complications include:

↑ PT/PTT
↓ Fibrinogen
Frothy sputum
Chest pain
Leukocytosis
Abdominal guarding
Bleeding
Bibasilar rales
Shortness of breath
Fever
Hemodynamic instability
Reaccumulation of ascites

9. **Mr. Garcia is receiving magnesium citrate and lactulose via the gastric aspiration port of the tube. What is the action of each of these medications?**

Magnesium citrate aids in purging the bowel of blood and fecal matter. As blood in the gut is degraded, protein metabolites and ammonia are released and absorbed into the blood stream. This can lead to an accumulation of ammonia and other toxins in the plasma, thus increasing the risk of hepatic encephalopathy.

Lactulose reaches the colon from the upper GI tract essentially unchanged. Once in the colon, enteric bacteria metabolize the lactulose into a mixture of organic acids. The acidification of the colonic contents causes the reduction of ammonia (NH_3) to the less diffusible ammonium ion (NH_4^+). Unable to traverse the gut wall, the ammonium is trapped and further absorption is prevented. Since the colon is now more acidic than the blood, ammonia may diffuse from the circulation to the colon and also be converted to ammonium, thus reducing plasma ammonia levels even further. Lactulose also causes an increase in stool water content, so it enhances removal of blood and fecal matter by promoting stool elimination.

10. **On day 5, the esophagogastric tube is pulled and the vasopressin is weaned. Mr. Garcia shows no evidence of rebleeding after 3 days. A total portal systemic shunt procedure is scheduled. What is the benefit of the shunt procedure? List the common surgical shunts presently performed.**

The major benefit of a shunt procedure is variceal decompression to prevent a further UGIB. Total portal systemic shunts are classified into two categories, end-to-side and side-to-side. End-to-side shunts decompress the splanchnic bed but not the liver. This occurs because the venous blood from the splanchnic organs now bypasses the liver and drains into the low-pressure vena cava. The pressure is lowered in the naturally occurring anastomoses and collaterals, such as the esophageal veins. Blood circulating in the liver bed cannot be shunted, because the portal vein is ligated in end-to-side procedures; therefore, sinusoidal hypertension remains.

In the side-to-side shunts, including mesocaval, portorenal, side-to-side portocaval, central splenorenal, and mesorenal, the portal vein is left intact. Both the splanchnic and liver beds are decompressed, because blood that meets high-pressure resistance flowing via the portal vein into the liver can now be shunted into the vessel that is surgically anastomosed to the portal vein (side-to-side). This lowers pressure in the liver bed as well as the splanchnic vasculature.

Selective shunts such as the distal splenorenal (Warren) shunt aid in decompressing esophageal varices without greatly affecting the portal hypertension in the splanchnic and hepatic vasculature. This hypertension is necessary to maintain portal perfusion and hepatic function in the cirrhotic liver.

Controversy regarding the effectiveness of shunt procedures is found in the literature. Although elective shunt procedures offer much better survival rates than emergency shunt procedures, long-term survival rates do not seem to be greatly different between shunted and nonshunted patients. Although UGIB may recur less often in the shunted group, hepatic encephalopathy and progressive hepatic failure occur sooner and more frequently.

11. **On postoperative day 3, Mr. Garcia becomes increasingly disoriented and lethargic. His ammonia levels are elevated, and he begins to show evidence of coagulopathies. What is occurring and why?**

Mr. Garcia is showing classic signs of hepatic encephalopathy and progressive liver failure. Because of the total portal systemic shunt procedure, Mr. Garcia's liver is receiving less perfusion. Blood from the GI tract, containing high levels of amino acids and other circulating metabolites, is not reaching the liver for adequate metabolism and detoxification. Plasma proteins and clotting factors are not synthesized by the failing liver in sufficient quantities. Ammonia levels rise as amino acids are inadequately metabolized, and urea synthesis and excretion decrease. Neomycin, lactulose, and a restriction of dietary protein intake may be used to reduce the level of nitrogenous wastes in the plasma that are exacerbating the encephalopathy.

12. What nursing diagnoses apply in this case?

> Alteration in fluid volume: excess related to renal retention of sodium and water and increased levels of aldosterone, renin, angiotensin II, and catecholamines
> Decreased cardiac output related to decreased venous return secondary to ascites, myocardial ischemia secondary to vasopressin, and hemorrhage secondary to UGIB and coagulopathies
> Anxiety related to severity of condition and therapeutic modalites
> Alteration in fluid volume: deficit related to hemorrhage and ascites formation
> Alteration in nutrition: less than body requirements related to alterations in hepatic metabolism, NPO status, nausea, and vomiting

SUGGESTED READINGS

Blei AT, Ganger D, Fung HL, Groszman R. Organic nitrates in portal hypertension. Eur Heart J 1988;9(Suppl A):205–211.

Brown MW. Gastroesophageal varices: management of hemorrhage in the cirrhotic patient. Prim Care 1988;15:175–186.

Henderson JM, Warren WD. Portal hypertension. Curr Probl Surg 1988;25:149–223.

Lancaster JR. Upper gastrointestinal bleeding. Primary Care 1988;15:31–41.

Levy M. Pathophysiology of ascites formation. In: Epstein M, ed. The kidney in liver disease. 3rd ed. Baltimore: Williams & Wilkins, 1988:209–243.

Panes J, Teres J, Bosch J, Rodes J. Efficacy of balloon tamponade in treatment of bleeding gastric and esophageal varices. Results in 151 consecutive episodes. Dig Dis Sci 1988;33:454–459.

Solomon J, Harrington D, Gogel HK. When the patient suffers from esophageal bleeding. RN 1987;50(2):24–27.

CHAPTER 48

Small Bowel Obstruction

Mary K. Roberts, RN, MSN, CCRN

Jeremy Tower is a 70-year-old retired schoolteacher who lives in the country on 10 acres of property. He is a bachelor who has always enjoyed good health except for having an appendectomy at age 13 and a cholecystectomy at age 50. Mr. Tower was taking a walk when he gradually began experiencing intermittent periumbilical cramping pain. Attributing his discomfort to something he ate, Mr. Tower continued with his daily activities. By the time he went to bed, the pain had increased in intensity and severity. During the night, he developed nausea and he vomited twice. Convinced that he had a flu virus, Mr. Tower stayed in bed the next day. During the day, he became increasingly uncomfortable and passed a small amount of flatus and stool without relief. Thirty-six hr after the initial onset of pain, he presented to the Emergency Department of his community hospital.

Physical examination on admission to the hospital revealed pertinent findings limited to the abdomen. Abdominal distention was noted with marked tenderness to palpation in the periumbilical area and right lower quadrant. Bowel sounds were markedly hyperactive with peristaltic rushes, tinkling bowel sounds, and borborygmi. His vital signs on admission were:

BP	100/60
HR	110
Resp	16
Temp	37.8°C

An IV administration of normal saline was started at 100 ml/hr, and a central venous line was inserted to monitor his fluid status. A nasogastric tube was inserted and connected to low wall suction. A Foley catheter was also inserted and connected to a urimeter. He was admitted to the Surgical ICU for further evaluation. One hr after his admission, relevant clinical and laboratory data included:

Vital Signs		CBC	
BP	100/50	WBC	11,800
HR	115	Differential	Neutrophilia with increased
Resp	18		number of bands
Urine output	30 ml/hr	Hct	52
Nasogastric output	200 ml		
CVP	4		

424

Electrolytes

Na	132
K	3.4
Cl	95
BUN	22

The arterial blood gas analysis, urinalysis, AP chest film, and electrocardiogram were normal. Abdominal x-rays revealed dilated loops of small bowel with air-fluid levels and no colonic gas. A diagnosis of mechanical small bowel obstruction was made.

The IV rate was increased to 175 ml/hr, and 20 mEq of potassium chloride was added to each liter of normal saline. Mr. Tower was taken to surgery where an exploratory laparotomy revealed a strangulated loop of ileum due to adhesions from his previous abdominal surgeries. After lysis of the adhesions, Mr. Tower was readmitted to the Surgical ICU for monitoring and continued gastric decompression.

QUESTIONS AND ANSWERS

1. **Mr. Tower was diagnosed with mechanical intestinal obstruction. What does this mean?**

   Mechanical intestinal obstruction refers to a physical barrier that blocks the intestinal lumen. In Mr. Tower's case, surgical adhesions from his two previous abdominal operations formed fibrous bands on the outside of the bowel and led to luminal obstruction. Adhesive bands are the most frequent cause of obstruction.

   Other mechanisms of mechanical obstruction include:

   > Intussusception
   > Impactions
   > Lesions of the bowel
   > Regional enteritis
   > Diverticulitis
   > Chronic ulcerative colitis
   > Strangulated hernia
   > Neoplasms
   > Abscesses and hematomas
   > Volvulus

2. **What does the term *strangulated obstruction* mean?**

   Strangulated obstruction refers to occlusion of the blood supply to a segment of bowel in addition to obstruction of the bowel lumen. Interference with the blood supply may occur from distention. As distention increases, there is an increased intraluminal pressure that compromises the circulation to the bowel layers. Interference with mesenteric blood supply by the mechanism that produced the obstruction can also lead to impaired blood flow and strangulation.

Extravasation of bloody fluid into the bowel and bowel wall occurs as a consequence of blockage of venous outflow from the strangulated segment. This occurs most frequently secondary to adhesive band obstruction, hernia, and volvulus.

3. **What physical manifestations of small bowel obstruction does Mr. Tower exhibit?**

   Acute onset
   Intermittent, severe cramp-like periumbilical pain
   Markedly hyperactive bowel sound with peristaltic rushes and tinkling bowel sounds
   Small amount or absence of flatus and feces
   Nausea and vomiting
   Abdominal distention

   Pain in small bowel obstruction is often diffuse and poorly localized. In high bowel obstruction, it is usually felt across the upper abdomen. Obstruction at the level of the ileocecal valve usually accounts for pain in the area of the umbilicus. The lower the obstruction, the longer the period of time between attacks of pain.

   In an attempt to push bowel contents past the obstruction, peristalsis becomes violent, producing markedly hyperactive bowel sounds. The peristaltic rushes are heard simultaneously with abdominal cramping. Peristaltic waves may be visible and are accompanied by tinkling sounds. These tinkling sounds are emitted from tiny gas bubbles that break through the surface of obstructed intestinal juices.

4. **How do the symptoms of large bowel obstruction differ from the above?**

   Large bowel obstruction has a progressive onset with the patient complaining of mild, steady pain. Abdominal distention is less severe, and the patient will complain of complete constipation but little or no vomiting. Bowel sounds are lower in pitch and last longer.

   Because the colon has little or no absorptive and secretory functions, fluid and electrolyte imbalances occur only if obstruction is prolonged.

5. **What diagnostic finding in Mr. Tower's case was highly suggestive of small bowel obstruction?**

   In the normal adult, there is little or no air visible in the small bowel on x-ray. Therefore, the gas-fluid levels seen in the upright x-ray film of Mr. Tower's abdomen were highly suggestive of intestinal obstruction. Additional radiographic studies are sometimes indicated. These include barium enema and administration of a contrast medium by mouth or nasogastric tube.

6. **Mr. Tower's admitting WBC count shows leukocytosis with a shift to the left. What does this mean?**

   The phrase "shift to the left" describes an increase in the immature neutrophils, known as bands or stabs, in comparison to the normal percentage, which is about 5–10%. The phrase evolved because the table of cells used in determining the differential count of WBC indicates the bands toward the left of the table and mature forms of neutrophils toward the right. The term *neutrophilia* indicates an increase in the percentage of neutrophils and is usually accompanied by some degree of shift to the left in acute infections. In strangulated bowel obstruction, there is a rapid proliferation of intestinal bacteria. Continued strangulation decreases the arterial blood supply, resulting in necrosis. If strangulation is not corrected, toxic materials leak into the peritoneal cavity, which can lead to peritonitis and sepsis.

   Mr. Tower's elevated WBC count, neutrophilia, and increased immature forms indicate a shift to the left and strangulation of the bowel.

   The WBC count is helpful in identifying those patients with strangulation. Simple mechanical obstruction usually leads to only a modest increase in neutrophils with some shift to the left. If the obstruction is strangulated, WBC counts are frequently elevated between 15,000 and 25,000/mm^3 with an increase in immature forms that could be as much as 25%.

7. **What are the gastrointestinal alterations causing abdominal distention in mechanical obstruction?**

   Blockage of bowel lumen
   Pooling of fluids and accumulation of intestinal gases
   Secretion of water and electrolytes into the obstructed lumen
   Inhibited absorptive ability of intestinal mucosa
   Bowel wall becoming edematous
   Continued secretion of water and electrolytes into obstructed segment
   Further compromise in motility
   Distention of successive loops of bowel proximally

8. **What is the importance of the nasogastric tube in Mr. Tower's preoperative and postoperative care?**

   The nasogastric tube is inserted preoperatively to empty and decompress the stomach. This minimizes the risk of aspiration and progression of abdominal distention from air swallowing. Decompression of the gastrointestinal tract is of primary importance in Mr. Tower's postoperative care. Normal bowel function will be delayed up to several days after the intestinal obstruction is released. The nasogastric tube will be maintained on low suction, and the tube must be kept patent. If the tube is accidentally pulled out, it must be replaced without delay. Once gastrointestinal motility is resumed, the nasogastric tube may be removed.

9. **What is the primary concern in the management of the patient with small bowel obstruction?**

Fluid and electrolyte balance is the primary concern in the preoperative as well as postoperative management of the patient with small bowel obstruction. Fluid and electrolyte exchange occurs through absorption and secretion processes across the small bowel mucosa. Normally, approximately 8 liters of electrolyte-rich fluid are delivered to the bowel per day. This fluid, consisting of saliva, gastric and intestinal juices, and biliary and pancreatic secretions, is mostly reabsorbed by the time it reaches the colon.

The abdominal distention that occurs in bowel obstruction alters the capacity of the small bowel to absorb this fluid, which leads to fluid and electrolyte loss.

A second factor contributing to fluid and electrolyte loss is an increase in intestinal secretions. This process is stimulated by the progressive distention and decreased absorption by the intestine.

A third and very important factor causing fluid and electrolyte depletion is third spacing of fluid through the bowel wall into the peritoneal cavity. Increased pressure within the distended bowel causes fluid to pass through the wall into the peritoneal cavity. The fluid sequestered in the peritoneal cavity is considered "third-space" fluid because it is physiologically unavailable to the circulation.

Finally, fluid and electrolytes can also be lost by vomiting or nasogastric suction. Considering all of these mechanisms, it is not uncommon for as much as 6 liters of extracellular fluid to be lost within 2 or 3 days following simple mechanical obstruction of the small bowel.

10. **What does Mr. Tower's hematocrit of 54% indicate about his fluid balance?**

The hematocrit expresses the volume percentage of red blood cells in whole blood. In bowel obstruction, the profound fluid loss leads to hemoconcentration and hypovolemia. The hematocrit rises roughly in proportion to the fluid loss and is therefore a reflection of the degree of hypovolemia.

11. **What other preoperative clinical findings indicate hypovolemia in Mr. Tower's case?**

The clinical indicators of hypovolemia and physiological explanation for each include:

> Tachycardia—decreased preload, resulting in decreased stroke volume, and heart rate increasing as a compensatory mechanism to maintain CO
>
> Decreased CVP—decreased right heart filling pressure
>
> Oliguria—decreased effective intravascular volume leading to decreased glomerulofiltration and oliguria
>
> Increased BUN—elevated due to dehydration and decreased renal perfusion

Restoring fluid balance is an important and challenging goal in managing bowel obstruction. Immediately following surgical correction of the obstruction, there is a large third space of sequestered fluid in the peritoneal cavity. Fluid replacement is essential to prevent hypovolemia and possibly even hypovolemic shock. Postoperatively, after a variable period, fluid moves back into the vascular compartment from the third space. Continual close monitoring of fluid balance is necessary to avoid volume overload. The CVP is the best index of the adequacy of volume replacement, with 4–6 mm Hg being the usual goal. Other indicators of adequate fluid replacement would include urine output of at least 0.5 ml/kg/hr, normal heart rate, and normal BUN and Hct values.

12. **What is the clinical significance of Mr. Tower's electrolyte values?**

Water can move across the intestinal wall through both secretion and absorption. The absorption of water is associated with the digestion of food materials. The chyme within the duodenum is brought to isotonicity by the secretion or absorption of water. Sodium can also move across the intestinal wall in both directions. Absorption of sodium occurs primarily in the jejunum. Potassium shows a net absorption in the small intestine. Chloride movement passively follows that of potassium in the duodenum and jejunum. Bicarbonate is both secreted and absorbed throughout the small intestine. In the large intestine, active absorption of chloride and active secretion of bicarbonate ions occur.

Mr. Tower exhibits hyponatremia, hypokalemia, and hypochloremia. These electrolytes are primarily absorbed and secreted in the small intestine. The three major factors contributing to his electrolyte depletion include vomiting, nasogastric suction, and third-space fluid accumulation. These factors lead to a loss of serum electrolytes.

Since Mr. Tower does exhibit a volume deficit, replacement of sodium can be accomplished through the intravenous administration of normal saline. Hypokalemia is associated with muscle weakness, dysrhythmias, and ECG changes, including flattened T-wave and depressed ST segments. The patient should be closely monitored for any symptoms. Until adequate urinary output is established, potassium must be given with extreme caution. Normal levels of sodium and potassium are also important to the gastrointestinal system. A deficit in either or both of these ions may result in prolonged paralysis of the gastrointestinal tract postoperatively. Chloride losses are often associated with sodium and potassium losses and are minimized by isotonic fluid replacement and the increased absorptive ability of the intestines after obstruction is removed.

13. **What acid-base imbalance might be present in the patient with bowel obstruction?**

    The acid-base disturbance that a patient might manifest depends heavily on the level of obstruction and the proportion of gastric juice, bile, or pancreatic juice lost by vomiting.

    A metabolic alkalosis can result from a very high obstruction if highly acid gastric juice is initially lost through vomiting.

    A metabolic acidosis is most common and occurs if the obstruction is near the lower end of the small intestine. Fecal material that is highly alkaline is eventually vomited, which leads to the loss of base.

14. **What is the nonoperative approach for small bowel obstruction?**

    In small bowel obstruction, an intestinal tube may be inserted to decompress the bowel and relieve obstruction. This is a controversial nonoperative treatment and is used only in mechanical obstruction, when there is no clinical evidence of strangulation. The double-lumen Miller-Abbott nasointestinal tube is most commonly used and has been successful in treating small bowel obstructions caused by adhesions. One lumen contains a soft rubber balloon, and the other is for suctioning. A mercury tip helps move the tube downward through the GI tract. Patients with this diagnosis may have already had previous surgery for lysis of adhesions. The function of this tube is decompression of the small bowel with subsequent relief of edema and return of intestinal peristalsis.

15. **What nursing diagnoses apply in this case?**

    Fluid deficit related to third spacing of sequestered fluid
    Alteration in comfort related to abdominal pain

Potential for impaired gas exchange related to shallow breathing secondary to abdominal distention and guarding

Anxiety related to hospitalization related to acute onset of illness

SUGGESTED READINGS

Broadwell DC. Gastrointestinal system. In: Thompson J, McFarland G, Hirsch J, Tucker S, Bowers A, eds. Clinical nursing. St Louis: CV Mosby, 1986.

Cargile N. Buying time when you face a bowel obstruction. RN 1985;48:August 40–44.

Greenberger NJ. Gastrointestinal disorders: a pathophysiologic approach. 3rd ed. Chicago: Year Book Medical Publishers, 1986.

Guyton AC. Textbook of medical physiology. 2nd ed. Philadelphia: WB Saunders, 1986.

McConnell EA. Meeting the challenge of intestinal obstruction. Nursing 87 1987; 17(7):34–41.

Schwartz SI, Storer EH. Manifestations of gastrointestinal disease. In: Schwartz SI, Shires GT, Spencer FC, Storer EH, eds. Principles of surgery. New York: McGraw-Hill, 1984:1021–1063.

Wolfson PJ, Bauer JJ, Gelernt IM, Kreel I, Cuifses AH. Use of the long tube in management of patients with small-intestinal obstruction due to adhesions. Arch Surg 1985;120:1001–1006.

Part VII

Multisystem Involvement

CHAPTER 49

Acquired Immune Deficiency Syndrome

Susan L. Oskins, RN, MS, CCRN, CS

Alan Hall is a 35-year-old man who presented to the Emergency Department complaining of severe shortness of breath and diffuse chest discomfort on deep inspiration. Two days prior to this admission, he had been to his private physician complaining of abdominal discomfort, nausea, vomiting, watery diarrhea, a recent weight loss of 10 pounds in 3 weeks, and chest pain. He was started on oral antibiotics, but his GI upset continued and his respiratory condition worsened, prompting him to seek help at the Emergency Department.

On admission, Mr. Hall's pulmonary assessment revealed equal breath sounds with inspiratory and expiratory wheezes but no crackles. His abdomen was very tender to palpation in the midepigastric area, and he had hyperactive bowel sounds. Vital signs included:

BP	130/78
HR	124
Resp	36 and labored
Temp	102.5°F

His medical history included a stab wound to the chest in 1984, requiring multiple blood transfusions. His psychosocial history indicated that he was a single, heterosexual male with multiple sex partners. He admitted to occasional use of marijuana, but denied intravenous drug use. He denied ever having had homosexual relations.

Mr. Hall was admitted to the general medical unit with a diagnosis of pneumonia and dehydration. The initial medical treatment plan included IV hydration; antibiotics; diagnostic cultures of blood, stool, sputum, and urine; oxygen therapy; and respiratory isolation. Despite this treatment, Mr. Hall's condition deteriorated over the next 24 hr. He developed sepsis and acute respiratory failure and was transferred to the Respiratory ICU.

In the ICU, Mr. Hall's severe hypoxemia was initially treated with high levels of oxygen per mask (80–100%) alternating every 2 hr with CPAP mask at 7.5 cm H_2O pressure. Due to extreme fatigue and ensuing total respiratory failure, he was intubated and treated with mechanical ventilation and PEEP. Clinical and laboratory data revealed significant immune dysfunction and uncontrolled sepsis. Bronchoscopy confirmed *Pneumocystis carinii* pneumonia (PCP). Oral and esophageal candidiasis was diagnosed and treated with nystatin and ketoconazole. Bactrim was used to treat the protozoal pneumonia, with Zinacef and erythromycin IV for antibacterial prophylaxis. Severe protein malnutrition was treated with TPN IV per central line.

After several days of aggressive treatment, Mr. Hall was weaned from the ventilator, extubated, and transferred to the medical floor receiving O_2 per nasal cannula. T- and B-cell laboratory analysis demonstrated a significant pattern of immune deficiency. Both HIV and Western blot tests were positive. Anergy panel and skin testing showed total lack of response. Opportunistic diseases of PCP and *Candida* were being treated. Mr. Hall was diagnosed with acquired immune deficiency syndrome (AIDS). After a full 2 weeks of IV Bactrim, Mr. Hall was weaned from oxygen and discharged. AZT therapy was begun 2 weeks later on an outpatient basis.

Significant Clinical and Laboratory Data

Blood Cell Count

Day:	3	6	9	13	16	Normal	Units
Hgb	10.7	10.5	12.5	12.9	12.6	13.5–17.5	gm/dl
Hct	31.3	30.9	36.7	28.4	38.8	41–53	%
ABS Lymph	0.7	0.5	0.4	0.5		2.7–3.3	K
ABS Mono	0.1	0.1	0.2	0.5		0.2–0.4	K
ABS Grans	11.3	3.8	0.2	4.9		3.9–4.7	K
Grans	93	87	91	84	71	50–70	%
Lymph	6	11	6	6.8	20	25–45	%
Mono	1	2	3	8	9	3–5	%
RBC	3.46	3.4	4.08	4.23	4.25	4.5–5.9	millions/mm^3
WBC	12.1	4.4	6.4	5.8	3.5	4.5–11.5	$\times 10^3$ cells/mm^3

Routine Chemistry

Day:	4	16	Normal	Units
NA	135	133	136–146	mEq/liter
K	3.4	4.7	3.5–5.1	mEq/liter
Cl	97	100	98–106	mEq/liter
CO_2	29	26	23–29	mEq/liter
Gluc	124	139	70–105	mg/dl
Creat	0.8	1.1	0.6–1.2	mg/dl
Albumin	1.7	2.6	3.5–5.0	gm/dl
BUN	4	9	7–18	mg/dl
Total protein	4.6	6.3	6.4–8.3	gm/dl

Microbiology

Day:	2	2	4	5	6
Specimen	Serum	Serum	Stool	Stool	Bronchial washings/lavage
Culture	HIV+	Western blot+	Light Yeast	Moderate Yeast	Negative AFB and Gram stain. Fungal positive for *Candida*. Silver stain positive for *Pneumocystis carnii* and yeast.

ABGs

Day:	1	2	3	5	6	10
pH	7.45	7.4	7.49	.5	7.48	7.46
$PaCO_2$	22	36	31	29	28	33
PaO_2	49	49	43	152	93	85
SaO_2	89%	84%	83%	99%	97%	96%
HCO_3	19	22	24	25	20	23
Mode				A/C	A/C	
Rate per vent				16	16	
FIO_2	0.21	0.5	1.0	1.0	0.5	0.5
Tidal volume				900	900	
PEEP				14	12	

Bronchoscopy

Day 6: Relatively normal bronchoscopy except for extensive thick mucoid secretions. Clinically patient has bilateral pneumonia. Studies pending.

Radiology/Chest X-Rays

Day:	2	5
CXR:	Minimal LLL infiltrate	Bilateral "ground glass" infiltrate
Day:	6	9
CXR:	ET/NG in place; bilateral pleural effusions	Lungs clear

Vital Signs

Day:	1	2	3	4	5	9	13
BP:	130/60	120/70	130/80	150/80	110/72	118/70	120/60
HR:	120	90	112	112	112	80	80
Temp:	101–103	99–103	100–103	100–102	100	98–99	98–102

Laboratory/Miscellaneous Immunology

T- and B-cell enumeration	(day 9)	Normal range
Total lymphocyte count	410	1000–4800 cells/mm^2
Absolute B-cell	98	70–816 cells/mm^2
Absolute T-cell	205	750–4368 cells/mm^2
Helper: suppressor ratio	0.07	1.3–2.7

QUESTIONS AND ANSWERS

1. What is AIDS?

In 1981, acquired immune deficiency syndrome (AIDS) was introduced as the descriptive term for an immune deficiency syndrome that was transmissible. Persons who were previously immunocompetent were noted to have diseases that were typically seen only in persons who were congenitally immunodeficient, receiving immunosuppressive therapy, or suffering from a disease known to be associated with immunosuppression, such as Hodgkin's lymphoma. Persons with AIDS and other immunodeficiency states are vulnerable to specific infections to which the immunocompetent individual is normally immune. Such infections are termed opportunistic and may be deadly to the immunosuppressed person who has AIDS. AIDS is an infectious disease transmitted via contact with body fluids, blood, or blood products. At this time, there is no cure for the immunodeficiency, but the opportunistic diseases can be identified and treated. Although patient mortality is high, AIDS is now considered a chronic, often progressive infection that requires long-term monitoring and treatment.

2. What causes AIDS?

AIDS is caused by a retrovirus called human immunodeficiency virus (HIV). While the usual mechanism of cellular genetic information processing is from DNA to RNA to protein, the retrovirus is able to reverse the process and make itself into a piece of DNA of the affected cell. The particular cell affected by the HIV virus is the T-lymphocyte, which normally coordinates the immune response.

3. How does AIDS affect the normal immune response?

Two types of immunity are recognized: (*a*) innate or natural and (*b*) acquired.

Innate or natural immunity is the inherent capacity of the body to resist invasion by foreign agents and includes the following:

The resistance of the skin to penetration by microorganisms
The secretion of acid by the stomach, which destroys many foreign
substances

The phagocytic capacity of leuokocytes and macrophages

The presence of natural antibodies and interferon substances, adding resistance to disease

Acquired immunity is the more specific capacity of the body to identify a substance as foreign (antigen). This type of immunity involves the following:

The development of antibodies toward these substances (humoral immunity)

The formation of blood lymphocytes to bind and destroy foreign substances (cellular immunity)

Interferon formation to inactivate viruses

Humoral immunity is brought about by the B-lymphocytes, and cellular immunity is accomplished by the T-lymphocytes. HIV retrovirus integrates itself primarily into the DNA cellular structure of the T4-lymphocyte. Upon stimulation of the infected T4-cell, the HIV virus replicates into other T4-cells. As the HIV virus continues to inactivate and destroy more T4-cells, the ratio of helper (T4-lymphocytes) to suppressor (T8-lymphocytes) becomes unbalanced, resulting in an inverted T4 : T8 or H : S ratio. The T8-suppressor cells inhibit any further B-cell production or activity and inhibit further T-cell production.

If the acquired immune system is damaged (such as in AIDS), the individual is susceptible to infections by viruses, parasites, and fungi. Lacking sufficient acquired immunity, the immune system does not recognize these antigens and the invading organisms overwhelm their host (opportunistic diseases). Normally, these organisms pose no threat to an immunocompetent individual.

4. **What type of activities are considered as high risk for contracting AIDS?**

The HIV virus that causes AIDS is passed from person to person through body secretions, such as semen and blood. The most common means of transmission are: (*a*) sexual contact involving the exchange of body fluids and (*b*) blood-to-blood contact through shared needles. AIDS is not transmitted through casual contact.

Persons highly susceptible for AIDS are those with any history of the following:

Male-to-male or bisexual activity with a high number of sexual partners

Intravenous drug use with needle sharing

Transfusion of blood or blood products, especially up to the spring of 1985 when universal screening of blood for HIV began

5. What factors in Mr. Hall's history put him at risk for AIDS?

Mr. Hall received blood in 1984 when HIV screening of blood was not routinely done, and he was promiscuous in his sexual behavior, having had many sexual partners whose sexual histories were unknown to him.

6. What tests are used to screen for HIV infection?

Two tests are used for screening: ELISA and the Western blot. These tests are used to detect the presence of antibodies elicited by the antigen-antibody reaction following exposure to HIV.

A wide range of incubation periods have been discussed concerning AIDS. The mean incubation period is 4.5 years. However, the length of time between the exposure to the virus and antibody conversion may be as short as 2 weeks. In 1985, a screening test, the enzyme-linked immunosorbent assay (ELISA) was distributed nationwide to screen all blood and blood products for the HIV antibody.

Because the ELISA (HIV antibody test) was developed to protect the blood supply, the cutoff between reactive and nonreactive values was set very low to capture all true positives. There is the possibility of false positives with this examination. When a positive result is obtained, it is necessary to repeat the ELISA. In patients with two positive ELISA results, the Western blot is conducted on the same or a new blood sample for confirmation of antibody reactivity.

7. What clinical indicators classified Mr. Hall as having AIDS, rather than ARC or just being HIV positive?

AIDS and ARC present with certain common patterns of subjective and objective data. Chief complaints frequently include a history of weeks to months of fatigue, feelings of general malaise, and low-grade fevers. The patient relates fever beginning in the afternoon and peaking in the evening, which finally breaks in the night, known as night sweats. Swollen lymph nodes in the neck or axillae are significant if over 1 cm in size. Weight loss of greater than 10% of baseline weight is seen. Patients may describe an upper respiratory infection occurring weeks before, but lingering on with a persistent dry cough and mild but progressive shortness of breath. Other patients report persistent diarrhea despite treatment. Episodes of oral thrush and herpes simplex or zoster are common. A variety of skin rashes or skin color change may be noted. The patient may also complain of headaches, stiff neck, confusion, or lack of ability to concentrate and short-term memory loss.

Persons with symptoms and signs suggestive of HIV infection, but without having an AIDS indicator disease, are said to have AIDS-related complex (ARC). The most common ARC symptoms are persistent generalized lymphadenopathy, idiopathic thrombocytopenic purpura, oral candidiasis, hairy leukoplakia, and flu-like syndrome.

The HIV antibody test shows if a person has made antibodies to HIV, thus indicating previous exposure. The test result (positive or negative) does not tell:

> If someone has AIDS or ARC
> If someone will develop AIDS or ARC in the future
> If someone is immune to AIDS or ARC

A positive test result simply indicates that antibodies to HIV are present in the blood, meaning that the individual has been infected with HIV and has produced antibodies. People with HIV antibodies have active virus in their bodies, and thus are contagious and capable of passing the virus on to others.

Mr. Hall's objective data fully met the criteria for AIDS with the following:

> Positive laboratory evidence of HIV infection (both with the ELISA and Western blot tests)
> PCP confirmed per silver stain with bronchoscopy
> Disseminated *Candida* identified in serum, bronchial washings, and stool culture
> Lymphocytopenia, leukocytopenia, anemia, inverted helper: suppressor lymphocyte ratio, and protein malnutrition

8. Of what significance is PCP in the immunosuppressed AIDS patient?

Organisms that are relatively nonvirulent to immunocompetent persons can cause severe, persistent, and life-threatening infections in AIDS. Pneumonia caused by PCP is the most common life-threatening illness in persons with AIDS.

9. How did the pulmonary diagnostics and Mr. Hall's symptoms indicate the need for transfer to the ICU?

The primary insult of PCP infection occurs in the alveolar wall, causing the alveolar spaces to fill with foamy protein exudate. The effects include intrapulmonary shunting, hypoxemia, and reduced lung compliance, with a clinical picture consistent with the adult respiratory distress syndrome (ARDS).

On admission, Mr. Hall had the usual symptoms of pneumonia with fever, dyspnea, and chest pain. Chest x-ray demonstrated minimal infiltration in the left lower lobe. Vital signs were essentially stable except for a fever of 103°F. Oxygen was required for treatment of hypoxemia.

As the PCP progressed, Mr. Hall developed refractory hypoxemia, and his chest x-ray revealed diffuse, bilateral pulmonary edema and bilateral pleural effusions. In such a life-threatening state, Mr. Hall required intensive care and aggressive respiratory treatment including intubation, mechanical ventilation, and PEEP therapy.

10. Which particular medical interventions in Mr. Hall's case were taken to ensure a successful outcome in the ICU?

Prior to ICU admission, Mr. Hall's permission was obtained for the ELISA and Western blot to be performed. These examinations were positive for presence of the HIV antibody. A fiberoptic bronchoscopy with a bronchoalveolar lavage was planned to rule out PCP as soon as the patient's condition permitted. Mr. Hall was given bolus doses of IV trimethoprim and sulfamethoxazole (Bactrim) followed by IV piggyback maintenance doses q 6 hr.

Upon entry into the ICU, Mr. Hall's noncardiogenic pulmonary edema was treated with continuous positive airway pressure (CPAP) at 7.5 cm H_2O per mask q 2 hr at 80% O_2 alternating with 100% oxygen per mask q 2 hr. Finally, Mr. Hall's ABGs revealed severe, refractory hypoxemia and he demonstrated signs and symptoms of overall respiratory muscle fatigue, requiring intubation and mechanical ventilation using PEEP up to 14 cm H_2O.

Fiberoptic bronchoscopy is the "gold" standard for diagnosis of PCP. This was performed and PCP was confirmed by culture and bronchial washings. Bactrim dosage was then increased and IV administration was maintained over a 14-day period. *Candida albicans* was also found in the bronchial washings, stool, and sputum cultures. Oral and esophageal candidiasis was treated with oral nystatin and ketoconazole. The opportunistic diseases were thus treated and controlled, as was the resultant life-threatening respiratory failure.

Mr. Hall's levels of albumin and total protein were low. With the high levels of stress, increased metabolism from sepsis and fever, and the GI distress from *Candida,* Mr. Hall required total parenteral nutrition. Any further muscle wasting was prevented and Mr. Hall's energy requirements were met.

If Bactrim had not been successful in controlling the PCP within 3–4 days, IV pentamidine isothionate would have been prescribed. A high incidence of drug toxicity has been seen for both drugs. Leukopenia, hepatic dysfunction, electrolyte and glucose imbalances, renal impairment, and severe skin rashes are some of the signs of toxicity. Other adverse reactions during drug therapy include hypotension, nausea and vomiting, phlebitis, distressing taste sensations, and mouth sores. Aerosol pentamidine is used to provide prophylaxis against repeat episodes of PCP.

11. How much risk is there of an ICU nurse getting AIDS from a critically ill AIDS patient?

The risk of acquiring AIDS from a patient is quite low. Only through improper handling of blood and body fluids by the health care worker does the possibility of AIDS transmission develop. Risk increases without the use of gloves in handling blood and body fluids of *all* patients, but especially by having any direct exposure of broken skin to HIV-positive body fluids.

The risk of acquiring HIV infection in health care–related activities is less than 1% at a 95% confidence level. Several research studies have been done recently as follow-up of health care workers who have sustained percutaneous, mucous membrane, or open wound exposure to blood of HIV-positive patients. In one such study, 883 health care workers were followed and only one became positive for HIV antibody. An NIH research study followed 332 health care workers with 453 needle-stick or mucous membrane exposures to HIV-positive blood and body fluids without a seroconversion seen. In the eight seroconversions of health care workers reported in 1987 by CDC, significant prolonged contact with blood and body fluids were identified by the workers without the use of gloves. Some of the affected workers had contact with HIV-infected body fluids through damaged unprotected skin (e.g., rash). Intact skin is protective against many infections, including HIV, but damaged or open skin is a serious risk factor. Areas of damaged skin provide a portal of entry to the virus, as well as easier access to T-cells for effective viral binding and adherence.

Some intensive care practitioners express concern about HIV exposure when suctioning secretions in patients with endotracheal tubes in place. Low titers of the virus have been found in some samples of saliva. Nurses should wear a mask and goggles when performing any procedure when the possibility for exposure through droplet or spray exists. HIV transmission by saliva has not been documented, but the lack of transmission has. In one exposure, two nurses gave mouth-to-mouth resuscitation to a patient with AIDS and neither has seroconverted. Nonetheless, mouth-to-mouth resuscitation is *not* recommended. Manual resuscitator bags should be strategically located and available for use in all parts of the hospital.

12. What infection control procedures should be followed in the care of the AIDS patient in the ICU?

Any patient diagnosed as HIV-positive or as having ARC or AIDS should be treated using "blood and body fluid precautions." A single room is recommended, but is not necessarily required. A single room with a separate bathroom should be provided for patients with poor personal hygiene practices, diarrhea, fecal incontinence, pulmonary TB, or noncompliant behavior.

Extraordinary care should be taken to prevent needle-stick injuries or trauma from sharp objects that are contaminated with potentially infectious material. Disposal of all used needles and sharps should be in an impervious container of plastic or metal. Recapping, bending, or clipping the needle before discarding is *not* recommended, since most needle-stick injuries are self-inflicted during cap replacement and bending or clipping facilitates aerosolization of the contents from the needle.

Body fluids, especially blood, of all patients should be considered potentially infectious regardless of the patient's diagnosis or HIV test results. HIV must enter the body via damaged skin or mucous membranes or through direct venous inoculation, i.e., shared needles. Intact or covered skin is the best protection against such penetration.

"Universal precautions" is a set of Centers for Disease Control (CDC) recommendations for prevention of HIV transmission in health care settings. In 1988 the United States Department of Labor, through its OSHA branch, made universal precautions a law. Please consult the infection control specialist at your institution for a full explanation of these precautions.

Overall, the universal precautions by CDC state:

Gloves should be worn for touching blood and body fluids, mucous membranes, or nonintact skin of *all* patients; for handling items or surfaces soiled with blood or body fluids; and for performing venipuncture and other vascular access procedures.

Gloves should be changed after contact with each patient. Masks and protective eyewear or face shields should be worn while performing procedures during which there is possible exposure of blood and body fluids to the mucous membranes of the mouth, nose, and eyes. Gowns are necessary if procedures are likely to generate splashes of blood or body fluids.

Hands or other skin surfaces should be washed immediately and thoroughly if contaminated with blood or body fluids. Hands should be washed immediately after gloves are removed.

13. What are some of the psychosocial interventions and comfort measures that the ICU nurse can use to support the critically ill AIDS patient and the family or significant others?

Patients with AIDS admitted to an ICU have a grave prognosis, particularly when requiring intubation and ventilator support. Often in the critical care setting, the AIDS patient is facing both a physiological crisis and a situational crisis. As a result, coping responses often include intense anxiety, denial, anger, depression, suicidal ideation, and feelings of abandonment by health care professionals, who might decide that continued treatment is futile. Friends, family, and significant others may fear contagion or social stigma.

As with all patients and families who are in crisis, the nurse can use this typical crisis intervention model in dealing with the critically ill AIDS patient and significant others.

> Identify the individual's perception concerning the illness, diagnosis, and prognosis. (Are they realistic and accurate?)
> Determine the individual's support systems prior to illness as well as at present.
> Identify the individual's coping mechanisms, both adaptive and maladaptive.
> Assist the individual in identifying alternative approaches to use for crisis (encourage patient to develop or decide possible strategies to resolve crisis).

14. **Which nursing diagnoses, collaborative problems, patient expected outcomes, and nursing orders could be identified in Mr. Hall's case?**

A. Impaired gas exchange related to refractory hypoxemia/acute respiratory failure secondary to uncontrolled PCP. Patient will achieve and maintain optimal gas exchange as evidenced by:

   –Absence of shortness of breath, tachypnea, cough, cyanosis
   –Return to baseline ABGs, oximetry, and vital signs
   –Return to baseline rate, depth, and pattern of respiration
   –Absence of adventitious breath sounds
   –Absence of anxiety or restlessness related to patient's ability to breathe
   –CXR results indicate clearing of infiltrates or effusion
   –Verbalization of relief from symptoms of dyspnea, air hunger, cough, and weakness

   1. Obtain a baseline assessment of respiratory function.
   2. Assess for signs of impaired gas exchange and hypoxemia such as tachycardia, cool extremities, cyanosis, anxiety, irritability, tachypnea, altered mental status, and changes in orientation.
   3. Reassess respiratory status q 2 hr or as necessary for increasing signs of respiratory failure, increasing hypoxemia, and respiratory muscle fatigue.
   4. Monitor CBC for anemia, ABGs for hypoxemia or hypercapnia, oximetry for decreasing O_2 saturation, CXR for changes in infiltration or effusion.

5. Suction as indicated; obtain specimens as ordered; carefully monitor laboratory results.
6. Administer antimicrobials on time as ordered; observe the patient carefully for side effects and toxicity.
7. Administer antipyretics to control fever; note their effect on temperature.
8. Administer antitussives or expectorants as ordered.
9. Monitor use and effectiveness of ordered therapies such as oxygen, mechanical ventilation, humidification, and medications.
10. Alert physician of significant changes in patient's respiratory status, laboratory studies, and diagnostic tests; modify ventilatory changes as ordered.
11. Assist the patient with clearance of secretions by effective coughing; prevent stasis of secretions by deep breathing, turning, or ambulation.
12. Assist patient to positions of comfort to aid in breathing.
13. Encourage fluid intake for secretion liquefaction.
14. Organize nursing care to permit periods of rest.
15. Administer narcotic analgesics and sedatives with caution; evaluate response.
16. Observe for postbronchoscopy complications such as bleeding, anxiety, drug reaction, ineffective airway clearance, or aspiration.

B. Potential for infection related to:

–Immunosuppression secondary to viral destruction of helper T4 lymphocytes (AIDS);
–Neutropenia related to medication, treatment, or infection;
–Knowledge deficit regarding infection control:
    Patient will be cared for using appropriate infection control guidelines;
    Patient will be monitored for early signs of infection;
    Patient will not be a source of contagion to staff, other patients, and visitors.

1. Monitor vital signs and laboratory tests for signs of possible infection.
2. Monitor skin integrity, including IV/puncture sites, oral mucosa, and perirectal area for signs of infection.
3. Administer antimicrobial therapy as ordered, carefully monitoring for side effects and toxicity.
4. Assess medication regimen to determine if it may be causing a low white blood cell count, necessitating dose adjustment or discontinuance of drug.

5. Follow universal precautions and blood and body fluid precautions as dictated per policy at all times.
6. Not necessary to wear gloves, gowns, or masks when entering the room to talk with the patient, take a blood pressure or temperature, administer oral medication, or deliver a meal tray.
7. Explain infection control procedures to patient, family, and visitors.
8. Instruct patient and caregivers on the disease process, prevention of infection, transmission of the AIDS virus, home management, and community resources by discharge.
9. Assist the patient and family in determining the extent of the disease evaluation and treatment measures desired if a new infection occurs.

C. Alteration in sexual patterns related to:

–Need for safe sex practices secondary to transmissibility of HIV;
–Changes in self-concept secondary to a life-threatening disease, changes in body image, social stigma, or potential rejection; and
–Physiologic limitations secondary to HIV disease process:
  Patient will identify how his or her sexual role has changed and understand its impact and significance on his or her life;
  Patient will explore and use alternative ways to meet sexual needs.

1. Elicit the patient's sexual history; assist him or her to verbalize the role or meaning of sex in his or her life.
2. Plan nursing care to permit time to assist the patient to express feelings, frustrations, or concerns about changes in sexual activity because of AIDS. Let the patient set the pace.
3. Provide information about alternative means of sexual expression and safe sex guidelines.
4. Instruct patient and any significant other or sexual partner regarding safe sex activity.
–Abstaining from sex with partners with any infection;
–Avoiding sex with partners whose sexual histories are unknown;
–Avoiding ingestion of or insemination with semen, blood, urine, or stool during sex; and
–Using a condom during all penetrating sex (oral, anal, or vaginal).
5. Provide emotional support for the patient's partner who may feel a threat to his or her own life because of the possible exposure.

SUGGESTED READINGS

Brock R. Caring for patients with AIDS: we've only just begun. Journal of Advanced Medical-Surgical Nursing 1989; 1(1):1–84.

Durham JD, Cohen FL. The person with AIDS: nursing perspectives. New York: Springer Publishing, 1987:1–265.

Gee G, Moran TA. AIDS: concepts in nursing practice. Baltimore: Williams & Wilkins, 1988:3–403.

Gurevich I. Acquired immunodeficiency syndrome: realistic concerns and appropriate precautions. Heart Lung 1989; 18(2):107–112.

Meredith T, Acierno LJ. Pulmonary complications of acquired immunodeficiency syndrome. Heart Lung 1988;17(2):173–178.

Nyamathi A, Van Servellin G. Maladaptive coping in the critically ill population with acquired immunodeficiency syndrome: nursing assessment and treatment. Heart Lung 1989;18(2):113–120.

CHAPTER 50

Air Transport of the Critically Ill

Lynda Lane, RN, MS

On a rainy night in west Texas, Leon Owens, a 47-year-old truck driver, jacknifed his 18-wheel rig. He was taken to the nearby community hospital and admitted to the 5-bed ICU. Mr. Owens had sustained a hyperflexion-hyperextension of his spine with a neurologic deficit at C4–C5, a flail chest on the right with three broken ribs, a fractured right tibia, and multiple abrasions.

Mr. Owens' neurologic examination revealed equal, weak hand grips and pedal pushes with diminished sensory response in his extremities. His cardiovascular status was stable with a sinus rhythm at 80 beats/min and a cuff blood pressure of 132/82. He had an IV of $D_5\frac{1}{2}NS$ infusing at 30ml/hr in his left arm. With his three fractured ribs, he had a flail chest and a hemothorax on the right, which required chest tube placement and volume ventilator support. He was orally intubated and connected to the MA-1 ventilator, with an FIO_2 of 0.40, tidal volume of 1100 ml, and assist control rate of 10. His breath sounds were equal bilaterally with good arterial blood gases, and there was minimal drainage from his chest tube. A clamped NG tube was in place, his abdomen was soft, and bowel sounds were present. A Foley catheter was in place draining clear, yellow urine in adequate amounts. He had a plaster cast on his right leg from his knee to his foot, with good capillary refill, intact sensory and motor response to his toes, and no edema.

On the 4th day after his accident, Mr. Owens' worker's compensation insurance nurse requested his early transfer to a neurologic rehabilitation center close to his home and family support in Dallas. Early rehabilitation would provide the best opportunity for regaining his motor and sensory loss. An air ambulance transfer was arranged by Lear jet (a pressurized aircraft with a cabin altitude of 6000–8000 feet), requiring a flying time of 1 hr.

QUESTIONS AND ANSWERS

1. **Mr. Owens is to be transported in a Lear jet with a cabin altitude of 6000–8000 feet. What does this mean, and what are the implications for his care?**

   The aircraft will be flying anywhere from 38,000 to 42,000 feet above sea level, but the barometric pressure within the cabin will be equivalent to the pressure found at 6,000–8,000 feet above sea level. This is accomplished by compressing air within the cabin, commonly referred to as "pressurizing." This is essential, since altitude determines barometric pressure, which in turn determines the partial pressure of oxygen in the ambient air. While the percentage of O_2 is 21% in ambient air regardless of altitude, the partial pressure of O_2 varies inversely with altitude. The higher the altitude, the lower the partial pressure. At sea level, the barometric pressure is 760 mm Hg, so the partial pressure of O_2 is 160 mm Hg (0.21 × 760 mm Hg = 160 mm Hg). At 8,000 feet, the barometric pressure is 550 mm Hg, so the partial pressure of O_2 is 116 mm Hg (0.21 × 550 mm Hg = 116 mm Hg). Therefore, the critically ill patient who is transported at a cabin altitude of 8,000 feet is subjected to a lower partial pressure of O_2 in the ambient air than occurs at sea level. Administration of O_2 is standard during air transport, and the FIO_2 is usually increased for the patient who was previously receiving oxygen.

When a patient is subjected to a substantially increased altitude, there is less atmospheric pressure impinging on the body. According to Boyle's law, the volume of a gas is inversely proportional to its pressure, providing the temperature remains constant. Therefore, when the pressure on the body decreases with altitude, gases trapped within the body expand and increase in volume. This applies to gas (air) in the middle ear, sinuses, GI tract, and dental cavities. Other possibilities include air introduced into cavities during diagnostic procedures (pneumoencephalogram, arthroscopy) and air introduced into tissue during trauma, pneumothorax, or penetrating eye injuries. In addition to gas trapped within the body itself, gas trapped in equipment spaces such as Foley catheter balloons, urine collection bags, tracheostomy cuffs, IV bags, orthopedic air splints, MASTs, or medication bottles will also expand at increased altitude. As air in the body spaces expands or contracts during ascent and descent, the patient may experience abdominal pain, toothache, or pain in the ears and sinuses. A pneumothorax that is not adequately evacuated may expand. If the gas in equipment spaces is not controlled, the gas expansion can lead to ruptured tracheostomy cuffs, ruptured Foley balloons, IV regulation problems, or air splints and MASTs that are too tight or too loose.

2. **In planning Mr. Owens' transport, what environmental factors should the flight nurse be aware of?**

    In addition to gas laws, there are other considerations in air ambulance transport. Fluid shifts, which occur with the acceleration of take-off, deceleration of landing, and tilting the stretcher while loading and unloading the patient in and out of the jet can have a detrimental influence on the hemodynamics of an unstable patient. Temperature changes can be rapid and extreme in the airborne environment, before and after landing, and during the ground transportation between the hospital and the airport. Noise, vibration, turbulence, a low cabin humidity (10–20%), and cramped cabin space are considerations during the in-flight phase of care. There are also considerations related to the available equipment space and power sources for equipment. The length of time on board the aircraft is important, and it must be understood that there are no opportunities to obtain supplies and no means of excretory elimination for the crew.

3. What information about Mr. Owens should the flight nurse obtain in preparation for transfer?

Data collection should include a thorough review of the chart, with special attention focused on medical history, recent progress notes, and current medication and treatment regime. Note should be taken of any recent diagnostic procedures. After receiving the report from the attending nurse, the flight nurse should perform a thorough systems assessment. Review of the flow sheet includes obtaining the most recent electrolyte, hemoglobin, hematocrit, and arterial blood gas reports. All life support equipment must be checked and all appropriate supplies and medicines obtained.

4. Mr. Owens is connected to the MA-1 ventilator. How will ventilation be accomplished in flight?

Mr. Owens will be placed on a small, pressure-cycled ventilator (Bird Mark 14) that does not require electricity. Time should be allowed for Mr. Owens to adapt to the change of ventilators before moving him from his bed to the stretcher. Arterial blood gases should be checked and reassurance should be offered as indicated.

5. Describe the nursing responsibilities involved in preparing Mr. Owens for transport.

Mr. Owens' multiple injuries required careful planning and in-flight management. Mr. Owens had an essentially negative medical history except for smoking. His life support equipment constituted the biggest challenge for his safe and comfortable transport. Equipment requiring special consideration included the endotracheal tube, ventilator, chest tube, IV fluids, NG tube, Foley catheter, and plaster cast. Once the flight nurse had completed her assessment and the respiratory therapist had stabilized Mr. Owens on the transport ventilator, he was moved directly to the air ambulance stretcher. Mr. Owens' cervical injury did not require traction but could have been aggravated by movement. The flight nurse placed sandbags on either side of Mr. Owens' head and secured a piece of tape across his forehead and onto the stretcher. His cardiovascular status was stable. The rate of IV fluid delivery was increased to 50 ml/hr to prevent dehydration caused by the low humidity in the aircraft. The IV fluid was in a plastic bag, and a portable IV infuser was connected to the IV bag. Mr. Owens' breath sounds were good and he was breathing comfortably on the transport ventilator. A Heimlich valve was placed between the chest tube and the water seal bottle, which was replaced with a drainage bag. The drainage bag was vented to allow for changes in barometric pressure and escaping air. The ETT was secured in place with additional tape, and proper position was verified. After instillation of Maalox, the NG tube was opened to air and a glove was taped to the opening to collect drainage. The tip of the tube was placed at the head of the bed. The connection between the Foley catheter and emptied drainage bag was taped securely. Mr. Owens' casted leg was warm with good capillary refill, pulses, and motor and sensory response. There was no swelling or edema. His leg was elevated during the transfer. If his extremity had had soft tissue swelling, the cast would have been bivalved to prevent injury caused by increased swelling at altitude.

6. **What special in-flight care was given to Mr. Owens?**

Mr. Owens was placed on the Lear jet. Normally, patients are positioned in the plane with the feet toward the nose of the plane and the head toward the rear of the plane. Just as when patients are transported on stretchers in the hospital, this position allows the patient to see where he or she is going and is less disorienting. The flight nurse made sure that all equipment was safely secured with the IV infusing, the chest tube and Foley catheter to dependent drainage, the NG tube open to atmosphere and at head level, and the casted extremity elevated. Prior to departure, the flight nurse connected a 10-ml syringe to Mr. Owens' Foley catheter and removed half of the volume of fluid from the balloon. She then connected a syringe to the cuff balloon of his endotracheal tube and took his vital signs. She explained to the patient the sensations he felt on take-off, and they began their 1-hr flight. At cruising altitude, the respiratory therapist and flight nurse deflated the ETT cuff and reinflated it with the minimal occlusive volume. Mr. Owens' vital signs were checked every 15–20 min and remained stable. Drainage from the NG tube increased and was greenish. The flight nurse was unable to hear bowel sounds, so she connected the NG tube to low suction to prevent abdominal distention and possible impairment of respiratory excursion or vomiting. Mr. Owens' casted foot was checked for swelling, which did not occur. Other than a possible ileus, the flight was uneventful. After landing, the flight nurse instilled fluid back into the Foley balloon and readjusted the ETT cuff volume.

7. **Shortly after take-off, the flight nurse noticed that the pressure within the ventilator oxygen tank had dropped substantially. Was this normal, or was it likely that the tank was malfunctioning?**

It is normal for the pressure in the oxygen tank to drop after take-off. This is a result of Charles' law, which states that if the volume of a gas remains constant, the pressure will vary directly with its temperature. Therefore, the pressure within an oxygen cylinder decreases if the temperature of the cylinder decreases. Since a temperature decrease of 2°C (3.5°F) per 1000 feet of ascent is expected, there would be a drop in indicated pressure on the O_2 tank gauge even if no O_2 had been used.

8. **What are the implications of Mr. Owens' air transport for the receiving nurse?**

Air travel can be very exhausting. The noise, turbulence, pressure changes, mild hypoxia, and general excitement associated with an air ambulance transfer is tiring. The patient may seem lethargic postflight. The cabin humidity is very low, and the patient may require additional hydration. Residual effects of being at altitude may be present, including gastrointestinal distention, toothache or sinus pain (if air is trapped in a cavity), ears that will not clear, joint pain, and other effects resulting from Boyle's law.

9. **What nursing diagnoses would apply to Mr. Owens' care?**

> Possible ETT cuff rupture related to atmospheric changes
> Possible hypoxia related to altitude
> Ileus related to gastric distention
> Fatigue related to air travel

10. **What kinds of clinical conditions require special consideration in patients being evaluated for air transport?**

Neurologic Disease

Head Injuries. The flight nurse must be watchful of increased intracranial pressure. If possible, the head of the bed should be elevated. If the patient's head must be kept flat, the flight nurse will want to position the patient's head toward the forward end of the plane. Patients with recent diagnostic air studies should only be flown if it is essential, and then only at a sea level cabin pressure. The pilot is able to provide a sea level flight by increasing the pressure within the cabin and flying at a lower altitude.

Spinal Cord Injuries. If the patient is in cervical traction, a means other than a weight and pulley system will have to be provided to maintain traction. A spring-loaded tension device that pulls on the tongs may be used. Sandbags on either side of the neck and tape across the patient's forehead will help prevent movement of the head and neck.

Unmanageable Psychiatric Problems. The critical care nurse and flight nurse must arrange for sedation prior to transport, and the flight nurse must sustain the sedation as needed.

Cardiovascular Disease

Atherosclerotic Heart Disease. Cardiac monitoring and supplemental O_2 should be provided. The FIO_2 should be increased above the hospital delivery percentage to compensate for a decreased O_2 partial pressure at altitude.

Recent Myocardial Infarction. Air travel is not recommended until 8 weeks after infarction, and then only in a cabin altitude of 6000 feet or less. Supplemental oxygen is essential with continuous cardiac monitoring and ACLS supplies and equipment.

Air Embolism. These patients are usually being transferred emergently to hyperbaric chambers and must be transported at a sea level cabin altitude. Exposure to high altitude (decreased barometric pressure) would increase the size of the embolus. The usual patient position (on left side with the right ventricle up) must be maintained during transfer.

Severe Anemia. Hypoxia can occur at low altitudes in anemic patients. If the anemia is due to blood loss from trauma, it is best to correct it preflight. The critical care nurse should advise the flight nurse of the patient's hematologic status. Supplemental oxygen and a low cabin altitude are important in transporting anemic patients.

Fluid Status. Prior to transfer, all patients must have a patent IV. The IV can be heparin locked if the patient is taking PO fluids. If an IV is running to assist fluid intake, the infusion rate will be increased to compensate for the very low humidity in the airborne environment. Plastic IV bags rather than glass bottles are recommended to prevent breakage and allow for expansion at altitude. The IV bag may require an infusion pump or have a pressure cuff placed around it to assist flow.

Pulmonary Disease

Respiratory Failure. If the patient is being mechanically ventilated, that support will need to continue during the air ambulance transport.

Often, the medical team at the transferring hospital, in an effort to make the transfer less cumbersome, tries to discontinue as much equipment as possible. However, most professional air ambulance providers can accommodate necessary life support equipment. It is much safer to transfer the patient on a ventilator than to risk early withdrawal from life support equipment. The air in the endotracheal tube or tracheostomy tube cuff will expand at altitude. The flight nurse should release air from the cuff at altitude and reinflate the cuff on landing. It is important that the ETT or tracheostomy tube be securely taped or tied in place.

Pulmonary Emphysema. Patients with pulmonary emphysema should be restricted to a cabin altitude of 4,000 to 6,000 feet and should be flown with supplemental oxygen provided by a Ventimask. With obstructive disease it is possible to rupture blebs at altitude.

Pulmonary Edema. Edema present preflight will expand at increased altitude. It may be advisable to provide intubation preflight. A sea level cabin altitude is essential.

Pneumo-hemothorax. The air in the intrapleural space will expand at altitude. This is another case in which the transferring facility must not remove equipment from the patient. Patients should not be flown for 72 hr after removal of a chest tube to allow for all intrapleural air to be reabsorbed and to ensure that the pneumo-hemothorax will not recur. Any air remaining in the intrapleural space will expand with altitude and could severely compromise ventilation. If the patient has a chest tube, it should be left in for the transfer. The flight nurse should place a Heimlich valve between the chest tube catheter and the drainage collection unit. A Heimlich valve is a one-way drainage valve that will allow fluid and air to escape from the chest tube yet will not allow air or fluid into the chest tube. It is best to avoid glass collection bottles, replace disposable drainage units with plastic bags, and securely tape all connections.

Gastrointestinal Problems

Intraabdominal Wounds or Recent Abdominal Surgery. With the expansion of abdominal air at altitude, the wound could be stressed. An NG tube is required to keep the stomach deflated during flight. The NG tube must be open to air and allowed to drain into a glove or gauze, or connected to suction if necessary.

Gastric Ulceration. If the patient has had GI bleeding, his or her hematocrit may be low, which will make him or her more prone to hypoxia. If active bleeding is likely, an NG tube for instilling iced saline is necessary. Transfers can be very stressful for the patient. To reduce gastric acidity and help reduce the likelihood of nausea and vomiting, Maalox may be instilled in the NG tube prophylactically.

Intestinal Obstruction. The air expansion that occurs at altitude will aggravate an intestinal obstruction. A partial obstruction can quickly become a complete obstruction or ileus with altitude. An NG tube must be placed to decompress the stomach and prevent distention, which could impair respiratory excursion. If an ileus is present, a means of draining gastric contents must be provided (a glove or small drainage bag). If a colostomy is present, the transferring nurse should provide extra bags and the patient should leave the transferring hospital with the colostomy bag empty.

Diet and Elimination. Some patients become air sick. It is advised that the transferring nurse hold tube feedings or provide a small bland diet for the patient prior to transfer. Maalox and Dramamine may be given to patients with documented intolerance to air travel. Generally, once air sickness begins, IV drugs (Phenergan) are required to relieve vomiting. There are no private commodes on most small planes. It is best for the patient, family members, and crew to make a "pit stop" prior to departure.

Urinary Problems

Foley Catheters. The balloon on a Foley catheter will expand at altitude and can rupture. The flight nurse should remove about half of the fluid in the balloon prior to take-off and should replace it on landing. The Foley catheter should be securely taped to the patient's leg or abdomen prior to transfer.

Musculoskeletal Problems

Maxillofacial Injuries. The possibility of free air in the sinuses can cause severe pain with pressure changes at altitude. In the case of a penetrating eye injury, air transportation is not recommended because the pressure changes with altitude can cause extrusion of global contents.

Skeletal Traction. See "Spinal Cord Injuries."

Casts. Tissue edema in a casted extremity will expand with altitude and can compromise blood flow and nerve function. If tissue edema is present, the cast will need to be bivalved prior to transfer. In flight, the casted extremity should be elevated and carefully monitored for blood flow and motor and sensory response.

Air Splints. Air splints are not recommended for air travel. The air in the splint will expand at altitude and needs to be closely monitored and adjusted. Conversely, if taking off from Denver where the altitude is 18,000 feet and traveling to Dallas, air will need to be added to the splint. It is very difficult to provide the correct amount of air in the splint for proper stabilization.

Air ambulance transport of a critically ill patient requires careful planning and an understanding of altitude physiology. The attending nurse, flight nurse, and receiving nurse have specific responsibilities in ensuring safe and comfortable transfer of the patient.

SUGGESTED READINGS

American College of Surgeons Committee on Trauma. Appendix C-2 to Hospital Resources Document. Air ambulance operations. Bull Am Coll Surg 1980;65:16–18.

DeHart RL, ed. Fundamentals of aerospace medicine. Philadelphia: Lea & Febiger, 1985.

Embry-Riddle Aeronautical University. Readings in flight physiology. Bunnell, FL: Embry-Riddle Printing Department, 1978.

Ernsting J, ed. Aviation medicine. London: Butterworths, 1988.

Federal Aviation Administration, U.S. Department of Transportation. Physiological training. Washington, D.C.: U.S. Government Printing Office, 1980.

Gaudinski MA. Coping with expanded nursing practice, knowledge, and technology. Aviat Space Environ Med 1979;59:1973–1975.

Hansen PJ. Air transport of the man who needs everything. Aviat Space Environ Med 1980;51:725–728.

McNeil EL. Airborne care of the ill and injured. New York: Springer-Verlag, 1983.

Oxer HF. Carriage by air of the seriously ill. Med J Aust 1977;537–540.

Parsons CJ, Bobechko WP. Aeromedical transport: its hidden problems. Can Med Assoc J 1982;126:237–243.

Stensrud RL. Hospital-based air ambulance service extends emergency care. Hosp Prog 1980;61:72–76.

CHAPTER 51

Bone Marrow Transplantation

Connie Glass, RN, MSN, CCRN

Mary Wells is a 23-year-old woman who was diagnosed with chronic myelogenous leukemia (CML) at the end of the 1st trimester of her second pregnancy. She was able to complete her pregnancy and delivered a healthy baby girl. Because she wanted to breastfeed her baby, treatment for CML was delayed. When her white blood cell count rose to 262,000 with a platelet count just under 1 million, she was started on hydroxyurea (Hydrea) 3 gm/day to stabilize her in preparation for possible transplantation. The baby was 5 months old at this point.

On January 23, Mary was admitted to the hospital for bone marrow transplant evaluation. She had been diagnosed 10 months earlier, and her CML was in a stable phase. Physical examination revealed a small, slightly pale young woman weighing 46.3 kg in no acute distress. Vital signs were stable. She had no bone pain, fever, or history of night sweats. Her spleen was palpable at the level of the umbilicus. She complained of gingival bleeding after recent dental work. A recent 3.6-kg weight loss was not associated with nausea, vomiting, or diarrhea. She had no cough, her lungs were clear, and there were no vision changes. Neurologic examination was normal.

January 23 Laboratory Values

Na	140	Hgb	7.8	Albumin	4.7
K	4.3	Hct	25	ALT	20
Cl	105	WBC	41,000	AST	23
CO_2	28	Plat	656,000	T Bilirubin	0.6
Gluc	92	PT	13/12	BUN	15
Creat	0.7	PTT	27/27		

Mary has no siblings and her parents were divorced when she was a young child. Her grandmother proved to be a good match and volunteered to be the bone marrow donor. Mary's husband has a very demanding job and was therefore unable to spend much time with his wife in the hospital. Mary's mother had agreed to care for her two small children. Her father and his second wife served as Mary's support system while she was hospitalized.

Once the evaluation was completed and Mary made the decision to have a bone marrow transplant, a double-lumen Hickman catheter was placed through the subclavian vein into the right atrium for medication administration and total parenteral nutrition (TPN). Busulfan (Myleran) was given for 4 days q 6 hr followed by cyclophosphamide (Cytoxan) 50 mg/kg/day for 4 days. Adequate hydration was maintained with D_5NS and $D_5\frac{1}{2}NS$. Urine remained negative for blood, protein, and glucose during this therapy. Mary experienced some nausea and vomiting during the course of her chemotherapy. Because she was 13 kg below her ideal body weight and was unable to maintain an adequate nutritional intake, TPN was begun on January 31. Cyclosporine (Sandimmune) was also begun on that day, which was 3 days before transplantation. (Often immunosuppression is not begun until the day before transplantation.) Ablation chemotherapy ended on February 1.

February 1 Laboratory Values

Na	134	CO_2	24	Hgb	7.6
K	4.4	Gluc	154	WBC	4,500
Cl	106	Creat	0.6	Plat	572,000

On February 3, 875 ml of her grandmother's marrow was infused intravenously over 3½ hr. There were no complications.

February 3 Vital Signs and Laboratory Values

BP	110/60	Hgb	5.9
HR	90	Hct	18.8
Resp	16	WBC	2,100
		Plat	432,000
		RBC	2.18

Mary felt well after her transplant, and even rode her exercise bicycle. Her anxiety before and during the transplant was replaced by a feeling of well-being.

During the days after her bone marrow transplant, Mary developed mucositis, manifesting as pain and ulceration in her mouth. She became febrile, spiking temperatures to 40–40.5°C. She developed a mild tachycardia, but her blood pressure remained stable and she had no respiratory problems. Cultures obtained from blood, sputum, throat, and stool were all negative. She was started on gentamicin, ceftazidime, and vancomycin. The vancomycin was discontinued after 1 dose because she developed generalized erythema. On February 9, 6 days after transplantation, her laboratory values were:

February 9 Laboratory Values

Hgb	8.8	Electrolytes within normal limits.
Hct	26.8	
WBC	200	
Plat	14,000	
RBC	3.14	

During this pancytopenic stage, Mary was given irradiated blood products to support her low hematocrit and platelet count. The erythema remained on her face, neck, and trunk, and she developed pruritis. Cyclosporine was discontinued and methylprednisolone 125 mg was given IV followed by 40 mg daily. Methotrexate was begun the following day. Antibiotics were changed when her temperature continued to spike and her skin rash spread to her legs and feet, covering the soles of her feet as well. No rash was present on her hands. Ten days after transplant, a skin biopsy showed mild lymphocytic interface dermatitis with few necrotic epidermal keratinocytes consistent with grade I or II graft versus host disease or postablation chemotherapy changes. On February 15, 12 days after transplantation, Mary's laboratory studies showed:

February 15 Laboratory Values

Hgb	9.1	Electrolytes within normal limits.
Hct	29.4	
WBC	300	
Plat	28,000	
RBC	3.10	

Her rash continued to wax and wane and her mouth remained very uncomfortable with large amounts of viscous saliva. Eating remained difficult because of mouth pain but she experienced no nausea, vomiting, or diarrhea and no elevation in liver function studies.

February 23 Laboratory Values

Hgb	12.9
Hct	37.2
WBC	1,100
Plat	77,000
RBC	4.32

She was allowed out of the laminar air flow room for the first time, which was a happy experience for her and her family. She weighed 42.2 kg and her steroid therapy was being tapered. Because of the continuing rash on her trunk, face, legs, and feet, she was believed to have low-grade graft versus host disease (GVHD). She continued to have low-grade temperature elevation, and antibiotics were continued until February 26. Her intake by mouth had improved with calorie counts showing 1500–1600 cal intake per day. As her weight increased, the TPN was decreased to 1 liter per day and on February 28 it was discontinued. At this point, Mary's diagnosis was acute low-grade GVHD of the skin with no GI or liver involvement. Her liver function studies remained normal and she was planning her discharge with great excitement.

On March 1, Mary's weight was 45 kg. She was on daily low-dose oral prednisone and methotrexate weekly.

March 1 Laboratory Values

Na	138	Hgb	10.7	Albumin	3.3
K	3.8	Hct	33	BUN	17
Cl	106	WBC	2,500	Chol	125
CO_2	26	Plat	137,000	T pro	51
Gluc	96	RBC	3.91		
Creat	0.5				

She was discharged the following day after thorough instruction on Hickman catheter care, incentive spirometry use, and medication administration times, effects, and side effects. Her progress was followed in the transplant clinic.

QUESTIONS AND ANSWERS

1. **Which diseases are currently being treated with bone marrow transplantation and at what stage is the treatment recommended?**

    Bone marrow transplantation is the treatment of choice for severe aplastic anemia, defined as granulocytes <500, platelets <20,000, reticulocytes <0.1%, and hypocellular bone marrow from more than one site. In less severe anemias, other therapies are recommended. Acute lymphoblastic leukemia (ALL) is initially treated with chemotherapy to produce remission. Bone marrow transplantation is usually recommended in the second remission or later remissions. Acute myeloid leukemia (AML) and other nonlymphoblastic leukemias are also initially treated with cytotoxic drug therapy to induce remission. When performed during the first remission, bone marrow transplantation can produce a 50% survival. Chronic myelogenous leukemia (CML) is not as common as ALL and AML. Transplantation offers the only hope for cure for CML. It is recommended early in the disease, because survival is decreased if blast crisis occurs. Blast crisis is a massive proliferation of immature blasts and promyelocytes. Also, a number of rare genetic disorders such as Wiscott-Aldrich syndrome, Fanconi's anemia, severe combined immunodeficiency disease (SCID) and thalassemia major can respond to bone marrow transplantation. In some centers, non-Hodgkin's lymphomas and other malignancies have been treated with bone marrow transplants.

2. **It was necessary to prepare Mary for her transplant. What is involved in this procedure?**

    Prior to her transplant, Mary was given a detailed description of each step of the transplantation procedure, including risks to herself and the donor. Clinical evaluation included a complete hematologic and biochemical workup, pulmonary function studies, nutritional consultation, and psychiatric and dental evaluations. After her eligibility was determined and a donor was identified, Mary made her final decision to receive the bone marrow transplant. Her long-term venous access was established with a double-lumen Hickman catheter. The main objectives of the patient's physical preparation are to eradicate residual disease and to condition the immune system to accept the graft. Although Mary received chemotherapy alone to eradicate the leukemic cells, other patients often receive both chemotherapy and total body irradiation (TBI) for several days. The TBI is usually given in divided doses, although it can be given as a single dose. In some centers, patients are given antibiotics to decrease the normal flora in the GI tract prior to transplantation. Mary was placed in a laminar air flow (LAF) room on the 3rd day of her ablation therapy. LAF provides a germ-free environment during the pancytopenic phase. Not all centers treat patients in a germ-free environment, but masks and strict handwashing are mandatory because of the patient's immunocompromised state. TPN was started when Mary could no longer maintain adequate caloric intake. Supportive care was given for stomatitis, nausea, vomiting, and diarrhea. Adequate hydration is imperative during preparation for transplantation. Immunosuppressive agents were given initially to help prevent graft rejection and later to minimize GVH disease. Mary was started on cyclosporine, but later switched to steroids and methotrexate.

3. How are nutritional needs determined?

Mary's nutritional needs were carefully assessed by the dietitian. Based on her height of 5 feet 4 inches (162.5 cm) and weight of 43.4 kg, Mary was approximately 16 kg below her ideal body weight of 59.5 kg. She had good visceral protein stores, demonstrated by an albumin of 4.7. Anthropometric measurements were made and it was calculated that Mary's needs for maintenance were 71 gm of protein and 1850 cal/day. Because the total WBC count was elevated, the lymphocyte count could not be used to evaluate Mary's nutritional status. Transferrin levels were followed, since these are useful with most patients.

4. During the pretransplant phase, what psychological concerns might Mary have?

Being separated from her two small children, aged 4 years and 10 months, was very difficult for Mary. She was unable to see her husband frequently because of his demanding job. Her father and stepmother gave her some support in the hospital setting, but she was very anxious about each part of the pretransplant procedure. She was often tearful, expressing her anger at having leukemia. She was concerned about being separated from her children and spoke of them often. The isolation of the LAF room was very confining and made her feel powerless. She was never willing to discuss the possibility of dying. Listening; allowing Mary to express her anger, fear and frustration; explaining procedures; teaching self-care; and keeping her informed of her progress and the goals of the therapy were helpful in caring for Mary during this time.

5. **What type of bone marrow transplant did Mary receive? Explain the three types of transplants in use and the advantages and disadvantages of each.**

Mary received an *allogeneic bone marrow transplant,* which is a graft from a donor not genetically identical to her. Typing is done for mixed (human) lymphocyte culture (MLC) nonreactivity. Her grandmother's blood was compatible for all HLA loci and was MLC nonreactive. ABO group incompatibility between donor and recipient is not a major problem, but Mary and her grandmother were ABO compatible. The disadvantage to allogeneic transplant is limited donor availability. Because there is a 25% chance of an HLA match for each sibling, only 35–40% of patients will have a match. Because Mary had no brothers or sisters, another compatible donor had to be found. Donor and recipient are not required to be related but in most centers family members serve as donors. Another major disadvantage of allogeneic transplantation is the probability of developing acute or chronic GVHD.

In a *syngeneic transplant* bone marrow is donated from an identical twin. The advantage of this type of transplant is the identical genetic makeup, which gives an identical match for all major loci and minor loci as well. GVHD cannot occur, therefore, in a syngeneic transplant. However, few people have identical twins. In addition, the rate of relapse in ALL and AML are higher with this type of transplant.

In an *autologous transplant,* the marrow is harvested from the transplant patient himself or herself, then stored and transplanted at a later date. This type of transplant may be done in a patient whose marrow is free from detectable tumor, who is able to tolerate the procedure of donating 10 ml/kg body weight, whose malignancy is at high risk for relapse from remission, and who is expected to be responsive to cytotoxic agents. The bone marrow is harvested, filtered, treated with a cryoprotective agent to prevent stem cell lysis when the marrow is frozen, and stored at $-40°C$ to $-50°C$. The advantages of this method are the assurance of compatibility, the availability of marrow when needed, and no GVHD. The disadvantages include the possibility of infusing undetected tumor cells along with the marrow; side effects from the cryoprotective agent causing nausea, vomiting, unpleasant odor and taste; hemoglobinuria from lysed RBCs; and fever from pyrogens released by lysed WBCs.

6. How is bone marrow harvested and prepared?

Bone marrow is usually harvested from the posterior iliac crest but can also be obtained from the anterior iliac crest or sternum. The donor is anesthetized in the Operating Room and multiple aspirations are performed to obtain approximately 10 ml/kg of recipient body weight. More important than volume is the number of stem cells collected. Stem cells are the primitive hemapoietic cells that differentiate into the various blood cell types. Bone marrow is collected in heparinized tissue culture media, filtered through metal screen filters into a single cell suspension, and administered within 3 hr of harvest. In some centers, randomly selected allogeneic bone marrow grafts are being treated with anti-T-cell monoclonal antibodies before administration in attempts to decrease the incidence of GVHD. However, this has been associated with an increased relapse rate.

7. Is there a danger to the donor?

Although the procedure is remarkably well tolerated by the donor, donors must be in good health. There is a small risk of infection or thrombosis. General anesthesia poses some risks, and spinal anesthesia is an option. The procedure usually requires approximately 30 min. Mary's grandmother was able to leave the hospital the day after she donated bone marrow, experiencing only soreness at the aspiration sites and slight weakness.

8. Describe the administration of the bone marrow transplant. What was Mary's response to her transplant?

The prepared bone marrow was infused unfiltered via a central IV line. In most centers, the transplant infusion is started by a physician and the patient is monitored closely by a nurse. The first 100–200 ml was given slowly, and when no adverse reaction occurred the remainder of the 875-ml infusion was given more rapidly. Vital signs were monitored frequently. Mary tolerated her transplant very well with no changes in vital signs and no symptoms of reaction. Psychologically, she displayed a sense of well-being with decreased anxiety after the transplant was completed.

9. Explain engraftment.

Engraftment is the repopulation of aplastic bone marrow by donor stem cells. The transplanted stem cells are able to restore hemopoietic function by differentiating into the various types of blood cells. Hemopoietic reconstruction is complete (including the lymphopoietic system) and permanent with successful engraftment. This is seen in increasing bone marrow cellularity and rising peripheral blood counts.

10. What problems did Mary experience during the posttransplant period?

Mary's cell counts continued to fall for the next 11 days to a WBC of 100 and platelet count of 12,000. She was at risk for bleeding and infection during the pancytopenic phase. Although no positive cultures were obtained, she was given broad spectrum antibiotics because of her temperature spikes. She received bacteria-free food and was cared for in a sterile environment in an attempt to decrease the risk of infection. Mucositis, pain, and oral ulcerations were treated with normal saline mouth rinses and dyclonine topical anesthetic. Oral care was done frequently and carefully to avoid bleeding. Because of her oral discomfort, she eventually received patient-controlled analgesia, which was very effective for her. The rash and accompanying pruritus were treated with calamine lotion, and she was placed on a foam mattress. Diphenhydramine was used to decrease itching. Because of her low blood counts, Mary was transfused several times with irradiated RBCs and platelets to maintain adequate hematocrit and platelet counts. Electrolytes were carefully monitored because of potential drug side effects. Mary's electrolytes remained within normal limits. Third spacing of fluid may occur as a result of decreased intravascular oncotic pressure from low albumin and protein. Intake and output were monitored to avoid dehydration or fluid overload.

11. Why are RBCs, platelets, and other blood products irradiated before being administered to a patient who has received a bone marrow transplant? What general parameters are used for giving blood and blood products to these patients?

Blood and blood products are irradiated prior to transfusion to prevent engraftment of donor peripheral stem cells from the transfusion. Packed red blood cells are given to keep the hematocrit around 30%. Platelets are given when the count is <20,000 or if an invasive procedure is necessary and the count is <50,000. Patients with persistent infections unresponsive to antibiotics will occasionally be transfused with granulocytes. With all blood products, the patient must be monitored very carefully for reaction. Most centers premedicate with diphenhydramine and acetaminophen.

12. **What are the possible causes of Mary's skin rash?**

Since the skin rash first appeared after her initial dose of vancomycin, drug reaction was suspected. After changes occurred in the rash and the medication had been discontinued, blood product reaction was considered. Association of the rash with her continued temperature spikes was questioned. Cultures were all negative. The dermatologic biopsy of the lesion on her back showed low-grade acute GVHD versus chemotherapeutic changes from ablation therapy. She was treated with immunosuppressant therapy to suppress the GVHD.

13. **When did Mary show evidence of engraftment? What criterion is used to judge engraftment and when can it be expected to occur?**

Evidence of early engraftment was shown on day 12 when Mary's WBC increased to 300 and her platelet count was up to 28,000. Engraftment usually occurs between day 14 and day 28 and is confirmed by the finding of active hemapoiesis on bone marrow aspiration. As peripheral blood counts continue to rise, engraftment is readily apparent.

14. **What is graft versus host disease (GVHD)?**

Graft versus host disease is a phenomenon occurring with allogeneic bone marrow transplants in which the T-lymphocyte cells in the grafted marrow attack and kill host cells as "foreign." Histocompatibility controls the degree of GVHD. Approximately half the recipients of HLA-identical sibling bone marrow develop acute GVHD. This is thought to be due to minor antigen incompatibility. The severity of GVHD increases with age, and recipients over 30 years of age are at greater risk of developing the disease. Attempts at prevention of GVHD include:

Selection of a histocompatible donor

Irradiation of all blood products to prevent lymphoid cell activity

Providing a protective environment. Studies show the incidence of GVHD decreases when a LAF environment is provided.

Immunosuppression. Prophylaxis with methotrexate is the standard, and steroids, antithymocyte globulin, and cyclosporine are also used.

T-cell depletion

15. **What organs are most frequently affected by acute GVHD and what symptoms occur?**

Acute graft versus host disease mainly affects the skin, liver, and GI tract. Symptoms vary according to the severity of the disease, which is graded on a scale of 1 to 4 depending on the damage to the target organs.

Skin. Itching, rash, blistering, and sloughing

Liver. Elevated liver function tests, icterus, painful abdomen, obstructive failure of the liver.

GI Tract. Nausea and vomiting, diarrhea, severe fluid and electrolyte losses; possible blood loss if ulceration occurs.

The prognosis worsens as GVHD involves more body systems.

16. **At what point after bone marrow transplantation is acute GVHD usually seen? How is this disease treated?**

The "window" for acute GVHD is usually considered to begin at day 15–20 and to extend to day 100 posttransplantation. Evidence of GVHD usually begins with a skin rash, which may be preceded by itching. Treatment of mild forms of GVHD with methylprednisolone and immunosuppressive drugs is often successful. Use of cyclosporine, ATG, and monoclonal T-cell antibodies have been effective in 35–50% of cases with grade 1 or 2 GVHD. Grade 3 or 4 disease seldom responds to treatment.

17. **What nursing diagnoses were useful in Mary's care?**

    Altered nutrition, less than body requirements
    Potential for infection related to immunocompromised state
    Potential for injury related to thrombocytopenia
    Altered oral mucous membranes related to mucositis
    Potential for impaired skin integrity
    Impaired social interactions related to LAF room and isolation
    Fatigue and impaired mobility related to anemia
    Body image disturbance related to chemotherapy
    Powerlessness
    Pain related to rash and mucositis
    Fear related to outcome of bone marrow transplant
    Anxiety related to separation from children

18. **Describe chronic GVHD.**

Chronic GVHD is later in onset, occurring after the first 100 days and up to 12–15 months after transplant. Chronic manifestations occur in the skin, oral mucosa, liver, eyes, joints, and occasionally muscles. Chronic GVHD can be compared to autoimmune connective tissue diseases such as scleroderma and systemic lupus erythematosis. Immunosuppressive drugs are used to treat this disease and outcomes are better if the disease is limited to the skin. Treatment is usually managed with steroids, azathioprine and cyclosporine. Prophylactic treatment is given with trimethoprim-sulfamethoxazole to prevent pneumocystis and pneumococcal infections. Sun-blocking creams, artificial tears, and chlorhexidine gluconate oral rinses are often helpful to the patient.

19. Describe long-term complications that may occur as a result of bone marrow transplantation.

High-dose chemotherapy, irradiation, and chronic GVHD can result in long-term problems for the bone marrow transplant patient.

Pulmonary Complications

Restrictive and obstructive pulmonary abnormalities occur. These patients have decreased total lung capacity, abnormal pulmonary function tests, and decreased ability to perform activities of daily living. Bronchodilators and teaching about effective cough, slow, deep breathing, and pursed-lip exhalation may be helpful.

Eye Complications

Cataracts may occur from 1 to 5 years after bone marrow transplantation, with most developing in the 3rd year. Patients should be taught to have an annual eye examination, since intraocular lens replacement may be effective in vision restoration.

Endocrine Dysfunction

Temporary or permanent sterility occurs in some patients, especially those who receive total body irradiation. Growth rate may be slowed in children who receive TBI.

Depression, anxiety, and fear of death are complications seen in some patients. These changes are more common in patients with GVHD or other long-term complications.

SUGGESTED READINGS

Burnett AK, McDonald GA. Bone marrow transplantation. In: Catto GRD, ed. Clinical Transplantation. Boston: MTP Press, 1987:171–197.

Cogliano-Shutta NA, Broda EJ, Gress JS. Bone marrow transplantation. Nurs Clin North Am 1985;20(1):49–66.

Corcoran-Buchsel P. Long-term complications of allogeneic bone marrow transplantation: nursing implications Oncology Nursing Forum 1986;13(6):61–70.

Gibson D. Bone marrow transplant—the process. Nursing Times 1987;83(3):36–38.

Krowka MJ, Rosenow EC, Hoagland HC. Pulmonary complications of bone marrow transplantation. Chest 1985;87(2):237–246.

Thomas ED, Sargur M. Bone marrow transplantation. In: Cerilli GJ, ed. Organ transplantation and replacement. Philadelphia: JB Lippincott Co. 1988:608–616.

CHAPTER 52

Burn Trauma

Lisa Morra Martin, RN, BSN, CCRN

Randy Marler, a 22-year-old engineering student, was home visiting his relatives for spring break. While working on the family car, Randy primed the carburetor and suddenly found his clothes in flames. While yelling for help, he immediately dropped to the ground and rolled in the dirt and grass. His brother heard the commotion, dashed outside, assisted Randy in smothering the flames, and then rushed to telephone an ambulance.

The accident occurred at 10:00 AM. At 10:30 AM Randy arrived in the Emergency Department of the regional burn center. He was awake and alert. A full history had been obtained en route by the paramedics. Randy described the circumstances surrounding the injury and stated that he was not presently taking any medications and has no history of preexisting diseases and no known allergies. He remembered receiving a tetanus immunization 3 years ago.

Randy's airway is evaluated. His respirations are 22/min and unlabored. His face and neck are burned and appear to be partial thickness. His nasal hairs, eyelashes, and eyebrows are singed. Forty percent oxygen is being administered via face mask. Other vital signs are temperature 97.2°F, heart rate 138, and BP 132/78.

All of Randy's clothing is removed and he is covered with a clean, dry sheet. No life-threatening injuries other than the burns are identified.

The burn injury is assessed and the percentage of total body surface area (TBSA) involved is estimated using the Rule of Nines. In addition to his facial burns, Randy is found to have circumferential full-thickness burns of both arms. He is also noted to have a combination of partial- and full-thickness burns covering the majority of his anterior and posterior chest. The TBSA burned is estimated at 53%. Bowel sounds are hypoactive. Tetanus toxoid 0.5 ml is given IM in Randy's right thigh.

A 16-gauge intravenous catheter placed by the paramedics is infusing Ringer's lactate. There are no signs of infiltration and the IV line is found to have a brisk blood return. A second IV catheter, size 14, is placed in Randy's right arm. Based on the percentage TBSA burned and Randy's weight of 83 kg, fluid resuscitation is calculated and Ringer's lactate is administered according to the Parkland (Baxter) formula. Laboratory tests including arterial blood gases, carboxyhemoglobin level, complete blood count, electrolytes, and type and crossmatch are drawn. A Foley catheter and nasogastric tube are inserted.

Peripheral circulation is evaluated and both radial and palmar arch pulses are barely palpable. However, Randy denies any numbness or tingling, and clinical evaluation reveals prompt capillary refill and no motor or sensory deficits.

At this point, fluid resuscitation is under way, and the physician decides to prophylactically intubate Randy to protect his airway from compromise secondary to edema. He is given 5 mg morphine sulfate and 5 mg Valium IV and he is nasally intubated with a size 7 endotracheal tube without complications. A chest x-ray confirms proper placement of the tube, and reflects no abnormal pulmonary findings.

At 12:00 PM Randy remains awake and alert, and his urine output for the last hour is 40 ml. His nasogastric tube is connected to low wall suction, and 75 ml of dark green drainage is noted in the canister. Vital signs remain stable with temperature 97°F, heart rate 130, BP 130/74, and respirations 20/min. The Burn Intensive Care Unit is notified that Randy will be transferred momentarily, and a full report is given to the nurse who will care for him.

Upon admission to the Burn ICU, Randy's vital signs are stable. He is transferred to the mobile scale and two safety belts are gently secured. He complains of pain and is given an additional 5 mg morphine sulfate intravenously over 5 min. The nurse checks his BP periodically during administration. The nurse also explains to Randy at this time that he will be taken down the hall where his wound care will be performed in a hydrotherapy tank. Upon completion of the tanking procedure, silver sulfadiazene (Silvadene) is applied to all burned areas. Both upper extremities are elevated on pillows.

At 1:00 PM Randy remains awake and alert and his urine output for the last hour is 40 ml. His vital signs are stable; however, during the assessment the nurse notes that she can no longer palpate Randy's radial or palmar arch pulses. Further assessment reveals that his pulses are audible by Doppler. When questioned, Randy nods his head affirming the numbness and tingling in his hands, which are cool to touch. He also complains of pain with movement of his fingers, and his capillary refill is sluggish. Randy's physicians are notified of these findings and the necessary materials and equipment are obtained for performance of escharotomies on Randy's arms.

QUESTIONS AND ANSWERS

1. What is burn shock?

Major burn injury causes a shifting of body fluids from the intravascular to the extravascular compartment. This translocation of body fluid occurs secondary to a dramatic increase in capillary permeability. As a result, plasma constituents move into the extravascular space and edema ensues. In addition, a great deal of fluid is lost from the exposed surface of the burn. Without adequate volume replacement, this hypovolemia leads to circulatory failure and burn shock.

2. **How is the depth of burn injury determined?**

A burn causes cellular damage and coagulation necrosis of the skin in varying degrees. The extent of the burn wound is determined by physical inspection. The depth of injury will depend on the intensity and duration of heat application, the thickness of the involved skin, and the conductivity of the tissues involved.

Traditionally, burns have been categorized as first, second, or third degree. First-degree burns are superficial, involving the epidermis only. There is local pain and erythema without blisters, and a mild to absent systemic response. Second-degree burns may be further divided into superficial and deep partial-thickness injuries. Superficial partial-thickness burns involve the epidermis and dermis, and appear red and moist with blister formation. The tactile and pain receptors remain intact, so these burns are very painful.

Deep partial-thickness burns extend further in depth than superficial partial-thickness burns, involving the epidermis and dermis and leaving only the hair follicles, sweat glands, and sebaceous glands (skin appendages) intact. It is often difficult to differentiate deep partial-thickness burns from full-thickness burns, yet they appear mottled, dry, and waxy white.

Third-degree burns involve the epidermis, dermis, and underlying subcutaneous tissue. They may also be referred to as full-thickness burns. The wounds appear white, cherry red, or black, and may or may not contain thrombosed veins and deep blisters. The wound is dry, hard, and leathery, since the elasticity of the dermis is destroyed. Finally, since the nerve endings are destroyed with full-thickness burns, there is little if any pain in these areas.

3. **What is the Rule of Nines?**

The Rule of Nines is a commonly used guide to estimate the extent of the burn. It divides the body surface into areas representing 9% or a multiple of 9% (with the exception of the perineum, which represents 1%). The rule does not apply to children, and first-degree burns are not included in estimations (Fig. 52.1).

4. **According to the Parkland (Baxter) formula, what would Randy's fluid requirements be for the first 24 hr after injury?**

4 ml Ringer's lactate × kg body wt × % total body surface burned
4 ml × 83 kg × 53% = 17,596 ml Ringer's lactate solution

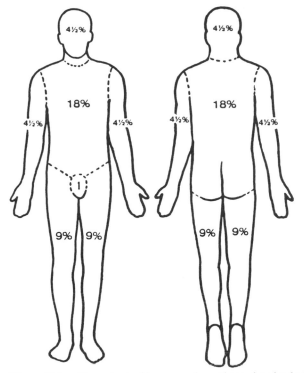

Figure 52.1. The extent of burn may be estimated and calculated by applying the Rule of Nines.

In the first 24 hr the Parkland formula calls for 4 ml Ringer's lactate solution per kilogram of body weight per percent total body surface area burned. Half of the total volume is administered in the first 8 hr (8798 ml), one-quarter in the second 8 hr (4399 ml), and one-quarter in the remaining 8 hr (4399 ml). It is essential to remember that the time is calculated from the time of injury, which in Randy's situation was 10:00 AM.

Fluid replacement on day 2 using the Parkland formula is calculated as follows:

24–32 hr after injury: Plasma 0.5 ml/kg of body weight per percent TBSA burned. In Randy's case: 0.5 ml × 83 kg × 53% = 2200 ml.

Following plasma infusion: D_5W titrated to the patient's urine output and electrolytes.

5. How can you determine if you are adequately resuscitating a patient with a major burn?

The adequacy of resuscitation can best be determined by evaluation of urine output and vital signs and by assessment of general mental and physical response. In adults, typical signs of adequate resuscitation include a urine output of 30–50 ml/hr, heart rate less than 110 beats/min, and a clear sensorium.

6. **What are the pathophysiologic changes associated with upper and lower inhalation injuries?**

Overall, an upper airway injury, or an inhalation injury above the glottis, is thermal and a lower airway injury, or an inhalation injury below the glottis, is chemical.

With the exception of a few rare occurrences, thermal injury to the respiratory tract is confined to the upper airways. The capacity of the respiratory tract to dissipate heat is so high that most heat absorption and damage occur in the pharynx and larynx above the true vocal cords.

As in Randy's situation, burns of the face, neck, and chest result in local edema after injury. Such swelling may actually be severe enough to result in upper airway obstruction. To avoid this complication and to provide airway control, Randy was electively intubated.

Chemical inhalation injury resulting from the inhalation of products of combustion may lead to several respiratory problems. Pathophysiologic changes associated with such an injury include:

Impaired ciliary action
Mucosal edema
Erythema
Bronchorrhea
Bronchospasm
Ulceration of mucous membranes

7. **What signs and symptoms are helpful in the diagnosis of an inhalation injury?**

Facial burns
Singed nasal hairs
Dyspnea
Tachypnea
Stridor
Hoarseness
Carbonaceous sputum
Erythema or swelling of the oropharynx or nasopharynx

8. **What other information may be obtained from the patient's history that might be helpful in the diagnosis of an inhalation injury?**

> Did the patient's injury occur in a closed space?
> Was the patient unconscious at any time?
> Was heavy smoke present at the scene?

9. **What is the pathophysiology of carbon monoxide poisoning?**

Carbon monoxide is a colorless, odorless, nonirritating gas that has an affinity for hemoglobin 250 times greater than that of oxygen. It produces carboxyhemoglobin, which blocks the oxygen binding sites on the hemoglobin molecule. In addition, it shifts the oxyhemoglobin dissociation curve to the left, increasing the affinity of hemoglobin for oxygen and potentially impairing oxygen release at the cellular level.

10. **What is considered to be a normal carboxyhemoglobin level?**

Less than 5% is considered normal in nonsmoking individuals; 5–10% is considered normal in smokers.

One must remember that carboxyhemoglobin levels obtained on admission will depend in part on the time interval between the injury and the examination of the patient. A low carboxyhemoglobin level does not necessarily exclude inhalation injury, while a high level denotes inhalation of combustive products and suggests one should observe for other associated inhalation injuries.

11. **As carboxyhemoglobin levels increase, what symptoms become evident?**

When carboxyhemoglobin levels increase to 20% in the blood, a mild headache may appear. At a 40% concentration, symptoms may progress to dizziness, confusion, irritability, nausea, vomiting, and fainting. When carboxyhemoglobin levels range from 60 to 80%, convulsions, coma, respiratory failure, and death may occur.

12. **Muscle relaxants such as succinylcholine are frequently used in the Emergency Department and ICU to induce muscle paralysis and facilitate intubation. Why was succinylcholine not used in Randy's situation?**

Succinylcholine, while an ideal depolarizing muscle relaxant in most emergency situations due to its rapid onset of action and each patient's quick spontaneous recovery from the drug, is contraindicated in the majority of burn victims. This contraindication stems from the potential for hyperkalemia induced by the drug, as succinyl choline can cause an efflux of potassium from the cell into the extracellular fluid. The hyperkalemia can be severe and lead to cardiac arrest. Overall, the larger the burn, the more likely the hyperkalemic response. In addition, the time after injury as well as the dose administered appears to affect the hyperkalemic response. The rise in potassium level begins within the 1st minute, peaks at 2 to 5 min, and then declines over the next 10 to 15 min.

There have been reports of succinylcholine being used in burn victims without cardiac arrest, yet it is recommended that this drug be avoided since its effects are unpredictable even in the early stage of burn trauma. In fact, indirect evidence suggests that an abnormal response may last up to 2 years after injury, therefore presenting danger long after complete healing of the burn wound.

13. What is eschar?

Eschar is the term used to describe the nonviable skin of the full-thickness burn.

14. What caused Randy to lose his pulses in his upper extremities?

Once fluid resuscitation is initiated in burn victims, swelling of the underlying tissues begins. Unburned skin is very elastic, allowing for a remarkable degree of stretch when necessary. In contrast, the full-thickness burns of Randy's upper extremities are very inelastic, preventing expansion of the underlying tissues. As his edema progressed, the tight eschar had a tourniquet effect and obstructed both venous return and arterial flow.

15. What is an escharotomy?

An escharotomy is an incision through the entire depth of the eschar, performed to relieve underlying pressure on the veins and arteries. Such an incision may also be necessary if constricting eschar in the chest area reduces chest excursion to the point of compromised ventilation.

16. How is the need for an escharotomy of an extremity determined?

Distal circulation is assessed by checking for progressive neurologic signs such as parasthesia, decreased sensation, deep tissue pain, or decreased motor activity. In addition, the affected extremity should be assessed for impaired capillary refill or absence of pulses by palpation or Doppler.

17. Why was Randy given an injection of tetanus toxoid?

All burn injuries are considered contaminated. As a result, unless the patient has been immunized within the previous year, tetanus prophylaxis is required. In addition, if the patient has not been immunized within 10 years prior to the burn injury, 250–500 units of tetanus human immunoglobulin should be administered at a second injection site.

18. Why did Randy require a nasogastric tube?

At some time during the first 24 hr after injury, most patients with greater than 20% TBSA burns will develop a paralytic ileus. This greatly increases the risk of vomiting and pulmonary aspiration, a complication that is associated with severe morbidity and high mortality. For this reason, insertion of a nasogastric tube is necessary to ensure decompression of the stomach until normal gastrointestinal motility resumes.

In addition, the placement of a nasogastric tube enables periodic inspection of the gastric contents. As a result of increased stress, patients with major burns are at a risk of Curling's ulcers (acute ulceration of duodenum or stomach) and hemorrhagic gastritis. With a nasogastric tube in place, gastric aspirate can be checked for the presence of blood, and gastric pH can be determined. The NG tube also provides a route to instill antacids as prophylaxis against erosion of the gastric mucosa.

19. What are the properties of the topical chemotherapeutic agent Silvadene?

Silvadene is effective against a wide variety of Gram-positive and Gram-negative organisms and *Candida albicans*. It is a nonstaining cream that is easily used with the open technique of burn would management. It has no major systemic effects nor does it cause electrolyte or acid-base abnormalities. It is soothing on application. The principal side effects include possible allergic reaction to sulfa (found in 5–7%), emergence of opportunistic infections, and delayed eschar separation.

20. What are the nursing considerations prior to administration of narcotics to major burn victims?

Partial-thickness burns may be quite painful initially, and pain from burn injuries may be increased substantially if the wound is exposed to a cold environment or handled roughly. A complete initial assessment is imperative to determine if associated injuries have occurred. Following the assessment, the wounds should be covered with a sheet and the patient kept warm. Heat shields may be indicated, depending on the patient's temperature and the presence or absence of shivering. These measures will minimize the pain from the burn sites, decreasing the need for analgesics. Prior to administration of sedatives and analgesics, hypoxia and hypovolemia should be excluded as the cause of anxiety or disorientation.

If the decision has been made to administer narcotics to a major burn victim, they should be given in small increments with dosages kept to an absolute minimum to prevent depression of cardiopulmonary function and to allow continued evaluation of the patient's sensorium. Finally, narcotics should always be administered intravenously during the first 4–5 days. The intramuscular and subcutaneous routes should not be used. Administration by these routes leads to erratic uptake of the drugs due to changes in fluid volume and decreased peripheral circulation to muscle and skin. Intravenous administration ensures rapid uptake of the drug and enables prediction of the drug concentration in the central nervous system.

21. What nursing diagnoses apply in Randy's case?

Potential fluid volume deficit related to capillary leak and fluid loss from the exposed surface of the burn

Potential for suffocation related to airway edema

Potential for aspiration related to lack of gastrointestinal motility

Altered peripheral tissue perfusion related to circumferential burns and burn wound edema

Potential for altered body temperature related to integumentary disruption

Potential for infection related to integumentary disruption

Pain related to burn injury

Impaired verbal communication related to presence of endotracheal tube

Fear of dying related to catastrophic injury

SUGGESTED READINGS

Boswick JA, Jr, ed. The art and science of burn care. Rockville, MD: Aspen Publications, 1987.

Curreri PW, Luterman A, Burns. In: Schwartz SI. Principles of surgery. 5th ed. New York: McGraw-Hill, 1989.

Desai MH. Inhalation injuries in burn victims. Crit Care Q 1984;7(3):1–7.

Fisher SV, Helm PA, eds. Comprehensive rehabilitation of burns. Baltimore: Williams & Wilkins, 1984.

Kenner CV. Burn injury. In: Kenner CV,

Guzetta CE, Dossey BM. Critical care nursing: body-mind-spirit. 2nd ed. Boston: Little, Brown, 1985.

Martyn J, Goldhill DR, Goudsouzian NG. Clinical pharmacology of muscle relaxants in patients with burns. J Clin Pharmacol 1986;26:680–685.

Mosley S. Inhalation injury: a review of the literature. Heart Lung 1988;17(1):3–9.

Surveyor J. Smoke inhalation injuries. Heart Lung 1980;9(5):825–832.

CHAPTER 53

The Critically Ill Child in the Adult ICU

Cathy H. Rosenthal, RN, MN, CCRN

Virginia is a 20-month-old child of 10 kg who has been admitted to the pediatric ward with a 1-day history of fever, cough, and rhinitis. After 24 hr and the development of progressive signs of respiratory distress, it is decided that Virginia should be admitted to an Intensive Care Unit. The Pediatric ICU is unfortunately full, so she is admitted to the adult Medical ICU for close observation. A percutaneous arterial blood gas study obtained on the pediatric ward prior to transfer revealed an acute respiratory alkalosis (pH 7.51, $PaCO_2$ 28, PaO_2 90, SaO_2 96%, HCO_3 21), perhaps due to the child's uncontrollable crying. All other chemistries and hematologic parameters are within normal range.

Upon physical examination, Virginia is wearing a 35% face mask and is irritable and cries when strangers approach her bedside. She withdraws and fights any physical contact with personnel. When left alone, Virginia pulls at her ECG electrodes and oxygen mask. She constantly hugs her stuffed yellow "Big Bird" and requests her "Mommy." At rest, her cardiac monitor reveals a heart rate of 145 beats/min without ectopy. She is warm and pink with a brisk capillary refill. Her temperature is 39.4°C.

Virginia has a frequent, nonproductive cough that awakens her during the night. Bilateral breath sounds are noted. Her respiratory rate is 42/min at rest and she is an abdominal breather. Slight substernal retractions are evident. A pulse oximeter is placed and reads an oxygen saturation of 95%. Virginia's chest x-ray reveals interstitial infiltrates in the upper lobes. Her abdomen is soft and protuberant with a palpable liver at 1 cm below the costal margin. Her peripheral intravenous line is located in her left antecubital space infusing D_5.45NS with 10 mEq KCl per liter at 42 ml/hr.

QUESTIONS AND ANSWERS

1. **Based on the clinical data and physical assessment, why does Virginia require close monitoring?**

    Infants and young children have immature anatomic and physiologic features that place them at risk for respiratory failure. Characteristics that place the infant and young child at risk for respiratory compromise include a compliant chest wall, immature accessory muscles, and small airways (1). The child's thoracic cavity is cartilaginous compared to the adult's. The ribs are also horizontally placed in relation to the sternum and vertebrae rather than at an angle as in the adult. With these characteristics, the infant or young child is predisposed to paradoxical chest movement. In other words, the chest wall may actually move inward rather than outward during inspiration (2). The child relies on diaphragmatic movement to assist thoracic movement. Anything compromising diaphragmatic movement can lead to respiratory failure (2). The small diameter of the child's airways also predisposes the child to respiratory failure. Even a small reduction in the airway diameter can lead to a substantial increase in airflow resistance (2).

These anatomic and physiologic differences complicate a child's response to a respiratory infection. In particular, children between the ages of 6 months and 3 years exhibit exaggerated symptoms of respiratory infection compared to older children (1). Virginia warrants close monitoring in an environment where immediate intervention is ensured in case of worsening respiratory distress.

2. **What safety precautions should be considered when caring for a pediatric patient in an adult intensive care unit?**

   As with any ICU patient, the nurse must ensure the presence of properly functioning emergency equipment. Appropriately sized equipment is vital in the care of the pediatric patient.

   The bedside of the pediatric patient should have an appropriately sized resuscitation bag and face mask. The resuscitation bag should be able to deliver a volume greater than or equal to the child's vital capacity. An adult-size resuscitation bag may not be appropriate for a young child and may place him or her at risk for barotrauma. The bag should be connected to a manometer to monitor delivered peak pressures (3). The manometer ensures that the mechanically ventilated child receives similiar pressures during manual and mechanical ventilation. Generally, most young children can be manually ventilated with peak pressures of 40 cm H_2O.

   Intubation equipment should also be present at the child's bedside. Specific pediatric equipment includes uncuffed and cuffed endotracheal tubes (sizes 2.5 to 7.0 mm internal diameter), Magill forceps, stylets, and laryngoscope blades (straight and curved) sizes 0, 1, 1.5, and 2 (3). In addition, appropriately sized suction catheters, blood pressure cuffs, and soft restraints are a necessity.

   Another safety precaution that should be in close proximity is a dose reference sheet for emergency or resuscitative medications, with the dosages calculated for the child's specific body weight. This sheet should be verified for accuracy by two nurses.

   Monitoring cardiac status via cardiac monitor is standard practice in most ICUs. Pediatric patients should have cardiac as well as respiratory status monitored via a cardiopulmonary monitor. Both cardiac and respiratory alarms should be on and have age-appropriate limits set.

The ICU bedside should be as child-proof as possible, with the side rails up and the bed in the position closest to the floor. In addition, no small objects should be placed on or dropped into the child's bed.

3. **What physical and behavioral parameters would be considered abnormal for Virginia?**

Temperature of 39.4°C. Body temperature is normally 37°C from birth to adulthood. Infections can cause a high and rapid increase in temperature in infants and young children, more so than in older children or adults. Infants and young children are also highly susceptible to temperature fluctuations. A rapid rise in temperature (40°C or higher) can precipitate a febrile convulsion of tonic-clonic nature.

Heart Rate of 145 beats/min. Virginia's heart rate should not be evaluated as a numerical value in isolation. When assessing a child's heart rate, considerations include the child's age, psychological and emotional state, level of activity and comfort, alteration in body temperature regulation (hypothermia or hyperthermia), and pathophysiologic state.

The toddler's normal heart rate ranges from 90 to 140 beats/min (refer to Table 53.1). It is vital to know the age-related normal values for heart rate to accurately distinguish between normal and abnormal. Tachycardia is a term reserved for significant and persistant increases in heart rate above the child's normal heart rate range (4), since the child is normally in a state of sinus tachycardia.

Virginia's heart rate was obtained at a time of rest, which is essential. The hospitalized child responds to the unfamiliar environment by changing his or her behavior and increasing heart rate and respiratory rate at the mere presence of a nurse at the bedside. The importance of observing the child from a "safe" distance and collecting assessment data during periods of rest and comfort cannot be overemphasized.

Tachycardia normally occurs during episodes of oxygen need, such as during a respiratory infection. Virginia is also hyperthermic, and for each centigrade degree of temperature elevation, the heart rate will generally increase 10 beats/min (4).

Respiratory Rate of 42. The same factors should be considered when assessing the child's respiratory rate as when assessing heart rate. It is important to be familiar with the age-related normal values for respiratory rate to accurately distinguish between normal and abnormal. The toddler's normal respiratory rate ranges from 24 to 40 breaths/min (see Table 53.1). Virginia's respiratory rate was obtained at rest. An ab-

Table 53.1. Normal pediatric ranges[a]

Age	Avg Wt (kg)	Normal BP[b] Syst/Diast	Heart Rate	ET Tube Size	Suction Catheter	Resp Rate	IV Maintenance (ml/hr)
Birth– 1 mo	4	60–90/120–60	120–160	3.5	6/8	30–60	17
3 mo	5	74–100/50–70	"	"	"	"	21
6 mo	7	"	"	3.5–4.0	8	"	29
9 mo	9	"	"	"	"	"	38
12 mo	10	80–112/50–80	90–140	"	"	24–40	42
15 mo	10.5	"	"	"	"	"	43
18 mo	11.5	"	"	4.0–4.5	8/10	"	45
21 mo	12	"	"	"	"	"	46
24 mo	12.5	"	"	5.0–5.5	10	"	47
30 mo	13.5	"	"	"	"	"	49
3 Yr	14.5	82–110/50–78	80–110	5.5–6.0	10/12	22–34	51
4 Yr	16.5	"	"	"	"	"	55
5 Yr	18	"	"	"	"	"	58
6 Yr	21	84–120/54–80	75–100	6.0–6.5	12	18–30	64
8 Yr	27	"	"	"	"	"	70
10 Yr	32	"	60–90	6.5–7.0	12/14	"	75
12 Yr	39	94–140/62–88	"	7.0–7.5	14	12–16	82
14 Yr	49	"	"	"	"	"	93
16 Yr	56	"	"	"	"	"	100

[a] From Curley MA, Vaughan SM. Assessment and resuscitation of the pediatric patient. Crit Care Nurse 1987;7(3):30.
[b] Blood pressure ranges include those in the 10 to 90 percentile.

normal respiratory rate obtained during a child's period of rest or sleep is more significant than one obtained during activity.

Virginia is expected to be tachypneic, since her respiratory infection places her in a state of imbalance between oxygen demand and supply. In addition, Virginia's respiratory rate is influenced by her hyperthermic state. For every centigrade degree of elevation in temperature, the respiratory rate increases 7 breaths/min (5).

Signs of Respiratory Distress. Virginia's signs of respiratory distress are abnormal and include tachypnea and presence of substernal retractions. Retractions occur because of the distinct immature features of the young child's compliant chest wall and poorly developed accessory muscles. Retractions are considered an early sign of increased respiratory effort (2).

An oxygen saturation of 95% is correlated to a partial oxygen pressure of approximately 85 mm Hg. Virginia's low PaO_2 levels and low saturations are products of her respiratory infection and resultant ventilation and perfusion mismatch. Virginia's abdominal breathing is considered normal for her age. Until middle childhood, all children are primarily abdominal breathers because of the immaturity of accessory muscles and compliant thoracic cavity (6).

Behavioral Responses. Virginia's behavioral parameters are equally important to assess. In a strange environment and without the presence of her family, Virginia resorts to only a few verbal statements. Communication, however, includes not only verbal communication, but also affective communication such as body language, behavior, play, etc.

The nurse must be familiar with the general developmental tasks and fears for the child's age group. The major developmental tasks for the toddler is the development of autonomy. Despite this need for independence, the toddler is very attached to and dependent on his or her parents.

Virginia's resistance to personnel and ICU equipment marks her attempt to assert independence and to gain control over her environment. In addition, Virginia's fear of separation is portrayed in her attachment to her stuffed bird and her requests for "Mommy." These behavioral manifestations are age appropriate and considered a normal reaction to the stresses of her hospitalization and ICU admission.

4. **What are the implications of Virginia's hyperthermia on her respiratory status?**

   Under normal conditions, rapid growth during childhood increases oxygen consumption up to twice that of an adult. In addition, for each degree of temperature elevation (centigrade), the child increases his or her basal metabolic rate by 12% (7), further increasing his or her oxygen requirements.

Virginia's hyperthermic state shifts the oxyhemoglobin dissociation curve to the right. Although this shift promotes the release of oxygen from hemoglobin, the hemoglobin has less affinity for oxygen. The result is less oxygen being picked up by the hemoglobin while passing through the pulmonary bed.

5. **What nursing interventions can be instituted to maintain a patent airway in a young child?**

The child's trachea is at risk for obstruction if hyperextended or hyperflexed (8). The young child has a trachea with poor cartilaginous support and benefits from positioning the head in a "sniffing" position using a small roll under the child's shoulders (8).

The child's respiratory effort can be supported by elevating the head of the bed. This measure assists gas exchange by lowering the diaphragm and abdominal contents and by facilitating chest expansion (6). This is especially important in the diaphragm-dependent young child with his or her normally protuberant abdomen.

Maintaining a patent airway can also be facilitated by chest physiotherapy and suctioning. The components of chest physiotherapy can be frightening to a child and should be modified, if possible, to ease the child's anxiety. The critical care nurse must attempt to diminish the child's anxiety and carefully assess him or her for signs of fatigue. Fatigue in a child with respiratory distress can have disastrous consequences, including respiratory arrest.

6. **Twenty-four hours later, Virginia is lying flat in her bed and is motionless, quiet, and calm. You note that her yellow bird is tossed to the opposite side of her bed. You are told that she has been a "good little patient." Virginia is pale and cool to touch. Her temperature remains at 39.8°C. Virginia quietly watches you as you continue to assess her. Her heart rate is 160/min without ectopy and her pulse oximeter is reading 91%. Her blood pressure is 92/64 via cuff. Respiratory rate is 50/min. Auscultation reveals quick, shallow, bilateral breaths with accompanied moist crackles in upper lobes. You note nasal flaring and grunting beneath her oxygen mask. Intercostal, substernal, and supraclavicular retractions are present. Chest x-ray reveals air trapping and patchy interstitial infiltrates in the upper lobes bilaterally. The abdomen remains protuberant and the liver is palpable at 2 cm below the costal margin. Urine output was 64 ml for the previous 8-hr shift via diaper. Sputum and Gram stain reveal *Haemophilus influenzae*.**

What physical and behavioral parameters indicate that Virginia is in distress?

Diminishing Peripheral Perfusion and Tachycardia. Virginia is pale and cool to touch despite her febrile state. The sympathetic nervous system has been activated as evidenced by Virginia's tachycardia and peripheral vasoconstriction. Urine output is diminished; an acceptable urine output in a child is 1 ml/kg/hr (10 ml/hr for Virginia). Her blood pressure remains within the normal range for her age group (see Table 53.1), although blood pressure changes will be a late sign of cardiac or respiratory decompensation.

Progressive Signs of Respiratory Distress. Virginia's signs of respiratory distress are blatant. She is tachypneic at rest. The presence of nasal flaring and intercostal and supraclavicular retractions indicate an increased work of breathing. The grunting heard beneath her face mask is an ominous sign of respiratory distress in the young child. It results from the child expiring against a closed glottis. Grunting attempts to increase end-expiratory pressure to maintain patency of small airways and promote gas exchange (6).

Behavioral Responses. Virginia's behavioral responses are worrisome. A 20-month-old child does not have the intellectual maturity to become compliant and cooperative during 24 hr. Virginia's behavior indicates a radical change from the day before and indicates an increase in respiratory compromise. Her expressionless facial features and motionless posture indicate that she is extremely ill. These behavioral changes should serve as a red flag of warning to the critical care nurse. Young children should, and normally do, respond to their environment and seek comfort in their security objects (i.e., "Big Bird") and significant caretakers during times of stress.

7.   **During the past 24 hr, Virginia has received 1008 ml of D$_5$.45NS with 10 mEq KCl per liter. Which of the following is a proper nursing diagnosis and why?**

   Fluid volume excess
   Fluid volume deficit
   Potential fluid volume excess
   Potential fluid volume deficit

In comparison to the adult, the child has a larger body surface area vulnerable to evaporative water loss, a higher metabolic rate, and greater insensible water losses. Each of these differences contributes to the child requiring more water per unit of body weight than the adult (2).

Despite the young child's increased need for water, the absolute amount of intravenous fluid required is relatively small. Maintenance fluid requirements are calculated based on body weight (refer to Table 53.2). Since Virginia weighs 10 kg, her maintenance fluid requirements

Table 53.2. Calculation of 24-hour
maintenance fluids in children[a]

Child's Weight	Kilogram Body Weight Formula
Newborns (0–72 hr old)	60–100 ml/kg
0–10 kg	100 ml/kg (may increase up to 150 ml if renal and cardiac function adequate)
11–20 kg	1000 ml for the first 10 kg + 50 ml/kg for each kg over 10 kg
21–30 kg	1500 ml for the first 20 kg + 25 ml/kg for each kg over 20 kg

[a] Reproduced by permission from Hazinski MF, ed.
Nursing Care of the Critically Ill Child. St. Louis, 1984,
The C.V. Mosby Co.

are 100 ml/kg or 1000 ml for a 24-hr period (approximately 42 ml/hr).
The critical care nurse can then modify fluid replacement based on the
child's actual clinical condition. Insensible water losses increase
approximately 10 ml/kg/°C/24 hr with an elevation in temperature
above 37°C (9). Virginia has had a temperature of 39°C for 24 hr, so
her daily fluid requirement would increase by 200 ml for the 24-hr
period (10 ml × 10 kg × 2°C).

Virginia's tachypneic state should also be considered. Tachypnea
can substantially increase the young child's insensible water losses.
The child may lose up to 15 ml/kg/24 hr from the lungs during normal
conditions (7).

Virginia has received only 1000 ml in the past 24 hr. Her requirement
includes 1000 ml for daily maintenance, 200 ml for supplementation of
her hyperthermic state, and 150 ml to replace normal insensible water
loss from the respiratory tract without considering tachypnea. She is
at risk for fluid volume deficit.

9. What other nursing diagnoses apply to Virginia?

> Altered tissue perfusion related to bradycardia and low oxygen content
> in the blood
> Impaired gas exchange related to ineffective airway clearance

Ineffective breathing pattern related to fatigue and respiratory inflammatory process

Hyperthermia related to *H. influenzae* inflammatory process

Anxiety related to separation from parents and presence in a strange environment

REFERENCES

1. Snow J. Pulmonary disorders. In: Hazinski MF, ed. Nursing care of the critically ill child. St. Louis: CV Mosby, 1984: 253–334.
2. Hazinski MF. Children are different. In: Hazinski MF, ed. Nursing care of the critically ill child. St. Louis: CV Mosby, 1984;1–11.
3. Escher-Neidig JR. Pediatric respiratory arrest: Emergency airway management in the critical care setting. Crit Care Nurse 1988;8(8):22–33.
4. Hazinski MF. Cardiovascular disorders. In: Hazinski MF, ed. Nursing care of the critically ill child. St. Louis: CV Mosby, 1984:63–253.
5. Whaley LF, Wong DL. Nursing care of infants and children. St. Louis: CV Mosby, 1979.
6. DeJong SB, McCandless SC. The respiratory system. In: Smith JB, ed. Pediatric Critical Care. New York: John Wiley & Sons, 1983:21–87.
7. Miller DR. Gastrointestinal disorders. In: Hazinski MF, ed. Nursing care of the critically ill child. St. Louis: CV Mosby, 1984:547–647.
8. Curley MAQ, Vaughan SM. Assessment and resuscitation of the pediatric patient. Crit Care Nurse 1987;7(3):26–42.
9. Hazinski MF. Understanding fluid balance in the seriously ill child. Pediatr Nurs 1988;14(3):231–236.

CHAPTER 54

Disseminated Intravascular Coagulation

Virginia Byrn Huddleston, RN, MSN, CCRN

Betty Dorsey, a 35-year-old multiparous woman, was admitted to the Labor and Delivery Department in active labor. She experienced tumultuous labor with tetanic contractions, and an emergency Cesarean section was performed. In the Recovery Room, Ms. Dorsey developed acute-onset respiratory distress. She became hemodynamically unstable with a blood pressure of 70/50 and a heart rate of 130. She was transferred to the ICU, where a pulmonary artery catheter and radial arterial line were placed. She was also intubated and connected to a ventilator. Laboratory values and vital signs taken upon admission to the unit revealed the following:

Hemodynamic Parameters		Laboratory Values		Ventilator Settings	
CVP	3	Hct	30	Mode	Assist control
PAP	40/22	Plat	80,000	Rate	12
PAWP	4	Fibrinogen	100	FIO$_2$	0.50
CO	3.2	FSP	50	Tidal volume	900
BP	80/62	PT	19	PEEP	5
HR	126	PTT	40		

A diagnosis of disseminated intravascular coagulation (DIC) secondary to amniotic fluid embolism was made. Assessment at that time revealed the following information. Ms. Dorsey was extremely anxious and restless. Auscultation of her chest revealed S$_1$, S$_2$, and bilateral breath sounds with inspiratory wheezes. Her skin was cool and diaphoretic. All peripheral pulses were weakly palpable and 2+ pitting edema was noted in both lower extremities. Capillary refill was greater than 5 sec in all extremities. Her abdomen was round and the uterine fundus was firm, although frank vaginal bleeding was present. Oozing was also noted at the incision site. A Foley catheter was draining blood-tinged urine. A heparin bolus was given, and an infusion was begun. Hemodynamic stability was restored with fresh frozen plasma, crystalloid, and dopamine at 8 µg/kg/min. Within 48 hr, hemorrhage was controlled and coagulation studies returned to normal. Ms. Dorsey was discharged from the unit, and the remainder of her postpartum course was uneventful.

QUESTIONS AND ANSWERS

1. **List the clinical conditions predisposing a patient to the development of DIC.**

Obstetric conditions	*Cardiovascular disorders*
Placental abruption	Shock
Placenta previa	Valvular heart disease
Amniotic fluid embolism	Abdominal aortic aneurysm
Retained dead fetus	Giant hemangioma
Preeclampsia	*Infections*
Septic abortion	Bacterial (Gram $-/+$)
Hemolytic and immune system	Viral
conditions	Parasitic
Transfusion reaction	*Neoplastic conditions*
Collagen disorders	Leukemia
Massive transfusion	Carcinomas
Extracorporeal circulation	Many others
Snake bite	*Miscellaneous conditions*
Anaphylaxis	Liver cirrhosis
AIDS	Pulmonary embolism
Tissue damage	Fat embolism
Trauma	Acute pancreatitis
Burns	Hypothermia
Prolonged surgery	Ascitic fluid reinfusion
Transplant rejection	

The abrupt onset, difficulty in management, significant mortality, and previous critical state of the patient make early identification of DIC crucial. Awareness of predisposing factors is critical in the prompt recognition of this syndrome. Observation of the early subtle signs of the process by the nurse at the bedside may prevent loss of valuable time during the course of treatment.

2. **Describe the pathophysiologic mechanism that occurs in DIC.**

DIC is not an independent disease entity but an intermediary mechanism of disease that presents secondarily to an underlying pathologic process. DIC represents a gross imbalance of the homeostatic mechanism involved in maintaining blood fluidity (Fig. 54.1).

An insult initiates the coagulation cascade via the intrinsic or extrinsic pathway. Excessive thrombin is generated, and fibrin deposition occurs primarily in the microvasculature. As the coagulation process continues, valuable clotting factors are consumed, thus the term "consumptive coagulopathy" is commonly applied to DIC. Concomitant with the initiation of the coagulation cascade at the time of injury, tissue-type plasminogen activator (t-PA), which catalyzes

486

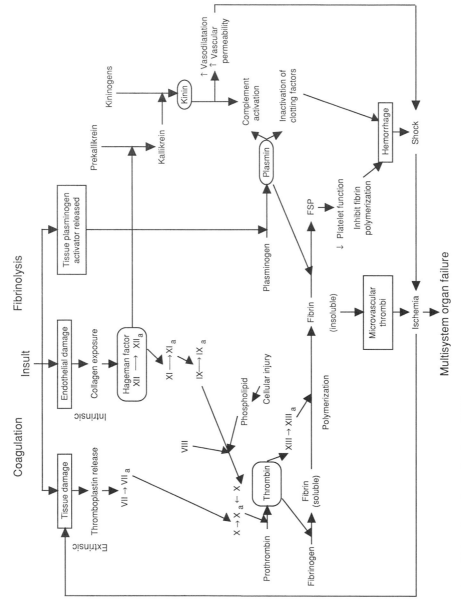

Figure 54.1. Cascade mechanism of DIC.

the conversion of plasminogen to plasmin, is also released. Plasmin degrades both fibrinogen and fibrin, releasing fibrin split (degradation) products (FSPs). FSPs inhibit fibrin polymerization and platelet function. These FSP effects operating in tandem with depleted circulating levels of coagulation components and plasmin-induced inactivation of clotting factors predispose the patient to significant hemorrhage.

Hageman factor (factor XII) assumes a key role in the development and progression of DIC. It initiates the intrinsic coagulation pathway following endothelial damage, converts prekallikrein to kallikrein, and indirectly leads to the activation of plasmin and complement. Increased vascular permeability and vasodilatation stimulated by the complement and kinin systems cause third spacing of fluid. This further volume loss potentiates the development of hemorrhagic shock, ischemia, and multisystem organ failure in a patient already at high risk for these complications secondary to diffuse microvascular thrombosis.

DIC represents a vicious, self-perpetuating cycle of accelerated coagulation, consumption of clotting factors, and secondary fibrinolysis. While hemorrhage is the most overt and distressing sign to the health care team, the thrombosis and potentiation of multisystem organ failure are actually the most life-threatening complications for the patient.

3. **What role does the endothelium play in the homeostasis of coagulation and the development of DIC?**

Recent research has identified numerous functions of the vascular endothelium. Although its primary role is that of permeability barrier, it serves active metabolic, humoral, and synthetic functions that significantly affect the inflammatory response and coagulation. The endothelium is the synthesis site of numerous bioactive substances, including prostacyclin, fibronectin, histamine, t-PA, and inhibitors and activators of platelet aggregation, blood coagulation, and fibrinolysis. Bradykinin, angiotensin, and serotonin are hydrolyzed by the vascular endothelium. Receptors for insulin, lipases, and lipoproteins on the enothelial cell surface influence both carbohydrate and lipid metabolism. The endothelial cell surface, the site of numerous antigens, is also susceptible to immunologic injury.

In DIC, damage to the endothelium by various etiologic insults not only exposes collagen (a potent activator of Hageman factor) but also may alter the synthesis and metabolism of various mediators involved in coagulation and fibrinolysis. For example, prostacyclin is a potent inhibitor of platelet aggregation. Alterations in the endothelium could thus affect platelet adhesion, aggregation, and clot formation. Thrombomodulin, a thrombin receptor on the endothelial cell surface, is involved in the conversion of thrombin (procoagulant) to a protein C activator (anticoagulant). This keeps the clot formation localized to the site of injury. If the endothelium is injured, this "buffer response" of thrombomodulin may be lost and thrombotic complications may ensue.

The endothelium is affected by numerous inflammatory mediators (endotoxin, interleukin-1, tumor necrosis factor, platelet activating factor, oxygen-free radicals, T-cells, PMNs, macrophages, complement, and kinins), and studies have shown an increased expression of thrombotic activity by the endothelium after exposure to the mediators. All these mediators (see Appendix F) have been implicated in many of the syndromes associated with DIC, such as sepsis, trauma, and multisystem organ failure.

4. **Why is the pregnant woman more at risk for developing DIC?**

Pregnant women are at a higher risk for the development of DIC for several reasons. Fibrin generation increases, fibrinolysis decreases, and the antithrombin III reserve is depleted during pregnancy, especially during the last trimester. The gravid woman is also susceptible to complications such as placental abruption and preeclampsia that initiate or potentiate coagulation abnormalities.

In amniotic fluid embolism, the maternal-placental barrier is disrupted and amniotic fluid enters the maternal circulation via the uterine venous sinuses. Amniotic fluid has a procoagulant effect by activating factor X. Amniotic debris leads to endothelial damage and activation of the intrinsic pathway, kinin, and complement systems in an already hypercoagulable host. Cardiovascular shock and DIC then ensue.

5. **What are the common sites of thrombus formation?**

Because the microvasculature is primarily affected in DIC, all organ systems are at risk for ischemia, organ dysfunction, and failure. The skin, kidneys, and lungs are the most commonly affected, followed by the heart, brain, liver, and organs of the GI tract.

6. **What conditions and clinical indicators are indicative of the thrombosis and fibrinolysis of DIC?**

The patient may present with signs and symptoms of thrombosis, hemorrhage, or both. The underlying disease process, previous patient condition, and extent of DIC progression all affect the clinical presentation (Table 54.1).

7. **Describe the common laboratory findings and their etiologies present in DIC.**

   Laboratory findings in DIC may be inconsistent and confusing. This is partially related to the heterogeneous clinical syndromes associated with DIC. Also, levels of the various factors depend on the rate of synthesis, activation, and degradation of the components by the bone marrow, liver, and reticuloendothelial system.

   Laboratory values must be interpreted in light of the patient's underlying condition. Ms. Dorsey shows a fibrinogen level close to normal limits, yet pregnant women usually have a high fibrinogen level. Ms. Dorsey's "normal" level is actually a low value for someone in her condition. This said, common laboratory findings are presented, but they are only guidelines, not hard and fast rules.

   > Decreased fibrinogen and platelets secondary to consumption in hypercoagulable state.
   >
   > Decreased assay levels of clotting factors secondary to consumption in hypercoagulable state.
   >
   > Increased PT/PTT secondary to consumption of clotting factors and platelets.
   >
   > Increased FSPs secondary to increased fibrinolytic activity.
   >
   > Decreased antithrombin III related to increased consumption secondary to increased thrombin activity.
   >
   > Decreased plasminogen secondary to increased fibrinolytic activity.
   >
   > Decreased hematocrit secondary to RBC destruction and hemorrhage.

8. **What therapeutic modalities are used in treating the patient with DIC?**

   Because the underlying processes and clinical presentations of DIC are so variable, management of the patient with DIC remains controversial. The cornerstone of therapy is the aggressive treatment of the primary pathology and intensive supportive care of the manifested derangements. Depending on the source, treatment may include surgical débridement, antibiotic coverage, evacuation of the uterus, or other modalities specific to the primary process.

   Treatment of the actual DIC process must also be based on the underlying disorder and clinical presentation. Heparin therapy may be indicated in amniotic fluid embolism but not in cerebral trauma, where it could precipitate intracranial hemorrhage.

   Blood component replacement has also received divided support in the literature. Some authors advocate replacement of clotting factors and volume in the form of fresh frozen plasma, cryoprecipitate, platelets, and packed RBCs. Others feel that replacement of components adds "fuel to the fire," although research provides minimal

Table 54.1. Conditions and Clinical Indicators of DIC

System	Thrombosis		Fibrinolysis	
	Condition	Indicators	Condition	Indicators
Neurologic	Cerebral infarct Spinal artery infarct	↓ LOC, headache, vision changes, ↑ BP, ↓ pulse, pupillary changes, paresthesias, paraplegia	Intracerebral hemorrhage	↓ LOC, headache, vision changes, ↑ BP, ↓ pulse, pupillary changes
Cardiovascular	Acute myocardial infarct Mural thrombi Arterial thrombi Deep vein thrombosis Pulmonary embolism LV dysfunction	Arrhythmias, ST changes, CV instability, shock, pain, edema, necrotic lesions, chest pain, shortness of breath, diaphoresis	Hemorrhage from wounds, venipuncture sites, invasive line sites, mucosal oozing	CV instability, ↓ BP, ↑ pulse, ↓ PAWP, shock, cool moist skin, weak pulses
Pulmonary	Microvascular thrombi Pulmonary embolism ARDS	Shortness of breath, hypoxemia, ↑ PAP, acidosis, chest pain, ↑ pulse, ↓ rate, ↓ static effective compliance, ↑ peak inspiratory pressure	Interstitial and intraalveolar edema	Atelectasis, shortness of breath, blood-tinged sputum, hypoxia, acidosis, ↑ peak inspiratory pressure, ↑ rate, ↓ static effective compliance

Renal	Renal artery/vein thrombi Acute renal failure Cortical necrosis	Hypertension, ↓ urine output, ↑ creatinine, ↑ BUN, ↑ K⁺, alterations in fluid and electrolytes	Bladder mucosal oozing or hemorrhage	Hematuria
Gastrointestinal	Mesenteric thrombosis Mucosal ischemia/infarct Hepatic necrosis	Abdominal pain, diarrhea, bright red blood from rectum, ↑ abdominal girth, alteration in metabolism and synthesis of protein, carbohydrate, and lipid; alteration in bile production and bilirubin metabolism	GI bleeding	Bright red blood or coffee ground aspirate from NGT, bright red blood or melena from rectum
Cutaneous	Microvascular thrombi	Distal necrosis, gangrene	Hemorrhage	Mucosal oozing and bleeding (oral, nasal, tracheal, gastric, bladder, rectal), ecchymosis, petechiae, pallor, epistaxis, SC hematomas

support for this premise. Heparin infusion has been recommended to decrease continued clotting while replacement therapy is being undertaken. Whatever treatment is employed, adequate oxygenation and perfusion are the key to maintaining organ viability and function. Serial laboratory studies and intense hemodynamic monitoring are indicated to assess the responses of specific organ systems to all modes of therapy.

Future therapy focuses on biochemical and immunologic modulation of the DIC process. Protein C and protein S (anticoagulants), tumor necrosis factor antisera, and antithrombin III concentrate infusions are currently being researched. Plasmapheresis to remove selected mediators is also being examined.

9. **Intravenous heparin is ordered at 1000 units/hr, following a 5000-unit bolus. Why is heparin given? What is its mechanism of action?**

The use of heparin in DIC remains extremely controversial. Few well-controlled prospective trials have been conducted. Heparin is more accepted in the treatment of amniotic fluid embolism because of the excessive thrombin known to be generated in this syndrome.

Heparin is given to prevent further generation of microvascular thrombi. It enhances the activity of antithrombin III, a major inhibitor of thrombin; therefore, thrombin activity is inhibited and thrombin-dependent cleavage of fibrinogen to fibrin is impeded when heparin is administered. Because levels of antithrombin III are often low in DIC, some clinicians now favor the administration of antithrombin III simultaneously with heparin, since the effects of heparin are dependent on the presence of antithrombin III.

The nurse caring for the patient must continuously monitor the patient for signs and symptoms of hemorrhage and shock. Serial PTTs, indicative of heparin-induced inhibition of the coagulation cascade, are monitored frequently. Standard precautions for bleeding such as padding the bed and side rails, avoiding shaving and toothbrushing, and minimizing venipunctures should be followed.

10. **What nursing diagnoses apply in this case?**

Alteration in tissue perfusion related to disseminated microvascular thrombi and decreased cardiac output secondary to hemorrhage

Fluid volume deficit related to hemorrhage

Impaired gas exchange related to pulmonary microvascular thrombi and alteration in capillary permeability secondary to circulating mediators

Anxiety related to severity of disease, status of baby, and invasive procedures

SUGGESTED READINGS

Baker WF. Clinical aspects of disseminated intravascular coagulation: a clinician's point of view. Semin Thromb Hemost 1989;15:1–57.

Bevilacqua MP, Gimbrone MA. Inducible endothelial functions in inflammation and coagulation. Semin Thromb Hemost 1988; 13:425–433.

Bick RL. Disseminated intravascular coagulation and related syndromes. Semin Thromb Hemost 1988;14:299–338.

Carr ME. Disseminated intravascular coagulation: pathogenesis, diagnosis, and therapy. J Emerg Med 1987;5:311–322.

Darovic G. Disseminated intravascular coagulation. Crit Care Nurs 1982;2(6):36–43, 46.

Feinstein DI. Treatment of disseminated intravascular coagulation. Semin Thromb Hemost 1988;14:351–362.

Fruchtman S, Aledort CM. Disseminated intravascular coagulation. J Am Coll Cardiol 1986;8(6 Suppl B):159B–167B.

Muller-Berghaus M. Pathophysiologic and biochemical events in disseminated intravascular coagulation: dysregulation of procoagulant and anticoagulant pathways. Semin Thromb Hemost 1989;15:58–87.

Weiner CP. The obstetric patient and disseminated intravascular coagulation. Clin Perinatol 1986;13:705–718.

CHAPTER 55

Multisystem Organ Failure

Virginia Byrn Huddleston, RN, MSN, CCRN

James Martin, a 24-year-old man, suffered massive crush injuries to both lower extremities when the car he was working underneath fell on him. On admission to the Emergency Department, he was hypotensive and unconscious but breathing spontaneously. Two large-bore IV lines were already in place infusing crystalloids at the maximum rate. He was taken to the Operating Room immediately, where he underwent vascular repair to his femoral and popliteal arteries and massive débridement of the lower extremities. External fixation devices were also applied to bilateral fractures of the tibia and fibula.

On admission to the ICU, Mr. Martin was arousable and following commands. He was in sinus tachycardia with palpable pulses distal to the injury in both lower extremities. He was extubated to a 40% face mask, and bilateral breath sounds were clear to auscultation. The NG tube was draining minimal green aspirate, and a Foley catheter was draining large amounts of blood-tinged urine.

On day 3, Mr. Martin's fever spiked to 103°F. Blood, urine, and sputum cultures were obtained. The next dressing change revealed numerous large areas of poor vascular supply and necrosis. Further surgical débridement was performed. Twelve hours postoperatively, Mr. Martin became hemodynamically unstable. A pulmonary artery catheter was inserted. On removal of the surgical dressing, new areas of extensive necrosis were discovered. Mr. Martin was returned to the Operating Room, where he underwent high bilateral above-the-knee amputations.

On arrival in the ICU, Mr. Martin remained hemodynamically labile. Refractory hypoxemia and poor ventilatory effort required ventilator assistance. Over the next 5 days, Mr. Martin developed fulminant sepsis, ARDS, and renal failure. Ventilator support was continued and hemodialysis was instituted. Evidence of subsequent liver failure was also present. Assessment at that time revealed:

Hemodynamic Parameters		Ventilator Settings		ABGs	
CVP	3	Mode	Assist Control	pH	7.29
PAP	15/7	Rate	16	$PaCO_2$	45
PAWP	4	FIO_2	0.60	PaO_2	70
CO	10	Tidal volume	900	SaO_2	82%
SVR	512	PEEP	15	HCO_3	20
BP	92/54				

Laboratory Results

K	5.8	Hgb	10.3
Ca	7.5	Hct	31
Creat	2.8	WBC	500
BUN	60	Plat	10,000
Albumin	1.5	APTT	35
AST	3500	Fibrinogen	100
SGPT	3200	FSP	50
D. Bili	1.8	PT	22
I. Bili	0.4		
T. Bili	2.8		

On postoperative day 10, Mr. Martin began oozing bright red blood from his NG tube, oral cavity, nares, rectum, and urethra. Fluid and blood replacement were inadequate to maintain hemodynamic stability, and vasopressor therapy was instituted. High-dose dopamine proved ineffective, and a Levophed was begun. Shortly thereafter, Mr. Martin suffered a cardiac arrest, and resuscitation attempts were unsuccessful.

QUESTIONS AND ANSWERS

1. **What was the cause of the large areas of necrosis discovered on day 3? Why did Mr. Martin become hemodynamically unstable 12 hr postoperatively?**

    Massive showering of septic emboli led to the development of the necrotic areas. Even after débridement, the systemic inflammatory response continued. Multiple mediators in a series of complex interactions continued to exert their effects on various target cells, thus causing hemodynamic instability (see question 7). Amputation of the legs was necessary because tissue damage was too extensive. Also, the septic source had to be removed to prevent further heightening of the inflammatory response and its concomitant damage to other organ systems.

2. **Define multisystem organ failure (MSOF).**

    Multisystem organ failure has been defined as the failure of three or more organ systems. Because the organs involved are often remote from the injury or source of sepsis, theories concerning the pathophysiologic mechanism involved in MSOF focus on common pathways and interactions between the organ systems, rather than isolated processes. Over 100 mediators have been implicated in the development and progression of the MSOF complex. Humoral, cellular, and biochemical interactions have been suggested. Despite the availability of high-tech equipment and the use of aggressive treatment modalities, the mortality rate of MSOF remains 60% to 80%.

MSOF constitutes the major cause of death following burn, traumatic, and septic insults.

3. What organ systems are at the greatest risk of failure?

Pulmonary	Renal
Cardiovascular	Hematologic
GI-hepatic	CNS

Different criteria are used by each institution to define dysfunction in the individual organ systems, so no criteria are presented here.

4. What clinical settings predispose the patient to MSOF?

Sepsis
Uncontrolled source of infection
Persistent hypermetabolic state
Perfusion deficit
Necrotic tissue
Injured tissue
Inflammatory process

5. What preexisting factors place the patient at added risk?

Age
Chronic disease states
Severity of initial insult
Immunosuppression

6. Briefly describe the pathophysiology and the proposed final common pathway in the development of MSOF.

Although sepsis is the most common predisposing factor to MSOF, other clinical syndromes can initiate the systemic inflammatory response, the final common pathway in the development of MSOF (see question 4). This host response, independent of the initiating factor, is now thought to be a result of the multiple mediator systems operating in tandem with each other (see question 7).

The original insult initiates the release or activation of various humoral and cellular components, including those of the complement, coagulation, and kinin cascades. These in turn activate or potentiate other biochemical mediators such as histamine, prostaglandins, leukotrienes, and immunologic factors. Alterations occur in vascular integrity (increased permeability and dilatation), and blood volume is maldistributed. Cardiac depression may also occur secondary to the influence of specific mediators such as myocardial depressant factor (MDF).

As these alterations progress, oxygen delivery to and use by the cells is impaired. The decreased ATP production, combined with changes in metabolic processes, leads to structural and functional damage of the various parenchyma. Pulmonary and hepatic abnormalities are usually the first to occur, followed by degeneration of the GI and renal systems.

7. **Discuss the role played by the common mediators implicated in the development and progression of the MSOF complex.**

The availability of more advanced biochemical instrumentation and techniques in recent years has provided the foundation for more extensive research into the processes associated with the MSOF complex. What was once thought to be a clinical presentation stemming solely from inadequate cardiac performance and oxygen delivery is now recognized as a problem occurring in the periphery, mediated by numerous systems, cells, and bioactive substances.

The mediator systems can be divided into two categories: humoral and cellular, with humoral usually preceding and probably activating the cellular system. These two systems can either release biochemical mediators or enhance specific bioactivity (see Appendix F). Interactions and effects may be on the systemic level or the cell-to-cell level (see Appendix F). Although the purpose of the mediator systems is to protect the organism, an extended acute response can eventually harm the organism by setting up the cascade of mechanisms that leads to the development and progression of the MSOF complex.

8. **Mr. Martin is receiving aggressive nutritional support with administration of TPN and lipids, but he demonstrates severe muscle wasting and metabolic signs of malnutrition. How does the hypermetabolic state differ from classic starvation? What is its significance to the development of MSOF?**

While much of the early research and literature focused on the clinical and physiologic hemodynamic alterations observed in sepsis and the resultant development of MSOF, current research is beginning to examine biochemical and metabolic processes coinciding with the progression of the MSOF complex.

The metabolic changes seen after insult are significantly different from the alterations observed in classic starvation. There is an increased energy expenditure in the hypermetabolic state, with an associated increase in the oxidation of major substrates (carbohydrate, protein, fat). A major difference in substrate oxidation lies in the percentage of each substrate used in the production of ATP. Protein becomes a major source of energy rather than the glucose and fat used in starvation. (Decreased glucose use may be related to decreased pyruvate dehydrogenase activity.) There is a reduction in total body protein synthesis, and gross autocannibalism of the skeletal muscle mass occurs, even beyond that accounted for by bed rest or starvation alone. Loss of lean body mass protein is followed by loss of visceral protein mass.

Energy expenditure, the respiratory quotient, gluconeogenesis, ureagenesis, and amino acid oxidation are much greater in the hypermetabolic state than in starvation, with the clinical signs of malnutrition developing much more quickly. The loss of autoregulation in the body itself through unresponsive feedback mechanisms and diminished responsiveness to exogenous administration of substrate make effective treatment much more difficult. These differences between starvation and hypermetabolism are felt to be mediator related, and future research and treatment will focus on manipulation of the mediator systems.

With extensive protein catabolism, decreased ATP production, and pathways refractory to feedback mechanisms, organ system integrity cannot be maintained. Toxic mediators continue to be released from damaged tissues, thus perpetuating the vicious cycle both locally and systemically.

9. **Describe the role the GI-hepatic system can play in perpetuation of MSOF syndrome.**

The hepatic macrophage is becoming the focus of attention in the literature for its role in the potentiation of MSOF. The release of bioactive substances from the various sources into the systemic circulation causes activation of the hepatic macrophage. Unfortunately, the hepatic macrophage can release its toxic by-products directly into the venous circulation, where they can further damage the pulmonary system and aggravate existing immune suppression. Excessive liberation of complement split products has been shown to desensitize PMNs, thereby decreasing their chemotactic, phagocytic, and bactericidal activity.

Although failure of the GI system has not usually been considered one of the most life-threatening of the MSOF complex, loss of mucosal integrity may lead to an exacerbation of the MSOF complex and increased mortality. Along with blood losses occurring secondary to GI bleeding, translocation of intestinal bacterial flora often produces secondary infection at sites distant from the original site of insult, such as the lungs or urinary tract. Further activation of the mediator systems and macrophages then results.

10. **What is the present focus of treatment? What future modalities are being researched?**

Aggressive attack on the underlying process and insult
Supportive care for organ systems involved

Newer modes of treatment will focus on:

Immunomodulation
Augmentation of the host's ability to contain infection
Biochemical manipulation of pathologic processes
Free radical inhibition
Prostaglandin administration or inhibition
Fibronectin administration
$MgCl_2$-ATP administration
Growth hormone administration
Alteration of hypermetabolic substrate use
Development of fuels that can reduce proteolysis
Methods to supply increased energy substrate that the hypermetabolic system will use

11. What nursing diagnoses apply in this case?

Alteration in tissue perfusion related to flow alterations and hypermetabolism secondary to mediator systems
Alteration in nutrition: less than body requirements related to hypermetabolism secondary to mediator systems
Anxiety related to ICU environment and severity of condition
Alteration in gas exchange related to atelectasis, decreased functional residual capacity, and intrapulmonary shunting secondary to ARDS
Fluid volume excess related to renal failure
Hyperthermia related to mediator systems
Fluid volume deficit related to third space fluid losses and blood losses secondary to vasodilatation, increased capillary permeability, and coagulopathies

SUGGESTED READINGS

Bengtson A, Heideman M. Anaphylatoxin formation in sepsis. Arch Surg 1988; 123:645–649.

Beutler B, Cerami A. Cachectin (tumor necrosis factor): a macrophage hormone governing cellular metabolism and inflammatory response. Endocr Rev 1988; 9:57–66.

Border JR. Hypothesis: sepsis, multiple systems organ failure, and the macrophage. Arch Surg 1988;123:285–286.

Cerra FB. Hypermetabolism, organ failure, and metabolic support. Surgery 1987; 101:1–14.

Cerra FB, West M, Keller G, Mazuski J, Simmons RL. Hypermetabolism/organ failure: the role of the activated macrophage as a metabolic regulator. Prog Clin Biol Res 1988,264:27–42.

Fry DE. Multiple system organ failure. Surg Clin North Am 1988;68:107–122.

Hyers TM, Gee M, Andreadis NA. Cellular interactions in the multiple organ injury syndrome. Am Rev Respir Dis 1987; 135:952–953.

Ninnemann JL. Prostaglandins, leukotrienes, and the immune response. New York: Cambridge University Press, 1988.

Rice, V. The clinical continuum of septic shock. Crit Care Nurs 1984;4(5):86–109.

Roitt I, Brostoff, J, Male D. Immunology. St. Louis: CV Mosby, 1985.

Schlag G, Redl H. Mediators in trauma. Acta Anaesthesiol Belg 1987;38.281–291.

CHAPTER 56

Septic Shock

Kathleen Martin, RN, MSN, CCRN

James Murphy is a 66-year-old man who was admitted to the Emergency Department after sustaining a gunshot wound to the abdomen. He was unconscious and hypotensive on arrival, and was receiving Ringer's lactate at the maximum rate via a 16-gauge catheter in the left forearm. A second 16-gauge catheter was quickly inserted in the right forearm, and a second liter of Ringer's lactate was started at maximum rate. Mr. Murphy was receiving 40% O_2 via face mask, his respiratory rate was 24/min, and he had clear breath sounds bilaterally. His heart rate was 130 and the monitor showed sinus tachycardia without ectopy. A Foley catheter was inserted and 300 ml of clear yellow urine was obtained.

Mr. Murphy's daughter arrived at the hospital shortly after he did. She stated that Mr. Murphy's medical history included a stab wound to the chest 3 years ago and a long history of alcohol abuse. He is retired and lives alone.

After 3 liters of Ringer's lactate was infused, Mr. Murphy's BP stabilized at 110/76 and he was taken to the Operating Room. During surgery it was noted that the bullet had traversed parts of the large bowel, small bowel, and vena cava. Bowel contents were seeded throughout the abdomen, so it was lavaged with cephalosporin solution. The injuries were repaired and a colostomy was performed. A fiberoptic pulmonary artery catheter was placed via the right subclavian vein, and a right radial arterial line was also inserted. The estimated blood loss was 2000 ml, and 8 units of whole blood was administered. The operative time was 6 hr, and Mr. Murphy was hypotensive during much of the procedure.

On arrival in the Surgical ICU, Mr. Murphy's clinical data included the following:

Ventilator Settings		ABGs		Laboratory Values	
Mode	Assist control	pH	7.42	Na	132
Rate	14	$PaCO_2$	38	K	4.8
FIO_2	0.40	PaO_2	85	Cl	98
Tidal volume	900	SaO_2	95%	Gluc	230
PEEP	0	HCO_3	25	Creat	1.8
				Hgb	12.1
				Hct	35
				WBC	12,000

Vital Signs		Hemodynamic Parameters	
BP	120/64	CVP	6
HR	124	PAP	25/10
Resp	14	PAWP	8
Temp	97°F	CO	6
		CI	3.5
		SVR	1027
		$S_{\bar{v}}O_2$	74%

Mr. Murphy was sleepy but easily arousable. He followed commands and complained of abdominal pain. His abdomen was distended but soft to palpation. No bowel sounds were audible, and a large midline dressing was dry and intact. He had a Jackson Pratt drain in the left lower abdominal quadrant and an NG tube in the right naris that was connected to low wall suction. His general appearance was of a thin, undernourished, elderly man in no acute distress.

Mr. Murphy was stable hemodynamically and received IV morphine sulfate for pain throughout the night. The next morning he was awake and cooperative with acceptable arterial blood gases. He was extubated and placed on 40% O_2 via face mask. He continued to improve until the 3rd postoperative day.

Septicemia—Postoperative Day 3

At this time, Mr. Murphy's level of consciousness decreased, his skin appeared warm, flushed, and dry, and his peripheral pulses were bounding. His clinical data included the following:

Vital Signs		Hemodynamic Parameters	
BP	128/68	CVP	2
HR	118	PAP	16/10
Resp	26	PAWP	7
Temp	103°F	CO	7
		CI	4.1
ABGs (on 40% face		SVR	983
mask)		$S_{\bar{v}}O_2$	72%
pH	7.47		
$PaCO_2$	32	**Laboratory Values**	
PaO_2	80	Hgb	10.2
SaO_2	95%	Hct	30
HCO_3	24	WBC	20,000
		Plat	150,000

Urine Output
20 ml/hr ×2 hr

A CT scan of the abdomen was performed, and a large intraabdominal fluid collection was located and percutaneously drained. Gram stain and cultures revealed Gram-negative organisms.

QUESTIONS AND ANSWERS

1. **Define sepsis. Would the term bacteremia, septicemia, or septic shock best describe Mr. Murphy's clinical state?**

   Sepsis is a pathologic state caused by bacteria, viruses, or fungi in the blood. It is a clinical continuum ranging from bacteremia through septicemia to septic shock.

   The term bacteremia merely implies the presence of bacteria in the blood. Septicemia refers to a systemic infection associated with pathogens or their toxins in the blood. Septic shock refers to a state of impaired cellular function and altered hemodynamics that develops secondary to sepsis. When septic shock occurs, it signifies that the body's defense mechanisms have failed. Septic shock is a clinical syndrome that occurs independently of the type of invading organism.

   Mr. Murphy is in the septicemia phase at present. His BP and CO are still in an acceptable range, but hormonal and chemical mediators are being released and causing physiologic changes.

2. **Mr. Murphy's WBC count is 20,000. Is this typical of septicemia?**

   Leukocytosis is common, with a typical WBC count being 15,000–30,000 with a shift to the left. This occurs secondary to demargination of WBCs in response to the infecting organisms and early release of immature forms from bone marrow. As the infectious process continues and septic shock develops, leukopenia may develop. This is because the WBCs are consumed. The bone marrow production cannot keep up with the demand, and the WBC count falls.

3. **What explanation could account for Mr. Murphy's serum glucose of 230 mg/dl?**

   When sepsis occurs, metabolic defects render the cells incapable of using glucose. This results in glucose intolerance, insulin resistance, and hyperglycemia. Gluconeogenesis occurs in the liver, since glucagon and catecholamines are released as part of the stress response.

4. **Mr. Murphy is malnourished and has a paralytic ileus. What form of nutrition would be most appropriate?**

   Early nutritional support is an essential aspect of caring for septic patients. The preferred route is enteral, but since Mr. Murphy has a paralytic ileus, the parenteral route must be used. Research has indicated that specific types of nutritional formulas, such as those high in branched-chain amino acids, may be of some benefit in this patient population. Branched-chain amino acids are metabolized by muscle rather than the liver. Research efforts continue to enhance the understanding of the metabolic machinery and the role of specific nutritional therapy.

Cultures were obtained of Mr. Murphy's surgical wound, blood, urine, and sputum. He was started on ampicillin, tobramycin, and Flagyl pending the sensitivity reports.

Normal saline was infused at 500 ml/hr for 3 hr until a PAWP of 12 mm Hg was achieved.

5. **Are steroids a useful form of therapy in sepsis?**

The use of steroids in sepsis is controversial. The theoretical advantages include decreased capillary permeability, decreased leukocytic aggregation, decreased formation of microemboli, decreased histamine release, and decreased coagulopathy. Steroids appear to be useful only when administered very early, as in anticipation of sepsis in a patient with massive contaminating injuries. Once septic shock occurs, the use of steroids is suspect.

6. **What are the potential side effects of aminoglycoside administration?**

Aminoglycosides are potentially nephrotoxic and ototoxic. The nephrotoxicity is increased when administered with a cephalosporin. Peak and trough levels should be obtained after the 3rd dose, and adjustments should be made to minimize toxicity. Creatinine should also be checked daily. Change in dosage or change in type of antibiotic may be necessary if the creatinine continues to rise.

Hyperdynamic Phase (Warm Septic Shock)— Postoperative Day 5

On postoperative day 5, Mr. Murphy's BP dropped and his respirations appeared shallow and labored, with marked use of accessory muscles. His clinical data included:

Vital Signs		Hemodynamic Parameters	
BP	82/58	CVP	2
HR	122	PAP	16/8
Resp	28	PAWP	5
Temp	103°F	CO	9
		CI	5.3
		SVR	569
		$S_{\bar{v}}O_2$	88%

ABGs (on 40% face mask)

pH	7.26
$PaCO_2$	35
PaO_2	55
SaO_2	88%
HCO_3	12

Mr. Murphy was intubated and connected to the Bennett 7200 ventilator with the following settings:

Mode	Assist control
Rate	14
FIO_2	0.50
Tidal Volume	800

7. **What risk factors for the development of septic shock are present in Mr. Murphy's case?**

Mr. Murphy's risk factors included:

Trauma
Age > 65 years
Malnutrition
Alcohol abuse
Possible hepatic dysfunction
Abdominal trauma/wound
Multiple invasive lines (Swan-Ganz catheter, arterial line, two peripheral IV lines, ET tube, Jackson Pratt drain, Foley catheter)

Other risk factors for septic shock include:

Age < 1 year
Debilitation
Cardiac disease
Renal disease
Diabetes mellitus
Pregnancy
Immunosuppression
Widespread use of antibiotics
Invasive diagnostic procedures
Burns
Urinary tract surgery

8. **Why is the patient with hepatic dysfunction at increased risk for septic shock?**

The Kupffer cells in the liver serve to phagocytize foreign particles in the bloodstream. When the activity of the Kupffer cells is depressed by hepatic dysfunction, microorganisms in the bloodstream are not effectively removed and the progression from bacteremia to septic shock is more likely.

9. **How does alcoholism predispose the patient to septic shock?**

   Alcoholism is frequently associated with liver dysfunction, general debilitation, and malnutrition, all of which decrease host defense mechanisms and facilitate the progression from bacteremia to septic shock.

10. **Immunosuppression has been identified as a risk factor for septic shock. List some treatments and conditions that cause immunosuppression.**

    Neoplasms
    Chemotherapy
    Radiation
    Cyclosporin
    Azathioprine (Imuran)
    AIDS
    Corticosteroids

11. **Is septic shock always caused by Gram-negative organisms?**

    No; although the greatest incidence of septic shock results from Gram-negative organisms, any type of microorganism (Gram-positive bacteria, viruses, fungi) can cause septic shock.

12. **What are the common causative organisms in sepsis?**

    Escherichia coli
    Klebsiella
    Enterobacter
    Serratia
    Pseudomonas aeruginosa
    Streptococcus pneumoniae
    Staphylococcus aureus
    Pneumococcus
    Viruses
    Fungi

13. **When Mr. Murphy's BP and SVR dropped on postoperative day 5, septic shock was suspected. What clinical indicators of septic shock did he demonstrate at that time? What is the physiologic explanation for each?**

Clinical Indicator	*Physiologic Explanation*
Decreased level of consciousness	Decreased cerebral perfusion
Warm, flushed, dry skin	Vasodilatation
Hypotension	Decreased systemic vascular resistance with inadequate cardiac compensation
Tachycardia	Compensatory response for hypotension
Tachypnea	Response to hypoxemia, endotoxins, stress
Fever	Pyrogens in bloodstream affecting the thermoregulatory center in the hypothalamus
Increased CI, increased CO	Compensatory response for vasodilatation
Decreased SVR	Massive vasodilatation
Increased $S_{\bar{v}}O_2$	Decreased tissue O_2 use due to cellular defect or peripheral shunts
Oliguria	Hypotension and renal vasoconstriction

14. What is the role of hormonal and chemical mediators in septic shock?

The cellular changes in septic shock are mediated by numerous hormonal and chemical mediators. (See Appendix F "Inflammatory Mediator Systems.")

15. What are the major pathophysiologic alterations in septic shock? Briefly explain how each occurs.

Peripheral Vasodilatation

Vasodilatation occurs in both the arterial and venous beds and is due to chemical mediators and vasoactive substances. As the arteriolar diameter increases, the SVR decreases and the BP drops. There is a compensatory increase in heart rate and cardiac output.

Maldistribution of Blood Volume

Blood flow through the pulmonary, renal, and splanchnic circulations decreases because of selective vasoconstriction. This vasoconstriction is mediated by chemicals such as catecholamines, angiotensin, prostaglandins, and myocardial depressant factor. This selective vasoconstriction causes pulmonary hypertension, reduced glomerular filtration, and decreased hepatic and pancreatic blood flow, possibly leading to release of myocardial depressant factor (MDF).

In addition to selective vasoconstriction, blood flow in some regions is reduced as a result of endothelial damage and microemboli. Microemboli form as a result of neutrophil aggregation, platelet aggregation, and clotting system activation. The blood flow is diverted away from the constricted vessels to the vessels with less resistance, resulting in overperfusion of some areas and inadequate perfusion of others. Cellular dysfunction is the result.

Several of the chemical mediators cause increased permeability of the capillary wall, so that fluid and protein move from the vascular bed into the interstitial space. This reduces the effective intravascular blood volume and exacerbates the effects of vasodilatation on preload. The increased blood viscosity leads to formation of microemboli.

Myocardial Depression

Even though cardiac output is generally elevated early in septic shock, studies have documented that myocardial depression is an important feature in septic shock. Factors contributing to this myocardial depression include complement activation, endorphin release, histamine release, and the possible release of myocardial depressant factor. A myocardial depressant factor has been isolated from the pancreas in an animal model, but its role in sepsis has not been clearly defined.

The explanation for an increased cardiac output in the setting of depressed myocardial contractility requires consideration of the four major determinants of cardiac output (preload, afterload, contractility, and heart rate). As previously described, the afterload is severely reduced by profound vasodilatation, and tachycardia occurs as a result of hypotension. These compensatory mechanisms allow for maintenance of a normal to elevated cardiac output even though myocardial contractility is depressed. The pathophysiologic alterations described above lead to hypotension, decreased tissue perfusion, altered biochemical function, and multisystem organ failure.

As previously discussed, profound vasodilatation and a leaky capillary endothelium lead to a relative hypovolemia and reduced preload in sepsis. This is reflected in reduced filling pressures (CVP, PAWP). Since myocardial contractility may be decreased, cautious volume loading is performed to maximize the Starling forces and maintain cardiac output. This usually requires a PAWP in the range of 12–16 mm Hg.

Vasoactive drugs such as dopamine and Levophed are also used, since vasodilatation is a major cause of hypotension. Positive inotropic drugs may be administered to treat the myocardial depression previously described.

Mr. Murphy continued to be dopamine dependent, tachycardic, and hypoxemic. A diagnosis of ARDS was made, and he was now requiring 15 cm of PEEP to keep his PaO_2 greater than 60 mm Hg and his SaO_2 above 90%. On his 8th postoperative day, his abdominal wound cultures were positive for *S. aureus*. *E. coli* and *P. aeruginosa* were present in cultures of both sputum and blood. Administration of cefotaxime sodium (Claforan) was started.

Hypodynamic Phase (Cold Septic Shock)

By the 10th postoperative day, Mr. Murphy's condition had deteriorated. The dopamine drip had been continually increased and was now at a rate of 22 μg/kg/min. He was pale, cool, diaphoretic, and anuric. He was having 2–5 PVCs/min, and an S_3 gallop was audible. He responded only to deep pain. His clinical data were as follows:

Vital Signs		Hemodynamic Parameters	
BP	74/58	CVP	7
HR	156	PAP	42/24
Resp	18	PAWP	22
Temp	96°F	CO	2.8
		SVR	1600
		$S_{\bar{v}}O_2$	50%

Laboratory Values		ABGs	
Na	150	pH	7.10
K	6.1	$PaCO_2$	50
Creat	3.5	PaO_2	45
Amylase	300	SaO_2	87%
AST	80	HCO_3	10
BUN	40		
Lipase	4.0		
SGPT	100		
FSP	40		
Plat	80,000		
PT	21		
PTT	97.5		

Mr. Murphy was now in the hypodynamic (cold) phase of septic shock. This phase is similar to the classic shock picture, characterized by decreased cardiac output, increased SVR, profound hypotension, and inadequate tissue perfusion.

16. **Why is the SVR increased in the hypodynamic phase of septic shock?**

    Profound hypotension resulting from heart failure causes an increase in circulating catecholamines and intense vasoconstriction. Prostaglandins released from damaged tissue also cause vasoconstriction.

17. **Why is the pulse pressure narrow in this phase?**

    While the systolic BP falls due to decreased stroke volume, the intense vasoconstriction elevates the diastolic pressure and narrows the pulse pressure.

18. **Mr. Murphy's temperature is 96°F. Is this common during the hypodynamic phase?**

    Yes, hypothermia is common during the hypodynamic (cold) phase. This is due to reduced metabolic activity and decreased heat production.

19. **What is the explanation for Mr. Murphy's decreased renal function?**

    Mr. Murphy's serum creatinine of 3.5, BUN 40, K 6.1, and Mg 4.2, are consistent with acute renal failure. Possible explanations include sustained hypoperfusion of the kidneys due to hypotension and high-dose dopamine administration, and nephrotoxicity resulting from aminoglycoside administration.

20. **Why are Mr. Murphy's liver and pancreatic enzyme levels elevated?**

    This reflects ischemia secondary to hypoperfusion of the liver and pancreas.

21. **What are the major therapeutic goals at this point?**

    Afterload reduction and myocardial support are crucial at this point. This may be attempted with vasodilators, such as Nipride, in combination with a positive inotrope such as dopamine or dobutamine. Cautious fluid administration with meticulous hemodynamic and physiologic monitoring is essential to provide normovolemia as the vascular capacitance increases.

22. **What nursing diagnoses are relevant in this case?**

    Fluid volume deficit related to massive vasodilatation and increased capillary permeability

    Alteration in tissue perfusion related to myocardial depression, maldistribution of blood volume, and altered cellular metabolism

    Decreased urinary output related to reduced renal cortical blood flow and hypotension

Ineffective thermoregulation related to the effect of endotoxins on the hypothalamic temperature regulating center

Impaired gas exchange related to decreased diffusion of oxygen secondary to interstitial edema

Alteration in nutrition; less than body requirements related to increased need for nutritional substrates secondary to increased metabolic rate

Potential for infection related to presence of invasive lines

Potential alteration in tissue perfusion: peripheral (hand), related to risk of impaired circulation secondary to presence of arterial catheter

Despite the aggressive management of Mr. Murphy, he died on postoperative day 12. Death was attributed to septic shock, complicated by DIC, ARDS, renal failure, and hepatic failure.

As this case illustrates, the pathophysiologic derangements in septic shock are complex and interrelated on various levels. Treatment is aimed at the elimination of the septic focus as soon as possible and the aggressive treatment of hypotension before metabolic derangements ensue.

For further inquiry into the sequelae of septic shock, see Chapter 54, "Disseminated Intravascular Coagulation"; Chapter 18, "Adult Respiratory Distress Syndrome"; and Chapter 55, "Multisystem Organ Failure."

SUGGESTED READINGS

Balk RA, Bone RC. The septic syndrome: definition and clinical implications. Critical Care Clinics Jan 1989;5(1):1–8.

Dhainaut JF. Myocardial depressant substances as mediators of early cardiac dysfunction in septic shock. J Crit Care 1982;4(1):1–2.

Keely BR. Septic shock. Crit Care Q 1985; 7(4):59–67.

Moorhouse M, Geissler A, Doenges M. Critical care plans. FA Davis, 1987:335–340.

Price M, Fox J. Hemodynamic monitoring. In: Price M, Fox J, eds. Critical Care Nurse. Rockville, MD: Aspen Publications, 1987:131–139.

Rice V. The clinical continuum of septic shock. Critical Care Nurse 1984;4(5):86–95.

Shoemaker W. Circulatory mechanisms of shock and their mediators. Crit Care Med 1987;15(8):787–793.

Swearingen PL, Sommers MS, Miller K. Manual of critical care applying nursing diagnoses to adult critical illness. St. Louis: CV Mosby, 1988.

Wilson RF, Wilson JA. Sepsis. In: Kinney M, Packa D, Dunbar SB, ed. AACN's clinical reference for critical care nursing 2nd ed. New York: McGraw-Hill, 1988: 1519–1555.

APPENDIX A

Units of Measurement and Normal Values

Unless otherwise specified, the units of measurement used in this book, along with normal values for each, are as listed below.

Hemodynamic Parameters

Parameter	Normal Value	Unit
BP	110–120/70–80	mm Hg
HR	60–100	beats/min
CVP	2–6	mm Hg
PAP	20–30/8–15	mm Hg
PAWP	6–12	mm Hg
CO	4–8	liters/min
CI	2.5–4	liters/min/m^2
SVR	900–1200	dyn/sec/cm^{-5}
LAP	8–12	mm Hg
MAP	70–105	mm Hg
PVR	<250	dyn/sec/cm^5

Laboratory Data

Parameter	Normal Value	Unit
	ARTERIAL AND MIXED VENOUS BLOOD GASES	
$PaCO_2$	35–45	mm Hg
PaO_2	80–100	mm Hg
SaO_2	≥95	%
HCO_3	22–26	mEq/liter
$P_{\bar{v}}CO_2$	41–51	mm Hg
$P_{\bar{v}}O_2$	35–40	mm Hg
$S_{\bar{v}}O_2$	60–80	%

Parameter	Normal Value	Unit
	ELECTROLYTES	
Sodium (Na)	136–146	mEq/liter
Potassium (K)	3.5–5.1	mEq/liter
Chloride (Cl)	98–106	mEq/liter
Carbon dioxide (CO_2 content)	23–29	mEq/liter
Calcium (Ca)	8.4–10.2	mg/dl
Magnesium (Mg)	1.3–2.1	mEq/liter
Phosphorus (Phos)	2.7–4.5	mg/dl
	HEMATOLOGY STUDIES	
Hgb		
Male	13.5–17.5	gm/dl
Female	12–16	
Hct		
Male	41–53	%
Female	36–46	
RBC		
Male	4.5–5.9	millions of cells/mm^3
Female	4.0–5.2	
WBC	4.5–11.5	$\times 10^3$ cells/mm^3
Platelets	150–400	$\times 10^3$ cells/mm^3
Prothrombin time (PT)	18–22	sec
Partial thromboplastin time (PTT)	60–85	sec
APTT	25–35	sec
Fibrinogen	200–400	mg/dl
FSP	<10	μg/ml
	NUTRITIONAL PARAMETERS	
Glucose	70–105	mg/dl
Total serum proteins	6.4–8.3	gm/dl
Albumin	3.5–5	gm/dl
	RENAL AND METABOLIC PARAMETERS	
BUN : creatinine ratio	10 : 1–15 : 1	
Prerenal azotemia	up to 40 : 1	
Intrarenal failure	10 : 1–15 : 1	
Creatinine		
Serum		
Male	0.6–1.2	mg/dl
Female	0.5–1.1	mg/dl
Urine, 24 hr		
Male	14–26	mg/kg/day
Female	11–20	mg/kg/day
Creatinine clearance		
Male	97–137	ml/min/1.73 m^2
Female	88–128	ml/min/1.73 m^2

Parameter	Normal Value	Unit

RENAL AND METABOLIC PARAMETERS (Continued)

Parameter	Normal Value	Unit
Osmolality		
Urine	50–1400	mOsm/kg
	(depending on fluid intake, with fluid restriction	
	>850 mOsm/kg)	
Serum	275–295	mOsm/kg
Urine specific gravity		
24 hr	1.002–1.030	
random	1.015–1.025	
Urea nitrogen		
BUN	7–18	mg/dl
Urine	12–20	gm/day
Urine protein		
24 hr	50–80 at rest	mg/day
Urinary sediment		
Casts		
Hyaline casts	Occasional (0-1)/HPF	
Red cell casts	None	
White cell casts	None	
Tubular epithelial	None	
Cells		
RBCs	0–2/HPF	
WBCs		
Male	0–3/HPF	
Female	0–5/HPF	
Epithelial	Few	
Urine sodium		
24 hr	40–220	mEq/day
Random	40–80	mEq/liter
Prerenal azotemia	<20–40	mEq/liter
Intrarenal failure	>40	mEq/liter

SERUM ENZYMES

Parameter	Normal Value	Unit
Alkaline phosphatase		
Male	62–176	U/liter
Female	56–155	U/liter
Amylase	25–125	U/liter
AST	10–30	U/liter
CK		
Male	38—174	U/liter
Female	96–140	U/liter
LDH	210–420	U/liter
Lipase	10–150	U/liter
SGOT	10–30	U/liter

APPENDIX B

Clinical Calculations

Cardiovascular and Hemodynamic

Parameter	Formula	Normal Value
Cardiac output (CO)	heart rate × stroke volume	4.0–8.0 liters/min
Cardiac index (CI)	$\dfrac{CO}{BSA}$	2.5–4.0 liters/min/m²
Cerebral perfusion pressure	MAP − ICP	80–100 mm Hg (average) 50–150 mm Hg (range)
Coronary perfusion pressure	diastolic BP − PAWP	60–70 mm Hg
Ejection fraction (EF)	$\dfrac{\text{stroke volume}}{\text{end diastolic volume}} \times 100$	>50%
Mean arterial pressure (MAP)	$\dfrac{\text{sys BP} - \text{dias BP}}{3} + \text{diastolic BP}$	70–105 mm Hg
Stroke volume (SV)	$\dfrac{CO \times 1000\ ml/liter}{\text{heart rate}}$	60–100 ml/beat
Systemic vascular resistance (SVR)	$\dfrac{MAP - CVP}{CO} \times 80$	900–1200 dyn/sec/cm⁻⁵
Pulmonary vascular resistance (PVR)	$\dfrac{\text{PA mean pressure} - PAWP}{CO} \times 80$	<250 dyn/sec/cm⁻⁵

Pulmonary and Oxygenation

Parameter	Formula	Normal Value
Arterial O_2 content (CaO_2)	$(Hgb \times 1.39 \times SaO_2) + (0.003 \times PaO_2)$[a]	20 ml/dl
$AVDO_2$	$CaO_2 - C_{\bar{v}}O_2$	3.5–5 ml
Dynamic compliance	$\dfrac{V_t}{PIP - PEEP}$	40–50 ml/cm
O_2 consumption	$CO \times Hgb \times 13.9 \times (SaO_2 - S_{\bar{v}}O_2)$	250–300 ml/min
O_2 transport	$CaO_2 \times CO \times 10$	900–1100 ml/min
Static effective compliance	$\dfrac{V_T}{\text{Plateau pressure} - PEEP}$	50 ml/cm H_2O

[a] An acceptable abbreviated formula is $(Hgb \times 1.39 \times SaO_2)$

Renal and Metabolic

Parameter	Formula	Normal Value
Anion gap	$Na^+ - (CO_2^- + Cl^-)$	≤ 15 mEq/liter
Creatinine clearance (GFR)[a]	$\dfrac{U \times \dot{V}}{P}$	
Estimated creatinine clearance	$\dfrac{1.0}{\text{Serum creatinine}} \times 100$	
Fractional excretion of sodium (FENa)[b]	$\dfrac{U_{Na} \times P_{Cr}}{U_{Cr} \times P_{Cr}} \times 100$	
Corrected total Ca	Total Ca + 0.8 (4.0 − albumin)	

[a] U, amount of creatinine in urine (mg/dl); $\dot{V}$, Urine flow in ml/min; P, Amount of creatinine in plasma (mg/dl).
[b] U_{Na}, urine sodium; U_{Cr}, urine creatinine; P_{Na}, plasma sodium; P_{Cr}, plasma creatinine.

APPENDIX C

Abbreviations

BSA	body surface area
CaO_2	arterial oxygen content
CI	cardiac index
CO	cardiac output
$C_{\bar{v}}O_2$	mixed venous oxygen content
CVP	central venous pressure
ICP	intracranial pressure
LAP	left atrial pressure
MAP	mean arterial pressure
PA	pulmonary artery
$PaCO_2$	partial pressure of carbon dioxide in arterial blood
PaO_2	partial pressure of oxygen in arterial blood
PAO_2	partial pressure of oxygen in alveolus
PAWP	pulmonary artery wedge pressure
PIP	peak inspiratory pressure
PVR	pulmonary vascular resistance
RAP	right atrial pressure
SaO_2	saturation of Hgb in arterial blood
$S_{\bar{v}}O_2$	saturation of Hgb in mixed venous blood
SV	stroke volume
SVR	systemic vacular resistance
V_T	tidal volume

APPENDIX D

Dubois Body Surface Area Nomogram

BODY SURFACE AREA OF ADULTS
Nomogram for determination of body surface area from height and weight

Find the patient's height in either feet or centimeters in the left column and the patient's weight in pounds or kilograms in the right column. Connect these two points with a ruler. The BSA is indicated at the point where the ruler crosses the middle column.

Height		BSA	Weight	
ft	cm	m²	lb	kg

Height (ft / cm):
8″
6′6″ — 200
4″
2″ — 190
6′0″
10″ — 180
8″
— 170
5′6″
4″ — 160
2″
5′0″ — 150
10″
8″ — 140
4′6″
4″ — 130
2″
4′0″ — 120
10″
8″ — 110
3′6″
4″ — 100
2″
— 95
3′0″ — 90
10″ — 85
8″ — 80
2′6″ — 75
4″ — 70
2″ — 65
2′0″ — 60
1′8″ — 55

BSA (m²):
2.8
2.6
2.4
2.2
2.0
1.8
1.6
1.4
1.2
1.0
0.9
0.8
0.7
0.6
0.5
0.4
0.3

Weight (lb / kg):
340 — 160
320 — 140
300
280 — 120
260
240
220 — 100
200 — 90
180 — 80
160 — 70
140 — 60
120 — 50
100 — 45
90 — 40
80 — 35
70 — 30
60 — 25
50
40 — 20
35 — 15
30
25 — 10
20
15 — 5
10

APPENDIX E

Glasgow Coma Scale and Scoring

Doris M. Gates, RN, MS, CCRN

The Glasgow Coma Scale (GCS) is one of the most widely used and accepted injury-severity indexes for assessment of level of consciousness and degree of coma. The GCS was developed in 1974 at the University of Glasgow, Scotland, and revised in 1977. The purpose of the scale was to standardize the terminology used to describe changes in level of consciousness (LOC). The GCS assesses and measures three aspects of LOC: eye-opening response, verbal response, and motor response. Scores are assigned based on the patient's best response to verbal or painful stimuli for each component. The scoring system is as follows:

Best eye-opening response:	Opens spontaneously	4
	Opens to verbal stimuli	3
	Opens to pain	2
	No response	1
Best verbal response:	Oriented	5
	Disoriented and confused	4
	Inappropriate words	3
	Incomprehensible sounds	2
	No response	1
Best motor response:	Obeys verbal commands	6
	Localizes to painful stimuli	5
	Withdraws to painful stimuli	4
	Abnormal flexion (decorticates)	3
	Abnormal extension (decerebrates)	2
	No response	1

The scores for each individual component are added together for a total score. Total GCS scores range from 3–15. A patient with a GCS score of 3 has no eye-opening response (E1), verbal response (V1), or motor response (M1). A patient with a GCS of 15 opens eyes spontaneously (E4), is oriented and converses (V5), and obeys commands (M6).

The GCS is simple to use and widely accepted as a standard assessment tool for neurologically impaired patients, especially head-injured patients. Changes in the patient's condition are easily identified by trending of the GCS data. However, the tool has limited applicability in certain populations of patients. The GCS supplies partial information in neurologically impaired patients who are hemiplegic, hemiparetic, aphasic, or who suffer from a spinal-cord injury. In addition, extreme periocular edema, intubation, or the presence of extremity immobilizers (i.e., casts, traction) interfere with eliciting the best response from patients. These patients' best response is not due to neurologic injury but to extraneous conditions. Although the overall score for these types of patients does not necessarily reflect the severity of injury or predict the mortality and morbidity for the patient, the assessment tool is still useful if these constraints are identified when interpreting the assessment results.

SUGGESTED READINGS

Ingersoll GL, Leyden DB. The Glasgow Coma Scale for patients with head injuries. Critical Care Nurse 1987;7(5):26–32.

Reimer M. Head-injured patients, How to detect early signs of trouble Nursing 89 1989;19(3):35–41.

APPENDIX F

Inflammatory Mediator Systems[a]

Virginia Byrn Huddleston, RN, MSN, CCRN

Table 1. Mediator systems—humoral

Component	Function	Source	Activated by	Action
Complement	Activation and enhancement of inflammatory/immune response Anaphylatoxin formation (C3a,C5a) May be direct mediator between tissue injury and PMN activation	Circulating pool-complex series of proteins and proteinases produced by cells of liver, small and large intestine, and macrophages	Alternative pathway: tissue trauma tissue ischemia cell debris kinins endotoxin bacterial cell debris Classic pathway: Antigen/antibody complex (IgM and IgG only)	PMN chemotaxis & phagocytosis PMN aggregation Stimulate PMN oxidative metabolism; provoke degranulation with release of lysosomal enzymes Vasodilatation ↑ vascular permeability Release of leukotrienes Stimulate release of mediators (histamine) Smooth muscle contraction Activate kinin system Opsonization Direct cytolysis Macrophage phagocytosis Neutralization of virus
Coagulation	Balance between hemorrhage and intravascular fibrin formation	Circulating pool—complex series of proteins operating in a cascade form; proteins produced by liver	Extrinsic pathway: tissue trauma long bone fractures → release of tissue thromboplastin → activates path via X and Xa Intrinsic pathway: Hageman factor (XII)	Coagulation

Fibrinolytic	Balance between hemorrhage and intravascular fibrin formation	Circulating pool—proteins produced by liver	Plasminogen → plasmin activated by: Tissue plasminogen activator (TPA) Thrombin Activated Hageman Kallikrein Lysosomal enzymes	Fibrinolysis
Kallikrein-kinin (Bradykinin)	Regulation of microvascular perfusion	Circulating pool—protein precursors produced in liver	Hageman factor Tissue trauma Complement split products PMNs	Potent vasodilatation ↑ capillary permeability PMN chemotaxis Stimulate PMN O_2 consumption and aerobic glycolysis Liberate elastase from PMN → ↑ PMN activity Smooth muscle contraction

Table 2. Mediator systems—cellular

Componenet	Function	Source	Activated by	Action

PMN	Inflammatory/immune response	Bone marrow
		Lymphatic tissue
		Marginal pool
		Circulating pool
			Complement
			Kinin system
			Tumor necrosis factor
			Interleukin-1
			Platelet activating factor
			Bacterial wall fragments
			Cell debris
			Elastase
				Phagocytosis
				Release mediators:
				  Platelet activating factor
				  Leukotrienes (LTB_4)
				  Prostaglandins
				  Oxygen radicals
				  Interleukin 1 & 2
				  Low molecular weight
				   macrophage stimulating
				   factor (LMW-MSF)
				  Proteinases (elastase,
				   collagenase)
				Stimulate T-cells

Macrophage	Inflammatory/immune response
	Antigen presentation to
	  lymphocytes
		Lymphatic tissue
		Marginal pool
		Peripheral tissue
		Alveolar
		Liver (Kupffer)
		Lymph nodes
		Spleen
		Bone marrow
		SQ (histiocyte)
			PMN by Il-1 type activity
			LMW-MSF
			Complement split products
			Activated T-cell lymphokines
			Monocyte chemotactants:
			  Complement fragments
			  PMN fragments
			  Bacterial fragments
			  Lymphokines
				Phagocytosis
				Release mediators:
				  Interleukin 1
				  TNF
				  Complement components
				  Prostaglandins
				  Coagulation factors
				  Colony stimulating factors
				  Plasminogen activator
				  Interferon
				  Oxygen radicals

Platelets	Inflammatory/immune response
	Coagulation
		Bone marrow
		Spleen
			Thrombin
			Platelet Activating
			  Factor released by PMN
			Aggregate secondary to
			  fibrin & exposed collagen
				Aggreation at endothelial
				  surface
				Enhance granulocytic,
				  aggregation, &
				  cytotoxicity
				Release mediators:
				  Thromboxane
				  Serotonin
				  Chemotactants
				  Complement activator

Table 3. Biochemical mediators

Mediator	Function	Source	Activated by	Action
Hageman factor	Activation of coagulation and kinin systems Link between coagulation and the inflammatory/immune response	Circulating pool Produced by the liver	Contact with damaged tissue Collagen Cartilage Endotoxin Basement membrane fragments Contact with Ag/Ab aggregates Contact with negatively charged particles	Convert prekallikrein to kallikrein Initiate intrinsic coagulation cascade
Histamine	Vasoactive amine	Mast cell Platelets Basophils	Complement binding Direct cell trauma	Vasodilatation ↑ capillary permeability Myocardial depression Smooth muscle contraction
Prostaglandins	Inflammatory/immune response	Cell membrane phospholipid (found in all cell types)	Cell membrane disruption by trauma or immune complexes → availability of phospholipid → arachidonic acid → cyclooxygenase pathway / lipoxygenase pathway → prostaglandins thromboxane / leukotrienes	

Mediator	Function	Source	Activated by	Action
PGE	Potentiate actions of proinflammatory mediators Feedback inhibition of macrophage response			Potent vasodilatation Induce suppressor T-cells Endogenous pyrogens Hyperalgesics Inhibit specific lymphocyte/ macrophage responses (Ag expression) Phagocytosis may be enhanced ↑ Il-1 release
PGI_2 (Prostacyclin)	Inflammatory/immune response			Vasodilatation Antiplatelet aggregation
PGF_{2a}	Antagonize effects of proinflammatory mediators			Pulmonary vasoconstriction ↑ vascular permeability
Thromboxane	Inflammatory/immune response Coagulation	Platelets Macrophages Arachidonic acid metabolite	Cell membrane disruption Arachidonic acid metabolism	Platelet aggregation Vasoconstriction
Leukotrienes (LTB_4, LTC_4)	Inflammatory/immune response	Arachidonic acid metabolite	Cell membrane disruption Arachidonic acid metabolism	↑ vascular permeability Activate phagocytosis Chemotactant Stimulate lymphocyte reactivity Potentiate inflammatory/ immune response Pulmonary vasoconstriction Prolonged contraction of selected smooth muscle

Interleukin-1 (Il-1)	Inflammatory/immune response	PMNs Macrophages Synovial fibroblasts B-lymphocytes Natural killer cells	T-cell lymphokines Phagocytosis of antigen and endotoxin	Leukocytosis Enhance T- & B-cell multiplication and activation Stimulate endothelium to express secondary inflammatory factors Stimulate production of acute phase reactants Fever (endogenous pyrogen) Synergistic with cytokines in stimulation of bone marrow hemapoiesis
Oxygen radicals	Intracellular killing of phagocytized microorganisms	PMN degranulation Reperfusion by-product	Shock states Hemorrhage Complement PMN phagocytosis	Endothelial damage Cell membrane damage ↑ capillary permeability Lipid peroxidation of membrane
Catabolic hormones: epinephrine glucagon hydrocortisone	Nonspecific response to mobilize substrate for hypermetabolism	Adrenal gland Pancreas	Trauma Shock states	Provoke hypermetabolism, hyperglycemia, and insulin resistance
Tumor necrosis factor (TNF)/cachectin	Stimulate acute phase reaction	Macrophages	Endotoxin activated macrophages	Pyrogenic Suppress lipoprolipase activity Enhance neutrophil and eosinophil function Fibroblast proliferation

527

Mediator	Function	Source	Activated by	Action
				Activate bone resorption ↑ oxygen radical production ↓ anticoagulant activity of endothelium Anorexia/wasting Endothelial damage Enhance macrophage function
GM-CSF	Enhance inflammatory/ immune response	T-cells Fibroblasts Macrophages Endothelial cells	Antigen Interleukin-1 Tumor necrosis factor	Enhance proliferation, phagocytosis, degranulation and cytotoxicity of PMN macrophage, and eosinophil Stimulate hemapoiesis
Opioids	Neuropeptides	CNS	Shock state	Stimulate central and peripheral receptors → vasodilatation and CV instability

Angiotensin	Regulation of sodium and water homeostasis	Circulating pool—produced in liver	Renin release stimulated by microorganisms and ↓ circulating volume	↑ release of catecholamines Potent vasoconstrictor Stimulate aldosterone → Na^+ & H_2O retention
Serotonin	Vasoactive amine Neurotransmitter	Intestinal tissue CNS Platelets	Stimulated platelets	Vasodilatation and vasoconstriction Inhibition of pain pathway
Elastase Collagenase	Proteinases	PMNs	Phagocytizing PMNs	Degradation of elastin and collagen → vascular damage
Platelet activating factor (PAF)	Inflammatory/immune response Coagulation	Mast cells Basophils Monocytes Macrophages PMNs	Stimulation of source cells	Change platelet shape → platelet aggregation Release serotonin Activate PMNs → oxidative metabolism and degranulation ↑ vascular permeability Smooth muscle contraction Vasodilatation and vasoconstriction

INDEX

Page numbers in italics denote figures; those followed by "t" denote tables.

Digital subtraction angiography, 45
Digitalis, 41–42
Digoxin, 56
 cardiac effects of, 56
 for congestive heart failure, 57
 furosemide and, 56
Dilantin. *See* Phenytoin
Diltiazem
 for acute MI, 24–25
 for cardiomyopathy, 42
 dose of, 171
 for non-Q wave myocardial infarction,
  129
2,3-Diphosphoglyceric acid
 effect on oxyhemoglobin dissociation
  curve, 357
 phosphorus and production of, 359–360
"Dirty dozen," 219
Disseminated intravascular coagulation,
  484–493
 case study of, 484
 conditions and clinical indicators of, 488,
  490t–491t
 conditions predisposing to, 485
 lab findings in, 489
 nursing diagnoses for, 493
 pathophysiology of, 485–487, *486*
 rhabdomyolysis and, 335
 risk in pregnancy of, 488
 role of endothelium in, 487–488
 sites of thrombus formation in, 488
 therapy for, 489, 492
  antithrombin III, 492
  blood component replacement, 492
  future methods, 492
  heparin, 492
Diuretics. *See also* specific drugs
 for acute renal failure, 298–299
 for closed head injury, 257–258
 for epidural bleeding, 265
Diverticular disease, 397–398
Dobutamine
 after cardiac transplantation, 14–15
 cardiac effects of, 57
 for cardiogenic shock, 29–30
 for congestive heart failure, 57–58
Dobutrex. *See* Dobutamine
Dopamine
 for cardiogenic shock, 28–30
 dose-related effects of, 56
 for myocardial depression of septic
  shock, 508, 509
 use of nitroprusside with, 5–6
Drift, 246
 assessment of, 246
 with a capture, 246
 frank, 246

 pronator, 246
Dura mater, 263–264
Dysrhythmias
 due to central venous pressure line, 88
 due to reperfusion, 147, 150
 in Prinzmetal's angina, 168

E

Edema, pulmonary. *See* Pulmonary edema
Effective arterial blood volume, 313–314
Ejection fraction, calculation of, 514t
Elastase, 539t
Electrocardiographic findings
 in anterior MI, 22
 in cardiomyopathy, 35
 in chronic obstructive pulmonary disease,
  189, *190*
 identification of normal intervals and
  segments, 117
 in left bundle branch block, 36
 in mitral stenosis, 115–117, *116–117*
 in multifocal atrial tachycardia, 189, *189*
 in myocardial infarction, *94–96*, 98–101,
  99
 in Prinzmetal's angina, 168
 in pulmonary embolism, 213
 in right bundle branch block, 36
 in status asthmaticus, 230
 in unstable angina, 159–160
 in ventricular hypertrophy, 35
Electrolyte imbalances
 in acute renal failure, 298–299
 after liver transplantation, 391
 in diabetic ketoacidosis, 359–360
 in prerenal azotemia, 316
 in rhabdomyolysis, 334
 in small bowel obstruction, 428–430
Electrolytes, normal values for, 512t
Embolectomy, for pulmonary embolism,
  215–216
Embolism
 air
  air transport for, 451
  due to CVP line, 87–88
 amniotic fluid, 488
 pulmonary, 208–216. *See also* Pulmonary
  embolism
Embolization, cerebral, 238
Emphysema
 air transport for, 452
 definition of, 187
 ECG findings in, 189, *190*
 paradoxical respirations in, 192
Empyema, 220
 definition of, 220
 signs and symptoms of, 220
 treatment of, 220